Tele-Audiology and the Optimization of Hearing Healthcare Delivery

Elaine Saunders
Blamey Saunders Hears, Australia

A volume in the Advances in Medical Technologies and Clinical Practice (AMTCP) Book Series

IGI Global
DISSEMINATOR OF KNOWLEDGE

Published in the United States of America by
IGI Global
Medical Information Science Reference (an imprint of IGI Global)
701 E. Chocolate Avenue
Hershey PA, USA 17033
Tel: 717-533-8845
Fax: 717-533-8661
E-mail: cust@igi-global.com
Web site: http://www.igi-global.com

Library of Congress Cataloging-in-Publication Data

Names: Saunders, Elaine, 1954- editor.
Title: Tele-audiology and the optimization of hearing health care delivery / Elaine Saunders, editor.
Description: Hershey PA : Medical Information Science Reference, [2019] | Includes bibliographical references.
Identifiers: LCCN 2018048529| ISBN 9781522581918 (hardcover) | ISBN 9781522581925 (ebook)
Subjects: | MESH: Correction of Hearing Impairment--methods | Telemedicine--methods | Delivery of Health Care--methods
Classification: LCC R119.95 | NLM WV 270 | DDC 610.285--dc23 LC record available at https://lccn.loc.gov/2018048529

This book is published in the IGI Global book series Advances in Medical Technologies and Clinical Practice (AMTCP) (ISSN: 2327-9354; eISSN: 2327-9370)

British Cataloguing in Publication Data
A Cataloguing in Publication record for this book is available from the British Library.

All work contributed to this book is new, previously-unpublished material.
The views expressed in this book are those of the authors, but not necessarily of the publisher.

For electronic access to this publication, please contact: eresources@igi-global.com.

Advances in Medical Technologies and Clinical Practice (AMTCP) Book Series

ISSN:2327-9354
EISSN:2327-9370

Editor-in-Chief: Srikanta Patnaik, SOA University, India & Priti Das, S.C.B. Medical College, India

MISSION

Medical technological innovation continues to provide avenues of research for faster and safer diagnosis and treatments for patients. Practitioners must stay up to date with these latest advancements to provide the best care for nursing and clinical practices.

The **Advances in Medical Technologies and Clinical Practice (AMTCP) Book Series** brings together the most recent research on the latest technology used in areas of nursing informatics, clinical technology, biomedicine, diagnostic technologies, and more. Researchers, students, and practitioners in this field will benefit from this fundamental coverage on the use of technology in clinical practices.

COVERAGE

- Medical informatics
- Telemedicine
- Clinical Nutrition
- Medical Imaging
- Nutrition
- E-Health
- Nursing Informatics
- Clinical High-Performance Computing
- Patient-Centered Care
- Biomechanics

The Advances in Medical Technologies and Clinical Practice (AMTCP) Book Series (ISSN 2327-9354) is published by IGI Global, 701 E. Chocolate Avenue, Hershey, PA 17033-1240, USA, www.igi-global.com. This series is composed of titles available for purchase individually; each title is edited to be contextually exclusive from any other title within the series. For pricing and ordering information please visit http://www.igi-global.com/book-series/advances-medical-technologies-clinical-practice/73682. Postmaster: Send all address changes to above address.

Titles in this Series

For a list of additional titles in this series, please visit:
https://www.igi-global.com/book-series/advances-medical-technologies-clinical-practice/73682

Histopathological Image Analysis in Medical Decison Making
Nilanjan Dey (Techno India College of Technology, India) Amira S. Ashour (Tanta University, Egypt) Harihar Kalia (Seemantha Engineering College, India) R.T. Goswami (Techno India College of Technology, India) and Himansu Das (KIIT University, India)
Medical Information Science Reference • ©2019 • 340pp • H/C (ISBN: 9781522563167) • US $265.00

Healing Through the Arts for Non-Clinical Practitioners
Jenny Bopp (Westtown School, USA) Amy M. Grebe (Zinnia Consulting and Design, USA) and Joanna Hope Denny (Pellisippi State Community College, USA)
Medical Information Science Reference • ©2019 • 309pp • H/C (ISBN: 9781522559818) • US $255.00

Medical Image Processing for Improved Clinical Diagnosis
A. Swarnambiga (Indian Institute of Technology Madras, India)
Medical Information Science Reference • ©2019 • 313pp • H/C (ISBN: 9781522558767) • US $245.00

Clinical Costing Techniques and Analysis in Modern Healthcare Systems
Ronald Ma (Austin Health, Australia)
Medical Information Science Reference • ©2019 • 265pp • H/C (ISBN: 9781522550822) • US $235.00

Optimized Genetic Programming Applications Emerging Research and Opportunities
Bahrudin Hrnjica (University of Bihac, Bosnia and Herzegovina) and Ali Danandeh Mehr (Antalya Bilim University, Turkey)
Medical Information Science Reference • ©2019 • 310pp • H/C (ISBN: 9781522560050) • US $225.00

For an entire list of titles in this series, please visit:
https://www.igi-global.com/book-series/advances-medical-technologies-clinical-practice/73682

IGI Global
DISSEMINATOR OF KNOWLEDGE

701 East Chocolate Avenue, Hershey, PA 17033, USA
Tel: 717-533-8845 x100 • Fax: 717-533-8661
E-Mail: cust@igi-global.com • www.igi-global.com

Table of Contents

Detailed Table of Contents

Leon Sterling, Swinburne University of Technology, Australia
Rachel Burrows, University of Melbourne, Australia
Belinda Barnet, Swinburne University of Technology, Australia
Simone Taffe, Swinburne University of Technology, Australia
Rachael McDonald, Swinburne University of Technology, Australia

The internet has created new possibilities for health practitioners to deliver services remotely. The potential for telemedicine is yet to be fully realized. Many factors hamper the uptake of telemedicine, including funding models and the availability of technology. This chapter concerns one important area often neglected by technology developers: considering the emotions of users interacting with systems and services. The authors believe that consideration of emotions is essential for the advocacy, adoption, and appropriation of telemedicine services by a wide range of stakeholders, who have diverse abilities and motivations. They consider one area of telemedicine: teleaudiology. The authors outline emotional factors that need to be considered in providing teleaudiology services drawing on research from software engineering developing agent-oriented models of socio-technical systems, as well as knowledge of assistive technology frameworks. They consider how emotional factors can be taken into consideration with respect to a specific teleaudiology service provided by a successful company.

This chapter aimed to estimate speech perception benefits in quiet for clients with different degrees of hearing loss. The difference between aided and unaided scores on a monosyllabic word test presented binaurally was used as the measure of benefit. Retrospective data for 492 hearing aid users with four-frequency pure-tone average hearing losses (PTA) ranging from 5 dB HL to 76 dB HL in the better ear were analyzed using nonlinear regression. The mean benefit for the perception of monosyllabic words in this group of clients was 22.3% and the maximum expected benefit was 33.6% for a PTA of 52 dB HL. The expected benefit can be expressed as a reduction of the error rate by about half for isolated words and about one quarter for sentences across the full range of PTA.

In the chapter, the authors address the prescient need to update accepted care models of cochlear implant (CI) fitting and long-term maintenance to better utilize self-care and tele-medicine possibilities, thus shifting the focus of CI maintenance to the recipient. There is a strong evidence base that such a move will better meet the needs of CI users, giving them greater control of and involvement in their hearing progress. Simultaneously, such an approach can better meet present shortcomings in the market acceptance and delivery of the benefit of cochlear implants, particularly in the elderly segment of the population, where device penetration of the market remains low (c. 7%). Such initiatives make it viable to reach many more users, as the present models are prohibitively expensive for such expansion. A case study of pilot software for CI maintenance based on tele-audiology is described with the inclusion of data collected from initial studies.

Tinnitus can be a debilitating hearing-related symptom. Access to evidence-based tinnitus interventions remain limited. Tele-audiology can assist by providing a clinically and cost-effective tinnitus management route. This chapter highlights how this is made possible by focusing on one form of tele-audiology, namely an internet-based intervention. Guidelines are provided for the development of such interventions. A framework outlining the various processes involved in evaluating newly developed interventions is also provided. The chapter closes by discussing factors that may facilitate or hamper the dissemination of new interventions into existing service delivery models. This well-defined outline for intervention development and evaluation can be applied and used to guide innovative intervention models by stakeholders.

This chapter provides a picture of the evolution of mobile applications (apps) for hearing health care (HHC) in terms of availability, variety, penetration, offered services, and target users. Special emphasis is given to newly developed methods that might assist audiologists and hearing professionals to get meaningful information and guidance for informed adoption of apps for themselves as well as for patients and their families. The chapter also shows how these novel methods can be used to characterize and compare a variety of apps across a wide range of services and target user groups. A representative sample of apps, assessed by using such a standardized framework, is analyzed to derive a multifaceted picture of apps for HHC. The chapter outlines and discusses emerging trends and needs in the area and highlights the open challenges as well as potential opportunities for professionals, researchers, developers, and stakeholders at large.

Security is a huge topic and not at all fun. It's hard to understand. It can be scary. It is always lurking. And poor security can bring down any system, regardless of how useful or important it is. Understanding the risks and vulnerabilities in systems and the motivations and methods of attackers is important in designing and operating secure and robust systems. This chapter aims to give a perspective on how to think about information technology (IT) security, how it applies to telehealth and audiology, and finally gives some recommendations about important considerations for tele-audiology systems that include devices, data housing, smartphone applications, and patient records.

Foreword

It is an honour to write the forward to Dr Saunders' timely book because it provides both practical and thought-provoking information about a topic that only relatively recently has come to the forefront of clinical practice.

The possibilities of tele-audiology, or more generally tele-medicine, are far-reaching. Tele-audiology has already proven its value to patients, practitioners, researchers and the hearing instrument industry alike. It gives easier clinical access for patients with geographical or health barriers, it can provide immediate access to specialists located far away, it opens the door to apps and mobile technology that enable self-monitoring of hearing and automated adjustment of hearing aid settings based on a location or sound environment, as well as allowing for development of diverse tools for self-management hearing, and much more - most of which has probably not yet been conceived of!

However, Tele-audiology can also raise a whole host of concerns and problems such as breaches of data privacy, ill-directed trust in unverified apps, and data ownership issues, to name a few. We live in an exciting but also somewhat disturbing age in which technology is ubiquitous and is critical to our daily function. Most of us rely on our computers to complete our work, our smartphones for navigation, entertainment and communication, and our smart watches and fitness trackers to monitor our health. Along with these conveniences and value-added services comes the potential for loss of autonomy and privacy, and disruption when the technology fails. It seems to me that the long-term successes and outcomes of tele-audiology will be dependent upon how it is used and the oversight provided.

A few years ago, I heard Elizabeth Krupinksi (Past President of the American Telemedicine Association) define tele-medicine (or tele-audiology) as 'The delivery of services and information via telecommunications technologies.' She pointed out something obvious - but which does not immediately come to mind - that tele-medicine (or tele-audiology) is not a separate subspecialty of medicine (or audiology), it is simply the use of technology as the means to an end. The important message, therefore, is that practitioners should expect to attain equivalent clinical outcomes to those attained via face-to-face service provision. Indeed, equivalent clinical outcomes should be a basic minimum need. On the other hand, one should rightly expect superior telehealth outcomes, i.e. outcomes resulting from providing clinical services via technology. Telehealth outcomes include metrics such as increased patient satisfaction with services received, increased provider satisfaction with service provision, decreased no-show rates, shorted wait times, decreased travel costs, increased completion of treatment regimens, decreased facility costs to the provider, etc. It is the attainment of outcomes such as these that should inspire the use of tele-audiology.

As a reader of this book, I am sure you will learn much and gain insights into both the benefits and limitations of tele-audiology. As you read, I encourage you to think about some of the following: First, how can we help clients navigate through the numerous online hearing-related materials, some of which provide accurate information, others of which do not? Second, in a similar light, what guidelines can we give consumers as regards the validity and reliability of hearing apps they may encounter in app stores? This is relatively new territory, for which there is no oversight or regulation. Is this a problem or is it the free market being free? Finally, if you are considering setting up a tele-audiology program, don't reinvent the wheel, instead make use of the extensive resources available from organizations such as the American Telemedicine Association (http://www.americantelemed.org/home), and Telehealth Resource Centers (https://www.telehealthresourcecenter.org/

At this point in time, the sky (or maybe the Cloud!) is the limit, and with continuing technological developments, even faster higher fidelity internet connections, and thoughtful oversight and considerations of pitfalls, we can all benefit from this new age of tele-audiology. I, for one, look forward to finding out what the future holds. I encourage you to do likewise.

Gabrielle H. Saunders
National Center for Rehabilitative Auditory Research (NCRAR), USA

Preface

The first thing we ought to recognize is that mobile is now part of the fabric—every day in everybody's life. So if you're not looking at mobile solutions, then you're not really looking at all solutions. (Mal Postings Global CTO — IT Advisory, Ernst & Young)

This book examines some aspects of tele-audiology, where tele-audiology is a blanket term for digital health solutions in audiology and auditory rehabilitation, including education and training. Tele-audiology is a rapidly evolving field which draws on new skills and enabling technologies to provide hearing healthcare at a distance, in a manner that provides appropriate outcomes and reduces delivery costs. Tele-audiology is part of a trend in health to greater user participation in decision making and personal empowerment. As in the rest of health, there are different considerations in different geographic locations and different economies.

For example, there have been several studies, and a resulting commercialization outcome in the area of remote audiometry, using a portable audiometer, with remote access and cloud based storage.

The introductory chapter delves into trends in digital health, but simplifying this up front, to understand how digital health is differentiated from IT enabled record keeping, it's useful to draw on the words of medical futurist, Bertalan Meskó (2018) who writes:

It's hard to draw a definitive line between health IT and digital health issues, although delineating a clear territory for them might help caregivers use new technologies to improve and expedite their job so that in the end they may spend more time with patients. The two areas are often intermingled while their nature and the solution they require are different on many scales. In a nutshell, IT issues impact physicians' everyday job the most but can be dealt with in the short term. Digital health has more impact on cultural changes and entails a long-term process.

The impetus for this book is that tele-audiology is gaining pace, partly driven by commercial developments in remote otoscopy, remote audiometry, and hearing aids that can be adjusted by a remote professional. The recurring theme in the literature is that audiologists are reluctant to use it. Increasingly, universities are beginning to incorporate aspects of tele-audiology into their audiology courses. This emerging field has provided the opportunity for hearing services professionals to re-think the service model, potentially with several tele-audiologists reporting to a more senior clinician, in order to make cost effective, scalable models of care. Clinicians using tele-audiology have the potential to expand their practices, and people in rural areas can be better served.

A change in service delivery model needs to be thought out with a clean slate (or digital document). If tele-audiology is completely based on digitizing current service models, we will reduce the potential impact and service efficiencies. There are examples in tele-audiology where a clinician uses video conferencing to work with a remote, intermediary professional such as a nurse. This model potentially increases rather than decreases the cost of service delivery, and does not deliver the goal of patient empowerment. There are also a number of audiology and hearing aid companies recruiting for positions in tele-audiology. The career qualifications are not yet agreed in Australia, though the American Speech-Language-Hearing Association (ASHA) in the USA has defined the role as a Tele-audiology Clinical Assistant:

Tele-audiology clinical technicians (TCTs) are persons who, after appropriate training and demonstration of competency, provide patient/equipment interface support under the supervision of an ASHA-certified and licensed audiologist using secure real time and/or "store and forward" audio/video technology to deliver audiology services from a site located at a distance from the actual patient testing site. A TCT may also be an audiology assistant or other health care professional (e.g., licensed vocational nurse, bachelor's-prepared nurse, master's prepared nurse, nurse practitioner, physician assistant, etc.) who has additional training to serve in the role as a TCT and support tele-audiology service delivery under the supervision of an ASHA-certified and licensed audiologist. TCTs are currently only utilized in the Veterans Administration health care system.

ASHA's definition is practical, and accommodates service scaling. Swinburne University in Australia is the first Australian university to offer training to meet this definition as a dedicated post graduate qualification, where they will graduate with the appropriate ICT and communication skills.

In an online editorial, Fabry and Groth (2017) cite one of Sergei Kochkin's studies in summarizing factors that affect the potential efficiencies of tele-audiology. These authors noted that, on average, approximately four office visits were required to successfully fit individuals with hearing aids in the USA. They also noted that visits for fine-tuning of hearing aids take a 28% share of the total number of visits to a clinician. If these adjustments are carried out, either by the client themselves, with a self-fit hearing aid, or with assistance using remote tele-audiology, the practice and the client use time and other resources more efficiently, potentially reducing the cost of service. For both the client and the clinician an implicit question is whether working remotely, and whether use of self-fit hearing aids works for everyone. A review of the literature in auditory rehabilitation and clinical experience would suggest not. This then raises the question of service planning, and the assumption that a blended service model of care is optimal. One such model, described in depth by Beckett, Saunders, and Blamey (2016), reports on 5 years of data using a blended service model. In the current volume, Saunders describes how a well-researched model of care has been adapted to implementing a blended model of face to face and tele-audiology care (Chapter 3: "Goldstein and Stephens Revisited and Extended to a Telehealth Model of Hearing Aid Optimization").

Audiology is a broad and multidisciplinary field, drawing on psychology, audiological sciences, sociology, engineering, clinical measurement, diagnostics, and sensory and speech perception. The practice of tele-audiology additionally requires a working, practical knowledge of common ICT systems, counselling and influencing skills and an ability to guide clients into the most suitable model of service and care. The current text assumes that future tele-audiologists will have a good understanding of audiological sciences, good counselling and influencing skills, and skill and confidence with enabling technology platforms. The tele-audiologist will in other ways act in a triage role, knowing when to refer to a specialist, be that a specialist hearing professional, primary care provider, or other. The tele-audiologist may go on to become a domain specialist, such as working with clients who have tinnitus, or vertigo, or with cochlear implants.

There are two chapters in this text addressing tele-audiology in specialist domains. Firstly, Vanpoucke, Stainsby and colleagues have contributed a study, "Empowering Cochlear Implant Users in Their Home Environment by eHealth Solutions" (Chapter 5). These authors draw on the clinical evidence around self-empowerment in healthcare to predict and investigate the potential importance of client buy-in during the rehabilitation process. Clinicians in the specialty of cochlear implantation have seen the potential for remote and self-enabled care from an early stage in tele-audiology. This chapter is an excellent example of a development in a specialist application in audiology. Another specialist area in audiology is the management of tinnitus. Beukes and colleagues have contributed "A Framework for Designing and Evaluating Internet Interventions to Improve Tinnitus Care" (Chapter 6). The title indicates that tele-audiology is being investigated, not just for economic reasons, but indeed to improve care. These authors use the term tele-audiology to describe telecommunication technologies to reach out to patients, to reduce barriers to care in underserved areas, improve user satisfaction and access to specialists, to help practitioners expand their practice reach, and to save patients from having to travel or be transported to receive high quality care. It is an important development in the future delivery of audiological services. This chapter highlights the potential benefits and some of the existing barriers to its implementation.

Tele-audiology is not all about the technology. Sterling and his colleagues (Chapter 1) hypothesize that the emotional interaction between both practitioners and recipients of such services is different to that experienced in face to face care. There have been barriers encountered in the implementation of telehealth and these authors note that focusing on technical issues while ignoring emotional factors may fail to get any technology used widely. Whilst other studies have considered attitudes to telehealth without investigating causal factors, these authors review the emotional aspects which may affect uptake.

However, studies on clinician attitudes towards tele-audiology, which are described in more depth in the Introductory chapter, indicate that practitioners need more understanding of the enabling technologies, in order to be more confident in providing services. This is not a book on ICT, but any educational program on tele-audiology should address this aspect. However, it's important that practitioners have a realistic understanding of the security risks that are present. The goal is not to create fear, but to create an awareness. Security experts Harvey and Mueller provide insights into this topic in Chapter 8, which they describe as *not fun*. This chapter gives a perspective on how to think about information technology (IT) security, how it applies to telehealth and audiology, and gives some recommendations about important considerations for tele-audiology systems that include devices, data housing, smartphone applications and patient records.

In common with security, as a topic underpinning telehealth, and not just tele-audiology, is the regulatory landscape. Hardacre, who is internationally successful in the field of client management systems, and her colleague Wheeler, address the changing world of regulations. As they point out, this is about more than just data jurisdiction, although that in itself is a complex area for cloud-based solutions in telehealth. Applying Hardacre and Wheeler's discussion to tele-audiology reveals a government program that appears wedded to procedures developed many years before the advent of telehealth. There are no obvious ways to adapt old regulations and procedures and nor is that necessarily desirable. Who would choose to use an Apple 1 rather than a recent Macbook Pro (other than a collector that is)? Hearing, and other medical devices have evolved significantly in the last 20 years, and some self-fit hearing aids, whilst proven effective in studies, don't fit in with the established government distribution requirements. Like all medical professionals, audiologists and teleaudiologists will need to understand the limitations and advantages of digital health systems, developing an awareness of privacy and data sharing considerations to assist their clients and their families to optimize their hearing care. A very obvious advantage is that digital health delivered at the client's home via tele-audiology is truly family-centred in a way that is rarely possible in the clinic setting.

Working in the client's home (and potentially elsewhere) requires different tools for the assessment of hearing, both aided and unaided, and for the fitting and adjustment of hearing aids. The chapter by Blamey (Chapter 4) describes the speech perception test tools and processes used by a successful blended audiology/ tele-audiology business in Australia in which about 55% of clients primarily use the teleaudiology services and 45% primarily use the face-to-face clinical services. Both client groups, clinic and online, derive significant speech perception benefits from the technology and services provided, and the speech perception test has been shown to provide benefits for clinical use as well as in online tele-audiology. Two important requirements of tools for tele-audiology are that they must not use jargon without explanation for the layperson, and they must provide the client with meaningful information about the quality of life improvements offered by the use of the tele-audiology services and technology. These requirements are essential to give the client confidence and trust in the tools, the teleadiology service, and the technology so that they are empowered to use them in a way that is largely "do-it-yourself". Blamey's chapter "The Expected Benefit of Hearing Aids in Quiet as a Function of Hearing Thresholds" describes how the speech perception test satisfies these requirements.

Tele-audiology also imposes new requirements on the software apps that are used for assessment and fitting of devices in terms of their usability and reliability in the hands of the end users. The apps must run on a wide range of platforms including PCs, smart phones, Windows, iOS and Android operating systems. Paglialonga and colleagues (Chapter 7) expand on this topic in "Apps for Hearing Healthcare: Trends, Challenges, and Potential Opportunities." In the background to this chapter, they note that the number of apps for smartphones is rapidly growing, covering a very wide range of functions and services for the different target user groups within hearing healthcare. These range from professional and patient education to hearing screening, from remote counselling to auditory training, from personal sound amplification to support tools for parents and significant others.

In short, the chapters in this book are written by expert practitioners in their fields, based on experience and not just academic research. The initial research that led to these expert practices and businesses may be several years old now, but the authors have been gathering evidence to support the initial research findings and refine them through real-world experience of teleaudiology and digital health with real clients. This is a snowball effect that will continue to grow at an ever-increasing rate as the digital health model generates data and learnings as it goes along, enabling practitioners to be at the cutting edge of research and innovation simultaneous with the cutting edge of clinical excellence and client satisfaction.

REFERENCES

American Speech-Language-Hearing Association (ASHA). (n.d.) *Teleaudiology Clinical Technicians.* Retrieved September 30, 2018 from https://www.asha.org/Practice-Portal/Professional-Issues/Audiology-Assistants/Teleaudiology-Clinical-Assistants

Beckett, R. C., Saunders, E., & Blamey, P. J. (2016). Optimizing Hearing Aid Utilisation using Telemedicine Tools. In I. M. Miranda, R. Martinho, & R. Rijo (Eds.), *Encyclopedia of E-Health and Telemedicine* (pp. 72–85). IGI Global. doi:10.4018/978-1-4666-9978-6.ch007

Fabry, D., & Groth, J. (2017). Teleaudiology: Friend or Foe in the Consumerism of Hearing Healthcare? *The Hearing Review.* Retrieved September 30, 2018 from http://www.hearingreview.com/2017/04/teleaudiology-friend-foe-consumerism-hearing-healthcare/

Meskó, B. (2018). *Health IT Or Digital Health? The Gary-Rule Helps!* Retrieved September 28, 2018 from https://www.linkedin.com/pulse/health-digital-gary-rule-helps-bertalan-mcsk%C3%B3-md-phd/

Introduction

TELE-AUDIOLOGY: AN INTRODUCTION

This text will take the reader into the world of Tele-audiology, which complements audiology as it has been practiced for the last 50 years. Hearing health can be optimized using the relatively new enabling technologies available to us, to provide services that are efficient, convenient and more client centered than has been possible until now. Software plays a major role in health management today. It's now seven years since Marc Andreessen's famous essay, *Why Software Is Eating the World* in the Wall Street Journal, and indeed as predicted, every business is in part a software business. The result is that there has probably never been such an exciting time to be a clinician as we gain tools and opportunities to work with our clients as never before.

Readers of this book may be audiologists, audiometrists, tele-audiologists, hearing therapists, speech pathologists, government agencies, medical practitioners, or students. The goal of this collection of chapters is to provide some insights into the possibilities of audiology and how it might enhance your practice. This is not a "How To" text – it's a text that draws on some of the latest work in digital health with specific examples in audiology, and additionally draws attention to the associated issues of data security, and regulatory confusion. The author-researchers come from both academia and industry, giving a broad outlook to the text.

Tele-audiology is a subset of digital health. The terminology in digital health is inconsistent and can be confusing. I have used the term "tele-audiology" although strictly it is "digitally enabled audiology" or "hearing healthcare at a distance". Tele-audiology is the utilization of telehealth to provide audiological services and can include almost the full scope of audiological practice. This means a change in thinking about audiological practice. The audiologist is the undisputed expert in audiologic differential diagnostic evaluation, auditory rehabilitation, vestibular evaluation and pediatric hearing evaluation. Potentially these are areas that lend themselves to use of a remote technician, or other personnel, under the remote guidance of an audiologist. However, other areas of hearing healthcare may be conducted remotely, directly with the empowered consumer.

Tele-audiology developments should be considered in the context of the changes that are sweeping through medicine and healthcare generally, including telehealth. Telehealth is well established in some countries; for example, in Canada, telehealth is having a major impact on access to services, on equity of service provision, on quality of outcomes, and is increasing productivity (Chien, Geffen, and Gordon, 2011). The Canadian report is one of many that show that the benefits arising from telehealth extend far beyond the facilitation of client/clinician communication at a distance. The report includes reference to over forty different medical and allied health disciplines using telehealth. Tele-audiology is not among them, reflecting that audiology has been slow to adopt telehealth.

Developments in tele-audiology aim to deliver similar impact and benefits to clients as other areas of telehealth. In Australia, a National strategy is under development and was documented by Gill, in 2011. The document draws on earlier work from the UK, and includes a quote from a report prepared for the UK National Health Scheme (Cruikshank, 2010, Page 75), that "The question around telehealth is not whether, but how and at what pace?" There is an international consensus that telehealth is ready for growth and will deliver widespread benefits to clinicians, consumer, and national healthcare programs, if formally incorporated into public and private models of health care. This forward-thinking must not exclude tele-audiology. Much of the technology and infrastructure developed for telehealth applications can be applied directly to tele-audiology, and specialist tele-audiology tools are available, but the speed of adoption is unlikely to be led by traditional medicine. As the wide public adoption of Uber and AirBnB demonstrate, it is the consumer leading digital change. Medicine is inherently conservative, and the structure has remained similar for hundreds of years. As Hilaire Belloc famously wrote in his Cautionary Tales for Children:

And always keep a-hold of Nurse

For fear of finding something worse

Of course, there is an appropriate approach to risk minimization in healthcare. The tension between regulation and smartphone healthcare is inevitable. As Silicon Valley physician and tech entrepreneur Jordan Shlain is quoted as saying, "the techie attitude of move fast and break things comes up against the medical attitude of move slowly and don't kill people" (Vize, 2017). We are at a unique juxtaposition of technology and healthcare, requiring health professionals to extend their skill set and be open to new ways of working: a change that will increase both access to services and consumer empowerment.

Coincident with the exciting telehealth developments, there are other social changes and technological developments that are relevant to the development and effectiveness of Tele-audiology. It is an ideal framework for client empowerment and truly client-centred care. It can also be an enabler of health empowered communities, based on distributed trust, as evidenced in virtual client communities (Eysenbach, 2008). People are becoming empowered to interact with one another and take more control of their own health management, as personified by e-Patient Dave (De Bronkart, 2013; Ziebland and Wyke, 2012), the *Journal of Participatory Medicine*, and the writing of Eric Topol, in particular, *The Patient Will See You Now* (2015). The patient is empowered and is becoming a consumer. Topol, a U.S. physician and futurist, upends healthcare as we know it, foreshadowing a future of 'bottom-up' medicine in which digitally empowered patients participate in and take charge of their own health and care. Electronic health records are a Top-Down approach to meet this movement.

National digital health agencies and electronic health records, such as the Australian My Health Record (https://www.myhealthrecord.gov.au/), have been established. Several recently published studies show that hearing aid users can be empowered to fit their own hearing aids with appropriate technology (e.g., Blamey, Blamey, and Saunders, 2015; Keidser and Convery, 2016) and that social networks can be effective adjuncts to the clinical management of children with cochlear implants (Aiello and Ferrari, 2015). These are exciting developments that indicate that tele-audiology may be catching up with some of the more advanced and established telehealth trends.

In Australia, telehealth is ideally placed to support major national programs associated with geographically remote hearing health care, dementia, mental health, diabetes and regional concerns related to rehabilitation, acute waiting list relief, and outpatient support.

Interconnectivity has become a feature of many devices, including hearing aids. Hearing aids are the most sophisticated body-worn ultra-low-power personal digital computing devices in the world. They connect directly or indirectly, via wires or wirelessly, with smartphones, computers, other digital devices, and with the internet. The most common reason to connect a hearing aid and a computer is for programming or personalizing the hearing aid to the user's hearing preferences. With the computer also connected to the internet, the situation is tailor-made for tele-audiology applications. For example, the client may fit the hearing aid themselves and transmit the data securely to a remote database (Blamey et al., 2015) or the clinician may program the device from a remote location (Wesarg et al., 2010; Kuzovkov, Yanov, Levin, Bovo, and Rosignoli, 2014). The continuous or regular connection of hearing devices to smartphones or the internet will enable new tele-audiology applications, so that hearing aids are stand-alone or part of a more holistic health management plan. For example, daily monitoring of the hours of hearing aid use may be a useful non-invasive measure of activity and alertness for aged care and treatment of mental or physical illness (Molini-Avejonas, Rondon-Melo, de La Higuera Amato, and Samelli, 2015). Other monitoring applications may be integrated, which has already given rise to the term "hearables". Research studies of outcomes in Tele-audiology and other areas of telehealth are important in informing both health and ICT infrastructure policy.

One of the consequences of burgeoning telehealth practices is that health and medical data are being exchanged electronically as a fundamental part of the process. It is a small step to store and accumulate these data in various repositories including electronic medical records and then a further step to analyze large volumes of data to gain new insights into health from diverse perspectives. This area of data science is generally referred to as health informatics. The study includes the incidence of various health problems, the delivery of health services, and perhaps most importantly the economic burden of disease and disability (Coiera, 2015). The availability of large quantities of audiological data for analysis is one of the major benefits of tele-audiology that will accelerate audiological research and its translation into practice. For example, there have been several large-scale tele-audiology studies on practical applications of remote audiology and data interrogation (Pross, Bourne, and Cheung, 2016; Blamey et al., 2015; Jacobs and Saunders, 2014).

Digital health is part of the digitization of everything. We are at a unique intersection of rapid advances in digital connectivity, access to Big Data, Industry 4.0 manufacturing, commoditization of mobile devices, robotics, personalized medicine, reducing manufacturing costs, but increasing health costs. In the history of healthcare there has never been such an opportunity for reform. But this will bring an end to the structures and hierarchies as we know them. This is inspiring. Highly qualified clinicians will be able to restore their status to global specialist experts, while the majority of people take a more active role in managing their own healthcare and wellness. A recent Government survey in Australia showed that, of 3,000 people surveyed, 2,000 wanted to manage their own health from their smartphone (Australian Digital Health Agency, 2018). This is consistent with the availability of mobile devices. Cisco Systems estimates that the number of devices connected to the Internet will reach 50 billion by 2020.

People want better access to mobile digital health services for the whole community – not just those who are experienced users of new technology. Australia is now implementing the first stages of its Digital Health Strategy, and all states and territories have prioritized digital health as key to improving service delivery and health outcomes. This is a worldwide trend; while health policies and priorities differ across countries, many nations aim to increase the quality and efficiency of care, reduce administrative and operating costs of the healthcare system, and/or enable new models of healthcare delivery through effective use of ICT. A 2010 OECD survey identified 4 objectives for health ICT implementation: "(1) Increase the quality and efficiency of care; (2) Reduce the operating costs of clinical services; (3) Reduce the administrative costs of the healthcare system; and (4) Enable entirely new models of healthcare delivery." (OECD, 2015, page 5).

As patients take advantage of the digital era, become more empowered and more like consumers, the term "Consumer e-health" is becoming commonly used. The Netherlands Council for Public Health and Health Care has provided a definition for consumer e-health "as information and communication technologies offered directly on the market to consumers without the intermediary of care providers, the aim of which is to support or improve users' health." (The Council for Public Health and Health Care, 2015, page 5).

The ways in which healthcare can become more effective and economically efficient are many. As previously discussed, digital information can be mined to provide the means to better health outcomes; the application of real-time monitoring helps individuals and their healthcare providers in decision making and gives more people the opportunity to have home-based care; sharing health information with family and with an ecosystem of carers results in significant benefits for consumers; there is compelling data that hospital admissions are reduced, there are fewer adverse drug events, reduced duplication of tests, better coordination of care for people with chronic and complex conditions, and better-informed treatment decisions.

Digital health makes it easier to improve healthcare availability and patient experience by putting the patient at the center of their healthcare and providing greater access to healthcare for people who are living in rural and remote areas, or are unable to physically access services.

Despite these trends, there is little research on whether people with hearing loss will be equipped to participate in managing their care from home. Given that it is well established that people with untreated hearing loss experience many downstream consequences that significantly reduce their quality of life, and add significantly to the healthcare cost burden, it seems an obvious imperative to establish tele-audiology within the digital health ecosystem.

The Editor's view is that there is a clinical need for tele-audiology. The World Health Organization (WHO, 2018) estimates that 466 million people (over 5% of the world population) have hearing loss that is disabling. Their estimate is based on a criterion for disability that most scholars would regard as quite conservative; that is, hearing loss greater than 40 decibels (dB) in the better hearing ear in adults and a hearing loss greater than 30 dB in the better hearing ear in children, measured over a four-frequency average. Current production of hearing aids meets less than 10% of the global need even with this criterion, but even if production could be accelerated, face-to-face services and audiological facilities are lacking.

In developed countries, adult acquired sensorineural hearing damage is the dominant cause of hearing loss, and if left unaddressed can lead to progressive auditory deprivation at the cortical level, leading to reduced speech recognition. This is of particular relevance in difficult environments where the signal to noise ratio is significantly weighted, in favour of noise. A reduced ability to detect, identify and localise speech sounds in various environments not only affects the lives of the individual with impaired hearing but also their significant others, as it can cause a breakdown in communication, or a barrier to accessing education and employment. A breakdown in effective communication may also lead to feelings of isolation, reduced social activity, and overall poorer quality of life. Acquired hearing loss is known to increase the likelihood of developing mental health and cognitive problems, including dementia (Lin et al., 2013; Arlinger, 2003). The sooner acquired hearing loss is rehabilitated the better the outcome. However, current services for hearing aid provision are not equal to the task of helping all people with hearing loss, and even where hearing aids are readily available, such as in Australia, where in 2006 and again in 2017 it was reported that fewer than one in five people who would benefit from hearing aids goes on to own and use them (Access Economics, 2006; Deloitte Access Economics for the Hearing Care Industry Association, 2017) may be inferred that these statistics suggest a need for more accessible and less costly audiology services and hearing aid fitting. Tele-audiology is a potential cost saving solution, reducing the need for expensive infrastructure at local sites, and overcoming the inadequate availability of appropriately trained professionals.

From a clinical perspective in developed countries, tele-audiology is a potential means to enable each service to structure a scalable and less costly service to attract more clients and achieve greater impact on the hearing health of the population. The proliferation of online hearing screening tests and questionnaires indicates that audiologists are well aware of this potential. Tele-audiology is also being used to provide face-to-face interactions with remote clients over the internet.

There is a shortage of trained clinicians in less developed countries. The WHO has taken the approach of trying to reduce the size of the problem and has provided strong guidance to try to reduce the prevalence of, particularly, childhood deafness, but there is likely to still be a shortage of trained clinicians for some time to come. There is thus both a need and an opportunity to change the audiology service delivery model.

As the chapters in this book demonstrate, there are diverse areas of tele-audiology and hearing care all aimed at reducing barriers, lowering costs, and bringing satisfaction to the consumer. Not all areas of tele-audiology have been included, as there are other texts addressing predominantly pediatric care or remote hearing screening. In audiology the benefits of telehealth are becoming apparent for both client and provider as evidence shows both diagnostic and treatment services can be done remotely, reducing barriers to access and resources, and as a result promoting a more client-centered approach to care delivery.

Tele-audiology can reduce some of the cost barriers to getting hearing aids or other hearing help. Cost impacts service seeking and uptake. Cost can create a barrier regardless of motivation, and remote service provision provides a path to cost reduction and easier access.

There are published reports of some of the savings and benefits, such as the work of Gabrielle Saunders (Saunders, 2014) of the National Center of Rehabilitative Audiology in the USA who, in a published presentation quoted results from the Alaskan Federal Health Access program where a program of remote audiology saved nearly 3 million miles in travel, reduced wait times, and provided strong consumer satisfaction. There are many pilot programs around the world making small wins like the Alaskan project, but despite the positive outcomes, tele-audiology has not been widely adopted.

In this Introduction, I have supplied some terms that are commonly used in digital health, all of which apply to Tele-audiology, and which can be described as follows:

- **Store and Forward:** Which may include photographs, including as captured by video otoscopy, and test results. The term is descriptive. It just refers to the capture of results which can then be forwarded to an expert.
- **Real-Time:** In contrast to *Store and forward*, and as described, this refers to live interaction with a remote expert. This could be Live chat, video consultation, remote testing, counselling, or hearing device tuning. In some cases, it might include guiding another health practitioner, such as a nurse, in carrying out audiological procedures.
- **Monitoring:** Perhaps one of the strongest advantages of connected health is the ability to monitor the user of the device, in order to identify changes that could potentially be posing health risks.
- **Mobile Apps:** There are thousands of Apps available for people with hearing loss, covering many topics. There is more on this topic in a later chapter.

The chapters in this book take the reader on a broader journey than "Does tele-audiology work?" to look at examples in diverse areas of hearing health and to introduce the readers to associate factors, such as security, the regulatory environment, and the emotional aspects of a new form of health delivery.

A key aspect of a tele-audiology model of service is that in order for the outcome to be successful, client empowerment and self-efficacy is key. In order to be achieve this, clinicians need to have access to appropriate information, support and resources.

In this book, a model of care is discussed which provides an example of incorporating tele-audiology with face-to-face services. In other chapters, important questions for the health provider are discussed including; considerations for information security, privacy in a shared model, maximizing communication in a digitally safe manner, and how to evaluate various aspects of a tele-audiology system.

The book starts with a topic on the Emotional Factors for Audiology in which the authors examine some of the factors that hamper the uptake of telemedicine, including funding models and the availability of technology. Leading off with an examination of the emotional factors is possible due to the already established evidence that many telehealth models work. There are still barriers to widespread uptake and the authors tackle the role that emotional factors contribute to the emotions of users interacting with systems and services. They look at the emotional factors that need to be considered in providing tele-audiology services drawing on information technology research. They also look at how emotional factors can be taken into consideration with respect to a specific tele-audiology service provided by a successful company. This same company is used in two other chapters as a source of data and practice, being an advanced tele-audiology service that has been running for 7 years.

Chapter 2 explores the regulatory aspects that must be considered in a telehealth environment. The authors point out that the regulatory issues are about much more than data jurisdiction, and touch on the challenges of payments in a system that spans jurisdictions.

Chapter 3 takes us into a blended channel hearing healthcare environment and examines the application of the robust Goldstein and Stephens model of Auditory Enablement. David Goldstein and Dai Stephens collaborated in the early 1980s to improve the integration of the various aspects of auditory enablement with the needs of patients. This led to the development of a ‘management model’ of audiological rehabilitation (Goldstein and Stephens, 1981). In the subsequent 35 years, there has been substantial research giving considerable evidence for their approach. Blamey & Saunders Hearing operates a blended model of care within a digital health hearing ecosystem, and the chapter explains the application of the Goldstein and Stephens model in applying consistent care and service across the channels.

An advantage of tele-audiology and cloud-based data is that it enables large data sets to be analyzed. Chapter 4 reports a study aimed to estimate speech perception benefits in quiet for clients with different degrees of hearing loss. The difference between aided and unaided scores on a monosyllabic word test presented binaurally was used as the measure of benefit. Retrospective data for 492 hearing aid users with four-frequency pure-tone average hearing losses (PTA) ranging from 5 dB HL to 76 dB HL in the better ear were analyzed using nonlinear regression. The mean benefit for the perception of monosyllabic words in this group of clients was

22.3% and the maximum expected benefit was 33.6% for a PTA of 52 dB HL. The expected benefit can be expressed as a reduction of the error rate by about half for isolated words and about three quarters for sentences across the full range of PTA.

Perhaps surprisingly, one of the most advanced areas in tele-audiology is in cochlear implants. In Chapter 5, the authors address the prescient need to update accepted care models of cochlear-implant (CI) fitting and long-term maintenance to better utilize Self-Care and Tele-Medicine possibilities, thus shifting the focus of CI maintenance to the recipient, which is consistent with the theme of empowerment that consistently recurs in this book. There is a strong evidence base that such a move will better meet the needs of CI users, giving them greater control of, and involvement in, their hearing progress. In the chapter, the authors describe a case study of pilot software for CI maintenance based on Tele-audiology with the inclusion of data collected from initial studies.

The 6th chapter was authored by a multidisciplinary team, with the stated aim of encouraging utilization of digital healthcare in the context of chronic conditions such as tinnitus. It provides a comprehensive and systematic framework for the design and evaluation of these interventions. The authors' aim is that the examples and guidelines can be applied by those interested in improving service delivery models such as clinicians, scientists, researchers, students, and government based workers.

The 7th chapter addresses the rapidly growing world of mobile apps in hearing health care (HHC) (mobile health or m-health). The authors review the recent evolution of apps for HHC and assesses the current scenario in terms of availability, variety, penetration, offered services, and target user groups. The chapter also shows how newly developed methods for app characterization and assessment can support audiologists and HHC professionals. These methods can enable them to get meaningful knowledge about apps, understand their peculiar features, and, in turn, help their patients to get increased benefit from informed, effective use of these solutions. Specifically, the chapter describes a recently developed method that is able to characterize apps for HHC, regardless of the operating system and hardware platform, by using a core set of features: the *ALFA4Hearing*. Then, the chapter describes the multifaceted picture obtained by using the *ALFA4Hearing* model on a representative sample of apps. Finally, the chapter discusses the main emerging trends and needs in this area and highlight the open challenges as well as some potential opportunities for professionals, researchers, developers, and stakeholders at large.

The final chapter addresses the flip-side of all the significant advances in technology, communications, business and social interactions of telehealth – that of security. The authors are data security experts. They note that for every new way that society finds to make use of technology for better efficiencies and outcomes, the bad guys find a way to abuse it. This is the reason why there seems to be an endless series of new cyber-attacks, privacy breaches and organizations being compromised.

Whilst not intended to deter people from tele-audiology, it's important that people are prepared and have a balanced view of the benefits and risks.

This collection of studies provides the reader with a broad view of the possibilities in tele-audiology. Students are encouraged to read more broadly in trends in digital health.

The world of healthcare is adapting and tele-audiology has been shown to have many service and client advantages. The book provides sufficient examples to demonstrate that tele-audiology is now part of hearing healthcare. Are you ready?

Elaine Saunders
Blamey Saunders Hears, Australia

REFERENCES

Access Economics. (2006). *Listen Hear!* The Economic Impact and Cost of Hearing Loss in Australia.

Aiello, C. P., & Ferrari, D. V. (2015). Teleaudiology: Efficacy assessment of an online social network as a support tool for parents of children candidates for cochlear implant. *CoDAS*, *27*(5). PMID:26648210

Arlinger, S. (2003). Negative consequences of uncorrected hearing loss - a review. *International Journal of Audiology*, *42*(2), S17–S20. doi:10.3109/14992020309074639 PMID:12918624

Australian Digital Health Agency. (2018). *What you told us.* Retrieved August 20, 2018 from https://conversation.digitalhealth.gov.au/what-does-australia-want-digital-health

Blamey, P. J., Blamey, J. K., & Saunders, E. (2015). Effectiveness of a teleaudiology approach to hearing aid fitting. *Journal of Telemedicine and Telecare*, *21*(8), 474–478. doi:10.1177/1357633X15611568 PMID:26556060

Chien, E., Geffen, M., & Gordon, D. (2011). *Telehealth Benefits and Adoption: Connecting People and Providers Across Canada.* A Study Commissioned by Canada Health Infoway. Retrieved August 18, 2018, from https://blogs.dal.ca/distmeded/files/2012/08/telehealth_report_summary_2011_en.pdf

Coiera, E. (2015). *Guide to health informatics*. London, UK: Taylor Francis.

Cruikshank, J. (2010*). HealthCare without Walls: A Framework for delivering telehealth at scale.* Retrieved August 18, 2018, from http://www.2020health.org/2020health/Publications/Publications-2010/telehealth.html

De Bronkart, D. (2013). *Let Patients Help*. CreateSpace Independent Publishing Platform. Retrieved April 10, 2018, from https://www.createspace.com/

Deloitte Access Economics for the Hearing Care Industry Association. (2017). *The Social and Economic Cost of Hearing Loss in Australia*. Retrieved August 22, 2018, from http://www.hcia.com.au/hcia-wp/wp-content/uploads/2015/05/Social-and-Economic-Cost-of-Hearing-Health-in-Australia_June-2017.pdf

Eysenbach, G. (2008). Medicine 2.0: Social networking, collaboration, participation, apomediation, and openness. *Journal of Medical Internet Research, 10*(3), e22. doi:10.2196/jmir.1030 PMID:18725354

Gill, M. A. (2011). *A National Telehealth Strategy For Australia - For Discussion*. Commissioned by Australian National Consultative Committee on Electronic Health (ANCCeH). Retrieved August 18, 2018, from http://www.who.int/goe/policies/countries/aus__support_tele.pdf

Goldstein, D. P., & Stephens, S. D. (1981). Audiological rehabilitation: Management model I. *Audiology, 20*(5), 432–452. doi:10.3109/00206098109072713 PMID:7271594

Jacobs, P. G., Saunders, G. H., Jacobs, P. G., & Saunders, G. H. (2014). New opportunities and challenges for teleaudiology within department of Veterans Affairs. *Journal Rehabilitative Research and Development., 51*(5), vii–xi. doi:10.1682/JRRD.2014.04.0093 PMID:25334005

Keidser, G., & Convery, E. (2016). Self-Fitting Hearing Aids: Status Quo and Future Predictions. *Trends in Hearing, 20*, 1–15. doi:10.1177/2331216516643284 PMID:27072929

Kuzovkov, V., Yanov, Y., Levin, S., Bovo, R., Rosignoli, M., Eskilsson, G., & Willbas, S. (2014). Remote programming of MED-EL cochlear implants: Users' and professionals' evaluation of the remote programming experience. *Acta Oto-Laryngologica, 134*(7), 709–716. doi:10.3109/00016489.2014.892212 PMID:24773208

Lin, F. R., Yaffe, K., Xia, J., Xue, Q., Harris, T. B., Purchase-Helzner, E., ... Simonsick, E. M. (2013). Hearing Loss and Cognitive Decline in Older Adults. *Journal American Medical Association Internal Medicine, 173*(4), 293–299. PMID:23337978

Molini-Avejonas, D. R., Rondon-Melo, S., de La Higuera Amato, C. A., & Samelli, G. A. (2015). A systematic review of the use of telehealth in speech, language and hearing sciences. *Journal of Telemedicine and Telecare, 21*(7), 367–376. doi:10.1177/1357633X15583215 PMID:26026181

Organisation for Economic Co-operative Development (OECD). (2015). *Draft OECD Guide to Measuring ICTs in the Health Sector.* Retrieved August 18, 2018 from https://www.oecd.org/health/health-systems/Draft-oecd-guide-to-measuring-icts-in-the-health-sector.pdf

Pross, S. E., Bourne, A. L., & Cheung, S. W. (2016). TeleAudiology in the Veterans Health Administration. *Otology & Neurotology, 37*(7), 847–850. doi:10.1097/MAO.0000000000001058 PMID:27273404

Saunders, G. (2014). *Teleaudiology: The future of audiology?* National Center for Rehabilitative Auditory Research. Retrieved August 22, 2018 from http://www.nationalacademies.org/hmd/~/media/Files/Activity%20Files/PublicHealth/HearingLossAging/1-13%20Saunders%20pdf.pdf

The Council for Public Health and Health Care. (2015). *Consumer e-Health.* Retrieved August 23, 2018 from https://www.raadrvs.nl/uploads/docs/Consumer_ehealth.pdf

Topol, E. (2015). *The Patient Will See You Now: The Future of Medicine Is in Your Hands*. New York: Basic Books.

Vize, W. (2017, September 8). The NHS must embrace digital services or risk being left behind. *The Guardian.* Retrieved August 22, 2018, from https://www.theguardian.com/healthcare-network/2017/sep/08/nhs-embrace-digital-services-risk-left-behind

Wesarg, T., Wasowski, A., Skarzynski, H., Ramos, A., Falcon Gonzalez, J. C., Kyriafinis, G., ... Laszig, R. (2010). Remote fitting in Nucleus cochlear implant recipients. *Acta Oto-Laryngologica, 130*(12), 1379–1388. doi:10.3109/00016489.2010.492480 PMID:20586675

World Health Organization. (2018). *Deafness and hearing loss*. Retrieved August 22, 2018, from http://www.who.int/mediacentre/factsheets/fs300/en/

Ziebland, S., & Wyke, S. (2012). Health and illness in a connected world: How might sharing experiences on the internet affect people's health? *The Milbank Quarterly, 90*(2), 219–249. doi:10.1111/j.1468-0009.2012.00662.x PMID:22709387

Chapter 1
Emotional Factors for Teleaudiology

Leon Sterling
Swinburne University of Technology, Australia

Rachel Burrows
University of Melbourne, Australia

Belinda Barnet
Swinburne University of Technology, Australia

Simone Taffe
Swinburne University of Technology, Australia

Rachael McDonald
Swinburne University of Technology, Australia

ABSTRACT

The internet has created new possibilities for health practitioners to deliver services remotely. The potential for telemedicine is yet to be fully realized. Many factors hamper the uptake of telemedicine, including funding models and the availability of technology. This chapter concerns one important area often neglected by technology developers: considering the emotions of users interacting with systems and services. The authors believe that consideration of emotions is essential for the advocacy, adoption, and appropriation of telemedicine services by a wide range of stakeholders, who have diverse abilities and motivations. They consider one area of telemedicine: teleaudiology. The authors outline emotional factors that need to be considered in providing teleaudiology services drawing on research from software engineering developing agent-oriented models of socio-technical systems, as well as knowledge of assistive technology frameworks. They consider how emotional factors can be taken into consideration with respect to a specific teleaudiology service provided by a successful company.

DOI: 10.4018/978-1-5225-8191-8.ch001

1. INTRODUCTION

The Internet and other technologies have created new possibilities for health practitioners to deliver services remotely, in order to address challenges such as access and geography, a phenomenon known as telemedicine or telehealth (WHO, 2011). The potential for telemedicine is yet to be fully realised. Many factors hamper the uptake of telemedicine, including funding models and the availability of technology. This paper concerns one important area often neglected by technology developers, considering the emotions of users interacting with systems and services.

Consideration of emotion, and the effect that emotion has on cognition, is essential for understanding and increasing the take up of telehealth services. Whether a service is adopted is affected by a wide-range of stakeholders, who typically have diverse abilities and motivations. Most computer software researchers focus on technical aspects when asked to develop software or systems for health. While technology can connect people in social domains and support people in their everyday lives, the technology is only valuable if it addresses and fulfills people's needs. Needs include cognitive and emotional needs, such as experiencing fun, feeling engaged or feeling valued (Prilleltensky, 2016).

When considering adoption of telehealth, the technology itself is an important factor. Factors such as reliability, trust and confidentiality, as well as access to appropriate software and hardware must be considered and must be correct. Without the reliability and validity of the technology itself, the person is unlikely to engage with the process. However the effective uptake and utilisation of telemedicine depends on the advocacy, adoption and appropriation of the software by a wide-range of stakeholders, who have diverse abilities and motivations.

Focussing on technical issues while ignoring emotional factors may fail to get any technology used widely (Mendoza et al, 2013). Further, lack of use of a technology effectively diminishes both the value of the investment in the technology and the significance in producing outcomes. The literature indicates that emotional expectations of the user are critical if users are to appropriate technology meaningfully into their lives (Boehner et al., 2007), which becomes even more complex when looking at health, healthcare and assistive technologies. Healthcare is always a highly emotional experience that involves intense emotions at all stages, including prior to intervention occurring (Berry, Davis and Wilmet, 2015).

The need for emotional design has been made cogently by Norman (2005). Norman refers to three levels of cognitive processing: visceral processing, associated with product "look and feel"; behavioral processing, associated with product characteristics such as performance and usability; and reflective processing, associated with the meaning of a product and its impact on self-image and satisfaction. Emotions play a role in all levels. While Norman's work seems not to have been adopted widely by software and app developers. However emotions have been discussed in the context of requirements engineering by (Bentley et al, 2002), (Ramos and Berry, 2005), and (Proynova et al, 2011) among others.

Given the highly emotive nature of health care, it is imperative that any changes or digitization be considered in the context of the emotion of the recipient. Emotion in the context of technology for assistive technologies, or innovation in supplying health care to address a deficit, mean that emotion must be at the centre of the process. Often, medical devices are designed with only functionality in mind. However, when providing healthcare technological innovations, there is a need to balance the needs as well as the abilities and limitations of a range of stakeholders, which includes the user, but also regulatory and funding bodies as well as the provider.

For take up and implementation of telehealth, it is important that the experience of using technology be considered. It has been purported with mainstream assistive technologies that poor design can reinforce negative feelings, such as isolation and stigmatization; and conversely, the technological experience of healthcare means that the affect of the experience of using the technological solution, combined with the meaning, and the feelings and emotions aroused must be considered. For this sort of health related technology to be successful, the intrinsic characteristics of the experience must be both successful as a functional outcome but also the emotions that are experienced by the end user (and the clinician).

This paper is concerned with one area of telemedicine, namely delivering audiology services over the Internet. Loss of hearing is an emotional issue for people, and the above discussion applies to teleaudiology. Given the importance of emotional factors in the success of uptake of new health services, we discuss the factors that are pertinent to consider when providing teleaudiology services. The emotional factors are explicitly represented in models, drawing on research from an area of software engineering encompassing agent-oriented modelling for socio-technical systems (Sterling and Taveter, 2009).

We use the term socio-technical systems to refer to systems that involve people and technology. Teleaudiology is a good example of a socio-technical system. To model the provision of audiology services over the Internet many stakeholders need to be considered: clients who have hearing concerns, audiologists who will assess hearing problems, customers who will pay for services, software developers who will develop any code that is needed, and people who will communicate the service. Each stakeholder has their own goals and objectives, and can be modelled as an agent. Agent models are well suited to describe socio-technical systems as will be illustrated in Section 4.

This paper is organised as follows. Section 2 discusses hearing services and how they can be met by teleaudiology. Section 3 discusses designing products that consider users' emotions. Section 4 presents motivational models that are used to depict emotional goals of socio-technical systems and presents a motivational model for teleaudiology. Section 5 presents a discussion of the emotional factors and how they can be manifest by looking at a particular teleaudiology service provided by Blamey Saunders Hears. Section 6 concludes.

2. HEARING SERVICES AND TELEAUDIOLOGY

Telemedicine is at least as old as the Internet, if not older. If one considers the use of the telegraph and telephone as a means to convey medical information, it could be said that it started in the mid-1800s (Krupinski, 2015). Teleaudiology is more recent, largely because the use of physiologic measures to test hearing did not become routine until the 1950s, and Audiology itself was not established as a discipline in Australia until the Office of Hearing Services (now called Audiology Australia) was created in 1997. It is now an established healthcare service, with certification for clinical competencies that are consistent with equivalent health professions.

Approximately one in six Australians are affected by hearing loss, expected to increase to one in four by 2060, with a cost of A$15.9 billion per year. Currently, hearing services in Australia require visiting an audiology practitioner and taking a series of audiology tests in a sound booth consisting of beeps at different frequencies to produce an audiogram. The audiogram, displaying the *softest* sounds you can hear across frequencies, shows your hearing thresholds. These thresholds tell the audiologist the degree of hearing loss you have and in many cases the type, conductive or sensorineural. The thresholds are used to program and dispense a hearing aid. The device must then be fitted – a mould is taken of the ear/s on one visit and the patient subsequently returns to have the device properly fitted. For adults the process can be completed in four visits, but for children, whose ear canal is growing rapidly, many more may be required. Fitting hearing aids is a largely unregulated industry. Only people who hold a healthcare card, or who are children/young people can have their hearing aid fitted for a reasonable cost. The focus has been on the devices themselves, but there is little attention paid to the rehabilitation and ongoing maintenance required for the hearing aid service to be successful. There are inadequate numbers of audiologists available; and so, the experience of attending an audiologist is coloured by this stretched service which costs the consumer a considerable sum.

Telemedicine is defined as "the use of medical information exchanged from one site to another via electronic communications to improve a patient's clinical health status. Telemedicine includes a growing variety of applications and services using two-way video, email, smart phones, wireless tools and other forms of telecommunications technology" (American Telemedicine Association, 2014). It is a new industry that aims in large part to dispense with the tedium of in-office visits. In the case of teleaudiology, it seeks to streamline the need to refine, fit, and dispense the device. Teleaudiology allows people from more diverse and rural areas to gain access to hearing services; rather than requiring proximity to a Hearing Australia office, which are concentrated in metropolitan regions.

It is difficult to conduct the full battery of hearing threshold tests over the Internet without an audiologist, and without using a sound booth for the patient. However new tests have been developed that allow audiological services and hearing devices to be dispensed over the internet. These tests can either be conducted synchronously, i.e. immediately, or asynchronously where the results are stored and later viewed by a healthcare professional. An example of such a test is the Blamey Saunders Hears speech perception test which uses the patient's *ability to hear words and speech sounds over the internet* rather than *threshold beeps in a sound booth* to determine the right settings for a hearing device. At the end of the speech perception test, conducted synchronously over the Internet, the patient can use the results to order a hearing device without needing to attend multiple in-office sessions.

Teleaudiology holds "much promise for improving access to health care and reducing the barriers that many people in both rural and urban environments face with respect to getting timely, appropriate, and expert care" (Krupinski, 2015). It is a growing discipline and requires practitioners who are both adept with technology and attuned to the needs of patients who use it. Here we argue that emotional needs need to be considered as well as the physiologic and technological needs.

Hearing loss and accessing hearing services is an inherently emotional topic. In children, hearing loss can delay language development and impact educational and social participation; in adults, a reduction in productive employment and social participation can be impaired. In the older population, or for people with other disaiblities, isolation and an increase in cognitive decline can result. Thus, teleaudiology has the promise to deliver real solutions to reduce isolation. All of the factors need to be considered in providing a teleaudiology service.

3. DESIGNING PRODUCTS THAT CONSIDER USERS' EMOTIONS

For many years designers have known that products and services elicit emotions in end-users. Designers accept that one of the barriers to the uptake of products and services is the design of a product itself. Norman's book '*Why we love or hate everyday objects*' highlights the designers' role in end-users' responses to products (2005). Books such as Funology (Blythe et al, 2004) and Love Marks (Roberts, 2005) provide explanations, tools and techniques for designers to consider the emotional aspects of the things they design.

It is acknowledged that designing for emotional response is not easy, as people have various goals for using a product on different days and in various contexts. Norman argues that while our understanding of emotions has advanced, tools for designers have been slow to develop.

Norman calls for more tools to be developed. The benefits considering emotions in the design process are identified as getting in-depth understanding of user emotions, determining the emotional impact of a product, keeping continuity of emotional intentions in communications, facilitating design creativity, strengthening emotional coherence and managing emotions within a product development team (Yoon, Pohlmeyer and Desmet, 2016). Previous research shows that it is possible to manipulate design features to elicit feelings in the end-user. For example, Kim and Moon's study was successful in designing a user interface for electronic commerce systems to evoke the feeling of trust for end-users (1998). Another study provides empirical evidence that the colour white elicits different emotional responses to other colours, confirming the importance for designers to consider emotional aspect of colour choices (Na and Suk 2014).

Desmet's book *Designing Emotions* provides a tool for studying end-users' emotional reaction to products across languages and cultures. His tool can be used to assess the emotional impact of a product and used as a guide for products to meet desired emotional requirements (2002). Desmet's tool relies on facial expression and body language that are universally understood. Desmet's tool is called PrEmo (short for Product Emotion) using one minute movies incorporating 14 animations, showing emotions through cartoon hand gestures and facial expressions. There are seven positive and seven negative emotions. He uses a 3-point scale for end-users to decide, 'I do, to some extent or do not feel the emotion expressed by this animation'. In 3 minutes, end-users respond to 14 emotions: Unpleasant, Indignation, Contempt, Disgust, Unpleasant Surprise, Dissatisfaction Disappointment Boredom Pleasant desire, Pleasant surprise, Inspiration, Amusement, Admiration, Satisfaction, Fascination.

Another study focusing on 'design for happiness' found design can foster social relationships and belongingness, create meaning in life, and helps consumers be active participants rather than passive observers ultimately contributing to profits and sales (Sääksjärvi and Hellén, 2013). While most authors discuss the role of positive emotions in design, more recently authors argue that designers can use negative emotions to enhance user-product interaction (Fokkinga and Desmet 2001). Fokkinga and Desmet show how designers can decide which negative emotion is naturally present within a user context, how and when this emotion is best detected or elicited, and how to apply this information to a concept design to create a rich user experience. Typically, designers understand that fear is evoked when something threatens a person, and sadness is evoked by a loss but designers can use these 'negative emotions' in reverse, to create the circumstances that elicit the chosen emotion in the user. Here we can imagine a teleaudiology interface that detects panic when the user can't hear people and adapts to promote relaxation that is achieved when the user can hear sounds clearly.

In understanding the emotional factors at play in the design and use of hearing aids, Kelly and Matthews (2014) identifies the feelings of stigma of the device, loneliness and isolation of the end-users and resistance to take advice of the healthcare professionals who are mistrusted as salespeople. In Kelly's study patients had concerns about hearing aids' visibility and level of comfort, doctors tried to give advice and allay fears at the same time. Audiologists have to confirm the fact of hearing loss and be a salesperson to persuade the patient to buy an expensive hearing aid, interfering with the patients' trust in the doctors to take up the device. In Kelly's study the patients tried to persuade the doctor they didn't need a hearing aid. Doctors can't convince patients of hearing aid benefits if they can't handle the patients' personal arguments against the devices (Kelly and Matthews, 2014). If a patient doesn't trust the healthcare practitioner, or understand their arguments, or are convinced by their motivations, they do not take up hearing aids.

People often think they are too young to wear a hearing aid, pointing to the stigma of ageing associated with hearing aids (Kelly and Matthews, 2014). Take the example of growing a beard for November which is a deliberate visible catalyst to start conversations and awareness about mens' health. Perhaps hearing aids could be designed with bright colours associated with sportswear or with high tech features, fitting in the music or gaming headphones category. Instead of designing with discretion, highly visible hearing aids could give people with hearing aids an identity with each other and a conversation starter to overcome potential problems of isolation and social withdrawal.

A recent project where emotions have been designed for explicitly is the development of the new hearing aid, Facett, by Blamey Saunders Hears. Leah Heiss, a designer from RMIT, spent 37 weeks with the engineering team to come up with a new generation of hearing aids (Heiss, 2018). In Heiss' words, "Research shows that when people accept their hearing loss and finally get hearing aids, the feelings of stigma around wearing them decreases. So that stigma is highest before they get the devices. The design of Facett is about helping people get over the line to take up a technology that could dramatically improve their health and wellbeing - to get them past that emotional barrier through great design." In an attempt to produce a beautiful design which would be aesthetically appealing, Heiss studied crystals at the Melbourne Museum. A picture of Facett, in its four different colours, is provided in Picture 1. We will say a little more about Facett and the emotional design process in Section 5.

4. AGENT-ORIENTED MODELLING, MOTIVATIONAL MODELS, AND EMOTIONAL GOALS

Software engineering is concerned with the development of complex systems involving people and technology. Methods have emerged that strive to simplify the task of building complicated software. Thinking about complexity led to research in intelligent agents. As expressed by Somerville, "*Agent-oriented technology is an effective way to construct socio-technical systems, which take into account organisational and human issues as well as technical issues. Agents are a useful abstraction that helps us think about how socio-technical systems deliver the services required by their users. We should think about this without regard to whether the agents that deliver these services are people or automated systems. Modeling a system as agents gives us a way of establishing flexible boundaries for the automated system that can be extended as our understanding of human tasks improve over time...*" (From foreword in Sterling and Taveter, 2009).

The essence of agent-oriented methods as described in Sterling and Taveter (2009) is to model a socio-technical system in terms of goals that need to be accomplished and roles with responsibilities and constraints which are undertaken by agents, which may be human or software, to achieve the goals. The goals are multi-faceted, encompassing both functional goals and quality goals. In recent years, research has highlighted the need to also consider emotional goals in software. One area where emotional factors have been considered in detail is providing emergency call services to older people living at home (Miller et al, 2015). Not focussing on emotional goals can greatly hinder uptake of technology (Mendoza et al., 2013)

Figure 1. Facett Hearing aid inspired by crystal designs

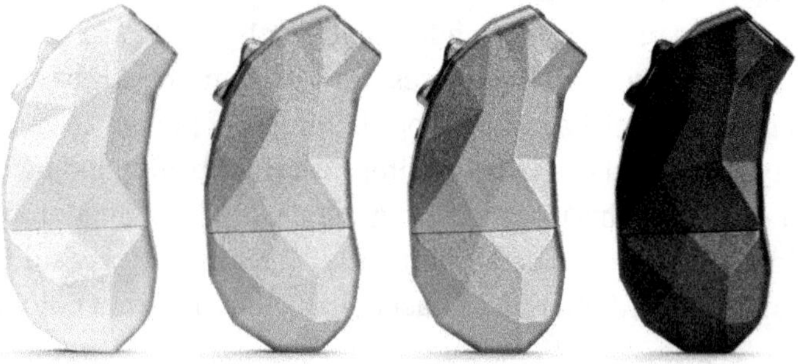

In Sterling and Taveter's work, models are described at three levels of abstraction. Models at the motivation level give the overall picture of what is trying to be achieved by the socio-technical system (a business brief in effect). Models at the design level describe which agents are needed, what tasks they perform, and what communication they need. Models at the implementation level specify the software that needs to be built and necessary interfaces. In this paper we solely discuss models from the motivational level.

Motivational models have been used extensively over the last several years. They are currently used routinely in teaching software engineering students at the University of Melbourne. Models have been developed for several research projects in the health domain, where emotional considerations are essential, including depression screening (Wachtler et al, 2018), mental health recovery (Thomas et al, 2016) and providing emergency care services for people in the home (Lopez-Lorca et al., 2014; Miller et al., 2015).

Motivational models are easy to generate with stakeholder workshop(s), and are easy to understand in our experience. The modelling process engenders useful conversations and allows people to agree on a high level understanding of the problem being solved or the service being provided. We have found these models can represent a common view for decision-makers within the company and consequently can support decision making disparate groups, such as service designers, developers or marketers. As can be seen with the model for tele-audiology described in this section in Figure 2, the models are (deliberately) not fully prescribed.

A motivational model is developed in response to a perceived business need that is often described with a motivational scenario. The scenario captures a shared understanding of a problem for which a socio-technical system will be (at least partially) developed.

Table 1 is a motivational scenario for one component of teleaudiology, assessing hearing online. A motivational scenario serves a similar purpose to a use case or a user story in more traditional software engineering. It has four components: a name, a description, a quality description, and an emotional description.

Table 1. Motivational scenario for assessing hearing online

Scenario name: Assess hearing online **Scenario Description:** A client accesses a Website providing a teleaudiology service and undertakes an online test. **Quality Description:** The test needs to be easy to take, valid and reliable, convenient for the client, and effective in its assessment of the hearing of the client. **Emotional Description:** The client needs to be reassured that the test is being conducted privately with appropriate care taken of private information. Furthermore the assessment needs to be a positive experience for the client, so that s/he feels empowered and in control.

Figure 2 contains a motivational model for an overall teleaudiology service. The model was developed in a standard requirements elicitation process with a range of stakeholders. There are four types of entities in the model. The parallelograms are goals which must be achieved by the overall socio-technical system which the teleaudiology service is addressing. Such goals loosely correspond to functional requirements. The people figures are roles which need to be undertaken within the socio-technical system. Roles, which are described through responsibilities and constraints, will be fulfilled by agents, either people or software agents. Clouds are quality goals, which are attributes the system is being designed to achieve, and are examples of non-functional requirements of the overall system. Finally hearts denote emotions, which are desirable emotions that agents should feel when interacting with the system.

Figure 2. Motivational model for teleaudiology

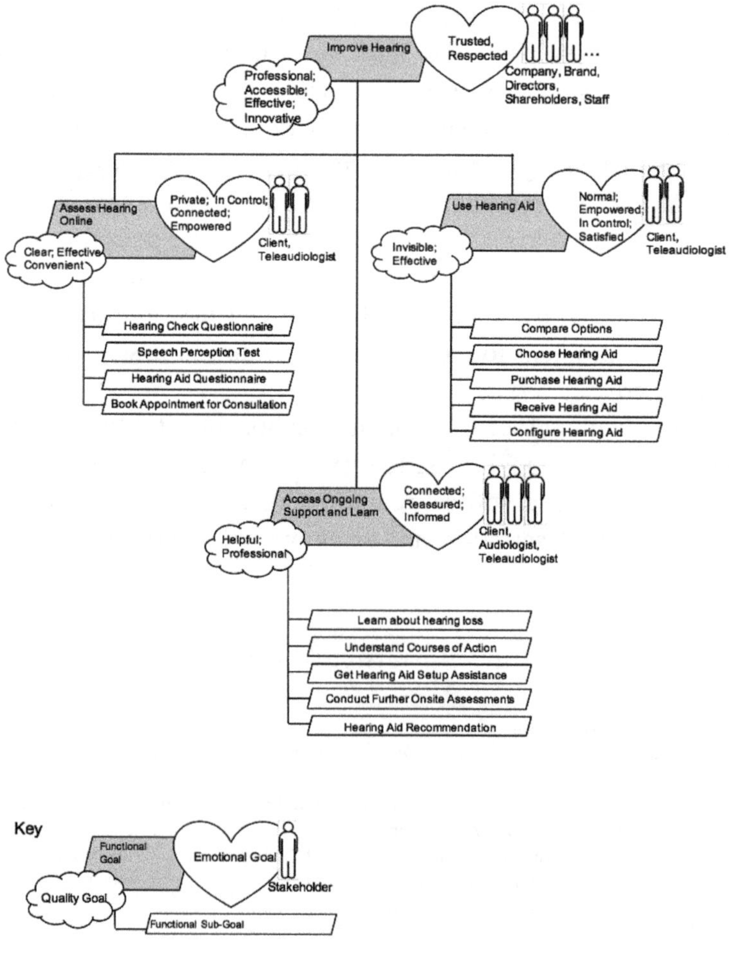

Let us explain Figure 2. The overall goal of the system, as depicted by the parallelogram at the top of the figure, is to improve hearing. The means to improve hearing, as noted in the quality goals in the cloud associated with the goal, must be accomplished professionally, accessibly, and efficiently. Such a service needs to embrace innovation. These qualities are the driver for teleaudiology where hearing services are often unavailable to people in remote areas or with inadequate transport. Emotionally the service needs to engender people involved with trust and respect. There are a large number of stakeholders involved with providing a teleaudiology service as indicated by the associated roles in the figure.

There are three subgoals of 'improve hearing' depicted in the motivational model. Let us consider each of these subgoals in turn along with its associated roles, quality goals and emotional goals.

The leftmost subgoal is 'assess hearing online.' There are two roles associated with the subgoal, that of client and teleaudiologist. While the role of client will be taken by a person, the role of teleaudiologist may be undertaken by software. This subgoal is associated with the motivating scenario in Table 1. The quality goals associated with the subgoal are that the test be clear, effective and convenient. The emotions expected of the client interaction when performing the hearing test is that s/he feels that the assessment is being conducted with sufficient privacy, and that the experience of performing the assessment is empowering with the client in control. Note that this subgoal has four subgoals of its own: a hearing check questionnaire, a speech perception test, a hearing aid questionnaire and the ability to book a consultation online for a follow up.

The next subgoal is using a hearing aid. It has the same two associated roles, that of client and teleaudiologist. It is desirable that the hearing aid is effective and invisible, and that the client feels satisfied and happy, while being empowered and in control and reassured of being normal. There are five subgoals of this subgoal given in the figure.

The final subgoal in Figure 2 concerns ongoing support and hearing. Here there are three associated roles: the client, the audiologist and the teleaudiologist. Note that some of the teleaidiologist role may be performed by software. It is important that the client feels connected, reassured and informed, and that the support is helpful and professional. The five subgoals of the ongoing support are given in the Figure, namely to learn about hearing loss, Understand Courses of Action, Get Hearing Aid Setup Assistance, Conduct Further Onsite Assessments, and receive a Hearing Aid Recommendation.

The process of constructing the goal model supports an understanding of how these goals may be supported different aspects of the service delivery process. Goals may increase the capability and/or opportunity for users to access teleaudiology services, both of which increase the motivation for users to do so (Michie, van

Stralen, and West, 2011). *Opportunity* to access telehealth-enabled services is realised by the physical and social factors of the surrounding socio-technical system. Whereas, the *capability* to improve hearing is enabled by the skills and knowledge delivered by the service itself. In the following we will consider the emotional and quality goals of 'assess hearing online'. As discussed previously, the goal of 'assess hearing online' should address the emotional goals of feeling in control, a sense of privacy, and empowerment. Fulfilling these emotional goals will directly increase the motivation of a user to engage with the service as it better addresses their needs.

The quality goal of being 'clear' supports the *capability* of a client to understand their own health situation. The information communicated through the website needs to be clear and provide the client with the necessary skills and knowledge. Clients need to have sufficient capability to conduct the online test and make appropriate decisions. This could relate to physical capability such as the ability to hear the words in the online test or the psychological capability to judge an appropriate course of action based on the results. Consequently, guidance and support may take a variety of different forms such as a website using chat mechanisms, over the phone, or by self-directed online learning. This shift in information provision creates new challenges and opportunities for a teleaudiology service as it empowers clients to take control of their learning online. The online accessibility of the hearing assessment functionality improves the *opportunity* for clients to feel empowered. This form of enablement removes the usual barrier of booking the hearing assessments in a clinic, thus saving time and money that some clients either don't have, or are not prepared to spend. Indirectly, it also increases the chance of clients recommending the service to family members due this service being informally accessed from home. This causes more information to be shared. At the end of the day, the other thing that needs to occur is that the end user needs to trust the assessment; that is, the result of their experience from the teleaudiometry should be as good, if not better than a visit to the clinic, in addition to the feeling of being in control.

5. CUSTOMISING THE MOTIVATIONAL MODEL

The core motivational model is a high level description of teleaudiology, a socio-technical system. In order to deliver a teleaudiology service, decisions need to be made with some of the goals expanded and possibly new quality and emotional goals added. This section describes some additional goals which pertain to the teleaudiology service provided by Blamey Saunders Hears, an innovative and award-winning small company in Melbourne, Australia. Figure 3 describes an expansion to the motivational model presented in Figure 2. There are two additional subgoals of the overall goal of improving hearing. We describe each in turn.

Figure 3. Additional motivational goals

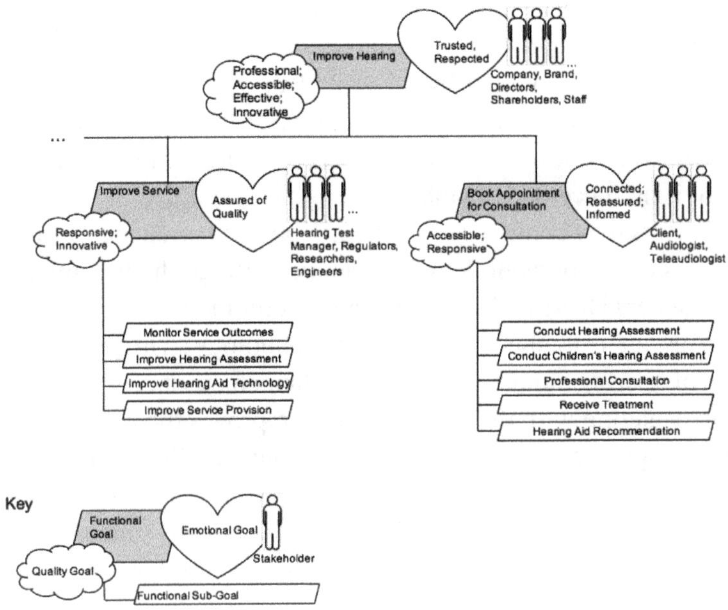

Blamey Saunders Hears allows for further consultation by allowing clients to book an appointment for an in-depth consultation following their initial interactions via the teleaudiology service. The associated roles are that of the client, audiologist and teleaudiologist. The process of scheduling the appointment should make the client feel reassured and informed, and connected to the service. There are five subgoals of booking a consultation appointment. The first three depicted in the figure are conducting a hearing assessment, conducting a child's hearing assessment, and booking an appointment for a professional consultation at a suitable time, while the remaining two are outcomes of the assessment, specifically receiving treatment and giving a recommendation for a hearing aid.

The other subgoal pertains to quality assurance. Part of the service is to ensure that what is provided is best practice and working correctly. Service improvement needs to be responsive and innovative. There are many roles associated with quality assurance including hearing test managers, regulators, researchers and engineers. Four areas of continuous improvement are identified in the figure: monitoring service outcomes, improving hearing assessment, improving hearing aid technology, and improving service provision.

Note that the subgoals in Figures 2 and 3 are not consistent, but are largely self-explanatory. It is an intended feature of the motivational models to be informal to allow conversations between stakeholders, rather than be a formal specification of a service. In our experience, fostering conversations is more important than formality.

It is also important to note that some of the goals are specific to Blamey Saunders Hears and might not be adopted by all providers of a teleaudiology service. For example, Blamey Saunders Hears desires to be an innovative company and has included 'innovative' in several of the quality goals. One can provide a teleaudiology service which is not necessarily innovative.

External factors may contribute to the emotional experience as well. To connect with new product development, let us re-mention Facett, the hearing aid launched by Blamey Saunders Hears in April 2018 the development of which was mentioned in Section 3 as an example of designing technology with emotions in mind. Testimonials of hearing aid users at a product launch event affirm that the positive experience in engaging with the device clearly improves the emotional experience of the teleaudiology experience. Thus the emotional/quality goal being innovative is partly met by ensuring that the hearing aid device is perceived to be innovative. Factors leading to the 'innovative feel' include the colour, shape, and ease of use in changing batteries (Picture 1). 'Hear Like never Before,' the slogan on the Facett marketing brochure is claiming innovation. Again, from the brochure, "giving you a new level of control on how you hear the world" which is intended to meet the "In control" emotional goal from Figure 2.

6. DISCUSSION

We have discussed models of a teleaudiology service that have explicitly included emotional factors, that is emotions that are desired for a person to feel when interacting with the service. Consideration of emotions is important if people are to adopt technology, especially in the case of hearing aids, which is an emotional topic for many people. Sustained engagement with a teleaudiology service is entirely voluntary, meaning that service providers must continually strive for a positive experience and ensure that potential clients have everything they need to use the service effectively.

The motivational model identifies the potential of a teleaudiology service to fulfil new stakeholder needs that were previously not possible to satisfy. These needs relate to the online hearing test, navigating information and accessing support, through to finding an effective hearing solution. Satisfying the emotional needs of clients in service design should ultimately increase their motivation towards using the service. For instance, a teleaudiology service should address the emotional goals of feeling in control, a sense of privacy, empowerment and connection, amongst others.

These opportunities also come with challenges as they place further requirements on the part of clients to comprehend the meaning of hearing test results. It is likely that these requirements will be wide-ranging which in turn necessitate that technology be able to cater for a wide range of user motivational models. Consequently, multiple methods of support and guidance need to be available.

It is clear that the impact of fulfilling these goals extends beyond individual user experience and relates to the wider support needed by the socio-technical system. Technology can be well designed and yet still be unused or rejected by potential clients. The technology is one part of a broader service delivery process and the support of multiple individuals and organisations is often necessary to ensure long-term success.

Yet it is not immediate that engineers consider emotional concerns when designing and implementing a service. While it is generally accepted that people should be consulted about their feelings, many people are surprised when confronted by the question: 'how do you want to feel when interacting with a service?' Despite the challenges in eliciting, modelling and incorporating emotional concerns in design there remains a wide acknowledgement that such considerations would be beneficial. The motivational models and the brainstorming process that produces them are one way these emotional factors can be considered and discussed explicitly.

To conclude, this paper came about from a meeting at a lunch between Elaine Saunders and Leon Sterling talking about research on 'Incorporating Emotions in Technology Development' being undertaken at Swinburne University of Technology. Elaine immediately recognised the relevance of the issue for teleaudiology. Some of the emotional factors have been listed here along with a way that they can be evaluated.

ACKNOWLEDGMENT

The research was partially supported through the ARC Discovery Project DP-160104083 'Catering for Individuals' Emotion'. The authors would like to thank Professor Peter Blamey and Dr Elaine Saunders of Blamey Saunders Hears for their help with the paper. The first author would like to thank Leah Heiss for a conversation about the involvement of design in the development of Facett.

REFERENCES

American Speech, Language and Hearing Association. (2014). Teleaudiology Clinical Technicians. Retrieved May 1, 2018, from https://www.asha.org/Practice-Portal/Professional-Issues/Audiology-Assistants/Teleaudiology-Clinical-Assistants/

Beirao, G., Den Ambtman, A., De Pourcq, K., De Regge, M., Simões do Carmo Dias, J., & Kandampully, J. (2016). *The healthcare experience : the supportive role of technology and people in the elderly care sector*. Presented at the Frontiers in Service 2016. Bergen, Norway

Bentley, T., Johnston, L., & Von Baggo, K. (2002). Putting some emotion into requirements engineering. *Proc. of the 7th Australian Workshop on Requirements Engineering*, 227-244. Melbourne, Australia

Berry, L. L., Davis, S. W., & Wilmet, J. (2015). When the customer is stressed. *Harvard Business Review*, *93*, 86–94.

Blamey & Saunders Hearing Pty Ltd. https://www.blameysaunders.com.au/ and http://www.scienceinpublic.com.au/media-releases/backgrounder

Blythe, M., Overbeeke, K., Monk, A., & Wright, P. (Eds.). (2004). *Funology: From Usability to Enjoyment*. The Netherlands: Springer.

Boehner, K., DePaula, R., Dourish, P., & Sengers, P. (2007). How emotion is made and measured. *International Journal of Human-Computer Studies*, *65*(4), 275–291. doi:10.1016/j.ijhcs.2006.11.016

Desmet, P. (2002). *Designing Emotions*. Delft University of Technology.

Fokkinga, S., & Desmet, P. (2001). Ten Ways to Design for Disgust, Sadness, and Other Enjoyments: A Design Approach to Enrich Product Experiences with Negative Emotions. *International Journal of Design*, *7*(1).

Heiss, L. (2018). *Designing Emotional Technologies - Collaborating across design, health and engineering to humanise wearable health technologies* (Ph.D. thesis). RMIT University.

Kelly, J., & Matthews, B. (2014). Displacing use: Exploring alternative relationships in a human-centred design process. *Design Studies*, *35*(4), 353–373.

Kim, J., & Moon, J. Y. (1998). Designing towards emotional usability in customer interfaces—trustworthiness of cyber-banking system interfaces. *Interacting with Computers*, *10*(1), 1–29. doi:10.1016/S0953-5438(97)00037-4

Krupinski, E. A. (2015). Innovations and possibilities in connected health. *Journal of the American Academy of Audiology*, *26*(9), 761–767. doi:10.3766/jaaa.14047 PMID:26415969

Lopez-Lorca, A. A., Miller, T., Pedell, S., Mendoza, A., Keirnan, A., & Sterling, L. (2014, November). One Size Doesn't Fit All: Diversifying "The User" using Personas and Emotional Scenarios. *6th International Workshop on Social Software Engineering*, pp. 25-32, Hong Kong, China.

Mendoza, A., Miller, T., Pedell, S., & Sterling, L. (2013). The role of users' emotions and associated quality goals on appropriation of systems: two case studies. In *24th Australasian Conference on Information Systems (ACIS)*. RMIT University.

Michie, S., van Stralen, M. M., & West, R. (2011). The behaviour change wheel: A new method for characterising and designing behaviour change interventions. *Implementation Science; IS*, *6*, 42. doi:10.1186/1748-5908-6-42

Miller, T., Pedell, S., Lopez-Lorca, A., Mendoza, A., Sterling, L., & Keirnan, A. (2015). Emotionally-driven models for people-oriented requirements engineering: The case study of emergency systems. *Journal of Systems and Software*, *105*, 54–71. doi:10.1016/j.jss.2015.03.044

Na, N., & Suk, H.-J. (2014). The Emotional Characteristics of White for Applications of Product Color Design. *International Journal of Design*, *8*(2).

Norman, D. (2005). *Emotional Design: Why We Love (or Hate) Everyday Things*. Academic Press.

Prilleltensky, I. (2016). *The Laughing Guide to Well-Being: Using Humor and Science to Become Happier and Healthier*. Routledge and Miffllin.

Proynova, R., Paech, B., Koch, S. H., Wicht, A., & Wetter, T. (2011). Investigating the influence of personal values on requirements for health care information systems. In *Proceedings of the 3rd Workshop on Software Engineering in Health Care*. Honolulu, USA. ACM. 10.1145/1987993.1988004

Ramos, I., & Berry, D. (2005). *Is emotion relevant to requirements engineering?* (Vol. 10). Requirements Engineering.

Roberts, K. (2005). *Love Marks: the future beyond brands*. Powerhouse Books.

Sääksjärvi, M., & Hellen, K. (2013). How Designers and Marketers Can Work Together to Support Consumers' Happiness. *International Journal of Design*, *7*(3).

Saunders, E. (2015). *Sound of Silence*. New Holland Publishers.

Sterling, L., & Taveter, K. (2009). *Art of Agent-Oriented Modelling*. MIT Press.

Thomas, N., Farhall, J., Foley, F., Leitan, N. D., Villagonzalo, K. A., Ladd, E., ... Kyrios, M. (2016). Promoting Personal Recovery in People with Persisting Psychotic Disorders: Development and Pilot Study of a Novel Digital Intervention. *Frontiers in Psychiatry*, *7*, 196. doi:10.3389/fpsyt.2016.00196

Wachtler, C., Coe, A., Davidson, S., Fletcher, S., Mendoza, A., Sterling, L., & Gunn, J. (2018). Development of a Mobile Clinical Prediction Tool to Estimate Future Depression Severity and Guide Treatment in Primary Care: A User Centered Design. *JMIR mHealth and uHealth*, *6*(4), e95. doi:10.2196/mhealth.9502 PMID:29685864

World Health Organization. (2011). Telemedicine - Opportunities and developments in Member States. Retrieved October 1, 2018, from http://www.who.int/goe/publications/ehealth_series_vol2/en/

Yoon, J. K., Pohlmeyer, A., & Desmet, P. (2016). When 'Feeling Good' is not Good Enough: Seven Key Opportunities for Emotional Granularity in Product Development. *International Journal of Design*, *10*(3).

Chapter 2
Regulatory Issues in Telehealth:
It's More Than Just About Data Jurisdiction

Alison Hardacre
Healthkit, Australia

Lachlan Wheeler
Healthkit, Australia

ABSTRACT

Telehealth and digital health more broadly have become two of the fastest growing IT sectors in the world. They have the potential to transform lives everywhere, often before regulation has had the chance to catch up to everyday reality in healthcare. This chapter is grounded in clinical practice occurring at the time of writing and discusses at a high level regulatory issues in telehealth. This chapter argues that complexities regarding regulation over clinical applicability, patient identification, bandwidth, and funding mechanisms, as well as data storage, jurisdiction, and usage should not prevent uptake of telehealth and digital health given the clinical benefits of telehealth in countries such as Australia and internationally.

DOI: 10.4018/978-1-5225-8191-8.ch002

INTRODUCTION AND BACKGROUND

Telehealth and digital health more broadly have significant potential to overcome shortcomings in the health system that affect people's lives through improving accessibility and efficiency of treatment, which ultimately improves effectiveness of treatment, as exemplified below in Table 1.

The regulatory issues affecting telehealth are myriad and ever-changing, and are further complicated by the fact that telehealth is already a reality in Australia: the internet is already facilitating the practitioner-patient relationship and treatment, such as online consultations as well as online medical records that are both practitioner- and patient- generated that necessarily facilitate online consultations as well as remote diagnosis and tracking. This chapter focuses on online consultations and to a lesser extent on remote health tracking. It leaves deeper consideration of broader telehealth areas, such as apps for diagnosis and treatment of conditions, to other areas of this book.

The growth of telehealth and digital health will only continue with improvements in IT privacy and security, increased internet access and bandwidth, cloud computing enabling rapid deployment, consumer push, and increased practitioner acceptance of technology driven by government and funding body incentives. For example, in the USA practitioners can claim up to $44,000 p.a. for using 'meaningful use certified software'. In Australia, practitioner computerization has been encouraged by Medicare's practice incentive payments (PIPs).

However, as with other technology-based industries, the technology – and its application – is ahead of the law and regulatory issues, but these regulatory considerations should not be considered as limitations curtailing the use of telehealth and digital health more broadly, given the significant health improvements achievable through telehealth.

Moreover, the very nature of healthcare and of health systems means that there will always be a high level of government involvement and regulation over the sector either through general regulation or through financial mechanisms, such as which services are – and are not – covered by rebates or other incentives.

This paper does not provide an in-depth summary of all laws relating to telehealth and digital health in Australia let alone globally; to do so would be a book in itself that would rapidly become obsolete particularly given that practice is ahead of regulation. Rather this paper is based on what the authors see in clinical practice. It discusses the issues to be considered in telehealth, and argues that many of the considerations are as applicable to face-to-face treatment and paper-based services, health monitoring and patient records, as they are applicable to telehealth, and highlights that regulatory issues in telehealth are more than just about clinical records and data storage. The online mode of treatment delivery, diagnosis and management

Table 1. Health system wide limitations that can be overcome by telehealth and digital health

Issue	Problem	Cause	Comments
Rural access	Rural people in Australia have up to 4 years less life expectancy than urban dwellers	Lack of access to health services in rural areas is a contributing factor	Online consultations overcome this barrier by enabling patients to see practitioners online through video conferencing facilities
Waiting times	Patients can wait months to see a practitioner of their choice in private practice and years for elective surgeries in public hospitals	The structure of the healthcare sector: most practitioners do not need more patients as they are busy enough with their existing patients, but waiting lists show patient populations need more treatment, with practitioners not necessarily located optimally to patient need	Practitioners can see more patients per day with efficiency tools such as: • Efficiency-driving electronic patient and practice management systems • Patient-driven personal health records enable patients to complete health tracking and administrative tasks which make each appointment more efficient • Apps that enable patients to self-diagnose and self-treat similarly ease pressure on private practice. • Online consultations can overcome mismatched practitioner-patient locations by making location obsolete where online consultations are practical and clinically effective
Emergency medical record access	Patients can have adverse reactions if treated by doctors who do not know their medical histories	Lack of access to patients' medical records with records held in multiple locations	Online medical records that are accessed in times of emergency overcome this by providing treating doctors with up to date medical histories of presenting patients
Dependence on service providers for medical devices	Patients have been dependent on pharmacists and practitioners to provide and to customise their devices, before patients can begin using them	Devices have had to be customised manually to each patient's needs and patients have not been able to do this themselves	A burgeoning opportunity is for patients to self-customise devices, saving patients money, practitioners time so they can treat more patients and enabling speedier use, thus ultimately easing pressure on the healthcare system

ensures that other practical considerations need to be reviewed, with the issues able to be broken down into two parts, also shown in Figure 1 below:

1. Practical factors, such as treatment payment, service delivery and clinical efficacy; and
2. Telehealth specific legal and compliance considerations, such as proof of patient identity, data storage and jurisdiction, and the implications – and opportunities – of practitioners and patients being in different countries.

Given this paper's focus on online consultations and to a lesser extent on health tracking rather than on the specific legislation regarding medical device regulatory approval through the Australian Federal government's Therapeutic Goods Administration (TGA) and the US Food and Drug Administration (FDA), consideration of these areas is limited.

Figure 1. Regulatory issues in the telehealth value chain

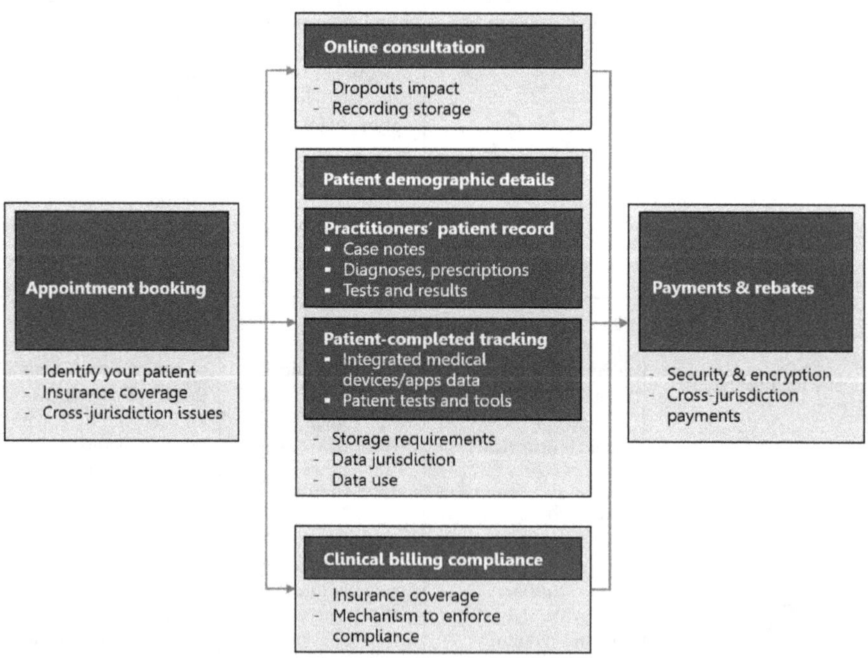

CLINICAL APPLICATION OF TELEHEALTH

Focusing firstly on online consultations, patients can be treated by practitioners over the internet using video conferencing facilities in a range of professions and for a range of modalities and purposes (and they are inapplicable in other circumstances).

Regardless of the availability of rebates directly available for online consultations (the absence of which could be a regulatory measure to limit and prevent the use of online consultations) and irrespective of the professional insurance implications for practitioners, online consultations and services are currently being used in Australia for:

- Mental health treatment, where online consultations are highly applicable given the lack of need for physical examination;
- Dermatology treatment, where – with the right quality visual technology – moles can be diagnosed as benign or as malignant through visual examination;
- Follow up appointments for surgeons to review progress after surgery or for physical therapists to review progress with patients between physically-based appointments; and
- To a lesser extent, medical certificates for acute, general conditions (such as colds) as well as regular prescriptions (such as contraception), with these consultation areas expected to increase, particularly if they are made rebatable.

Medical indemnity insurance policies generally limit indemnity insurance coverage to consultations where the practitioner and the patient are in the same country. However, anecdotally there are instances of practitioners in Australia of specific ethno-linguistic backgrounds treating patients overseas particularly where that country may lack medical or clinical services in their field.

The very nature of online consultations where the patient is not physically present in a practitioner's office makes them readily applicable to online consultations. However, this in turn means that online consultations will most likely only ever be a smaller proportion of consultations than face-to-face consultations. Therefore face-to-face consultations will always be the mainstay of medical practice, but online consultations will become more readily used in the above circumstances, necessitating ethical standards and possible regulation in these areas.

Ethical standards have already been developed for online consultations in the mental health sector in the United States, see for example: the American Academy of Child and Adolescent Psychiatry (AACAP) Committee on Telepsychiatry and AACAP Committee on Quality Issues, (2017). However such standards can become rapidly dated – for example, it is unlikely that in ten years the expectation will be that all patients and practitioners will have met face-to-face prior to beginning online consultations, as online technologies will overcome dropout risk and be as crisp as real life so that rapport can be built as easily as in face to face consultations.

Beyond online consultations, remote health tracking can range from:

- Fitness performance tracking such as wearables (e.g., Fitbit and other wearable tracking devices that can track heart rate, steps taken and other metrics), which may also be applicable in a rehabilitation context;
- Blood glucose monitors and medical devices that integrate into personal health records so that patients can track for example glucose levels over a period of time, which can also be remotely monitored by patients' practitioners to track health and medication efficacy; and
- Patient self-monitoring through phone-based apps, which is self-reported and requires active entry of data (rather than passive data entry in the case of integrated blood glucose monitors that automatically upload data into health records for tracking purposes).

Although consumer uptake is rapidly growing, the use of this data by practitioners for healthcare purposes and for telemedicine is still nascent in its adoption and often has been limited in Australia to pilot programs that have not had long term funding. As such this paper focuses primarily on online consultations.

The Implications of Dropouts and Bandwidth

Whereas the only interruptions to face-to-face consultations are interruptions that occur external to the actual clinical treatment (e.g., a person entering the consultation room, or a telephone call) which are also applicable to online consultations, online consultations can also be interrupted by functions essential to the consultation itself: internet connection/bandwidth and hardware at the practitioner site and the patient site. For example:

- If the internet drops out during a mental health consultation, the consultation does not occur for the length of time of the dropout; and

- If the camera hardware is not of sufficient quality at the patient end or the practitioner end for a mole check, the assessment of the mole may not be accurate.

Improvements to internet speed and bandwidth, combined with increasing accessibility of high quality hardware will reduce dropouts and hardware risks. However, these issues are currently considerations for online consultations highlighting that online consultations are currently a "last resort" where face-to-face consultations are not available or viable, or where transportation to a face-to-face consultation is out of the question due to distance or to the infirm health of the patient.

In the meantime, questions need to be asked about the effect of the dropout on a consultation. If there is a complete dropout for only 1% of the consultation, does this have any effect on the efficacy of a consultation? Arguably not. What if there was a complete dropout for 25% of the consultation, or low bandwidth for 40% of the consultation – did the consultation fully occur? Arguably not. Where should the line be drawn?

The implications of this are profound for patients, practitioners and funding bodies, as well as legislators. For patients in rural areas, poor internet or hardware may mean that there is little clinical benefit in treatment via online consultation. For funding bodies, paying rebates, subsidies and incentives for ineffective or sub-optimal online consultations may be a financial imposition on budgets that they are not willing to take. For practitioners, the choice over whether to treat patients online is one of clinical efficacy and prioritisation: should a practitioner treat a patient face-to-face knowing that the only issue affecting clinical outcomes is within their control versus treating a patient online knowing that the patient outcome may be affected by issues outside their control, for which they may be held responsible by medical insurance authorities.

The Requirement to Know Your Patient

Practitioners may be less likely to meet their ethical and regulatory obligations to identify their patients correctly, which is rooted in their obligation to provide the correct clinical diagnosis and treatment to specific patients. If a patient attends a face-to-face appointment for the first time, the patient usually completes a patient intake form with their contact details and Medicare/private health insurance card details, which if required, can be verified with photo identification. With online consultations, this process *can be* completed electronically but without the comfort of identification being completed in person, practitioners and funding bodies may have less confidence that this obligation is met.

However, the power of technology means that confirmation of patient identity can be easier and more accurately completed than in person, because identity including visual identity can be completed electronically by verifying identity information with social media (without any information being posted publicly). This in fact makes it harder for people to fake their identity to a practitioner, meaning practitioners may well be more likely to meet their obligation to correctly identify their patient. As comfort with the use of technology grows, practitioners' *perception* of this risk will reduce in line with the actual risk having been reduced.

With the expected growth in the uptake of shared patient record systems such as My Health Record, it is expected that protocols will be developed for patient identification in online consultations. Such protocols are also expected in the future for the integration of health tracking devices - i.e., protocols that enable confirmation that the health device and health data tracked belongs to the patient into whose records the data is integrated).

Practical implications of Telehealth: Payments and Rebates

The very nature of the above consultation types and modalities mean that patient appointment fees must be paid remotely, just as the appointment is held remotely. Without remote patient appointment fee payment processing and also rebates processing capabilities being directly integrated into video consultations platforms, practitioners have no guarantee of being paid appointment fees, which creates reluctance to use online consultations facilities, and was a key reason why online consultations failed to get uptake prior to the introduction of Medicare rebates for some online consultations services (HealthKit Team Analysis, 2009-2018).

Anecdotally some practitioners do treat patients online and receive Medicare rebates for online consultations using the rebate available for face-to-face consultations, and have done so for 10 years. However, in July 2011, Medicare introduced rebates and incentives for online consultations for some medical specialists (dermatologists and psychiatrists) and general practitioners (refer Department of Human Services, *MBS and telehealth*), consisting of (refer Table 2):

The low take-up of online consultations meant these rebate amounts have been reduced and removed over time. In November 2017, rebates were extended to patients in highly rural areas being treated online for some mental health conditions, with $9M allocated over three years (Department of Human Services, 2017).

Although patient appointment fee payments can be paid through internet transfer from the patient to the practitioner, there is no guarantee that payment will be made given the lack of physical relationship and proximity between the patient and practitioner. Only by solving this issue, through card payment storage and enabling automatic patient appointment fee payment processing at the time of appointment

Table 2. Medicare rebates and incentive payments for online consultations

Rebate	Purpose	Requirements	Comments
Up to $6,000	Hardware (e.g. big screen televisions)	• Practitioner must complete 1 online consultation in the quarter that they buy the hardware • No requirement to return rebates or hardware if they did not complete online consultations in other quarters	Considered a rort in the sector
Per consult	Incentivise consultations	• Rebate paid in addition to the ordinary rebate already being paid • Patient cannot login from home; they must login to the consultation in a rural GP practice and be supported by a nurse in the practice (who also receives a rebate)	Impractical requirements Limited use of online consultations

without any trigger from patients or practitioners, has HealthKit removed this barrier for practitioners to treat patients through online consultations.

The net effect of payments being essential to online consultations is that practitioners and software applications must adhere to payments regulations in addition to health data and service delivery regulatory standards.

Data Storage

When people think of telehealth and digital health, it is often assumed that the key – and sometimes the only – issue to consider is health data storage. However, one of the most baffling issues in telehealth regulation is that the regulation and management requirements for processing payments are more settled than equivalent regulation for health data. This disparity traces back to the lack of history of digitisation of healthcare as well as the country-specific nature of healthcare meaning that international protocols have not been established in the way that they have been for payments management. In fact, in the absence of direct, national, well-recognised legislation governing health data storage and usage, the authors' business, HealthKit, has received queries from practitioners in Australia (and elsewhere) asking whether Healthkit is HIPAA (Health Insurance Portability and Accountability Act of 1996) compliant. HIPAA is United States legislation that provides data privacy and security provisions for safeguarding medical information, one of the requirements of which is that data is stored in America, and so is not applicable to Australia (refer U.S. Department of Health and Human Services, *Summary of HIPAA Privacy Rule*).

Beyond the Australian Privacy Principles, there are health data-specific laws regarding the storage and use of health data by practitioners and other services. Of course, health data incorporates patient health records, case notes and clinical diagnoses. However in healthcare privacy goes beyond the obvious case notes taken during an appointment. Even someone's name attaches to it a greater significance: if that person is seeing a mental health practitioner online for a mental health condition or for any other service, there is potential for adverse judgment against that person which could have significantly more negative consequences than that person's name being disclosed as a client of, for example, a bank.

With telehealth, online consultation data also constitutes health data and can span metadata of the consultation through to an actual recording of the online consultation, which leads to further consideration of regulation regarding consent to the recording and storage from both the patient and the practitioner.

There has been significant focus on the country where data is stored. Under the Australian Privacy Principles, data can be stored outside of Australia so long as the jurisdiction where data is stored is disclosed in companies' terms and conditions. However, there is additional legislation governing where health-specific data can be stored and, frustratingly, these laws differ by state, and there are different opinions about whether health data can be stored outside of Australia.

Medicare Australia has sought to overcome these ambiguities by requiring through its Cloud Computing Policy that for Medicare rebates to be claimed, "Medicare claiming data" is to be stored in Australia. This is narrower than the scope of Medicare Australia's original draft Cloud Computing Policy which proposed that Medicare rebates would only be able to claimed if all health data in the cloud-based software were stored in Australia. The background to this change reflects the complications of defining what health data is where technology is further advanced than the law such as in the case of medical devices and apps as well as online consultation data where data is stored overseas, and where approval of medical devices may be required by the TGA or FDA (see above).

For example, a patient could track his/her blood glucose levels through a medical device where glucose level data is aggregated and can be fed into practitioners' clinical records software enabling remote glucose level monitoring, which in some circumstances may have life saving outcomes for some patients. The data from the medical device may be stored in the USA and not in Australia, and yet the data is integral to the patient's health record and to their clinical treatment. This example highlights the tension between health data jurisdiction and the realities of clinical technologies in the speed with which they develop in this technological era, which even legislation in much larger jurisdictions than Australia (such as the European Union under the General Data Protection Regulation) have yet to fully grapple with.

Moreover the real issue with health data is not data jurisdiction (although it is important as it governs which laws apply to its use), but rather confidentiality of the data held in the software, which comes down to data security measures discussed in Chapter 8, to prevent database hacking, and to the design of the actual software holding the health data to prevent every day, likely inadvertent breaches of confidentiality. For example, HealthKit's practice and patient management software covers this through:

- Extensive user access levels, with four levels for practitioners and three levels for administrative staff; including a number of specific options within each level dependent upon the particular user;
- Hiding of sensitive information within patient profiles and clinical notes (e.g. users cannot immediately see clinical notes when they open a patient's profile); and
- Anonymisation of invoices and financial reports, so that you can provide invoices and reports to funding bodies and accountants without breaching confidentiality.

Other software may use similar techniques to support confidentiality.

Data Use and Health Informatics

A burgeoning area of telehealth and healthcare IT more broadly is health data analytics which has been enabled by cloud-based software, meaning that health data can be gathered, anonymised and analysed at an aggregate level for the benefit of participating patients and wider patient populations. For example, the anti-inflammatory drug Vioxx killed 27,000 people over five years (and caused heart disease in 140,000 others), typically 18 months after use (Cockburn, 2012). Noted epidemiologist, Dr Fiona Stanley AC, says linked health data could have detected the risk of heart disease years earlier, but such data was not accessible (Prime Minister's Science, Engineering and Innovation Council Working Group on Data in Science, 2006, Page 56). In fact, Dr Stanley argues that using data even without consent is required given its potential to save lives (Stanley, 2010). Whilst we would not go so far, this statement does highlight the power of health data.

In fact, HIPAA reinforces this concept and recognises the power of health data by providing an exception to non-data usage where the data is anonymised and being used for research purposes, where research is defined as, "a systematic investigation, including research development, testing, and evaluation, designed to develop or contribute to generalizable knowledge" (U.S. Department of Health & Human Services, 2003).

We expect to hear more about health data analytics in the coming years, both positive insights and intense controversies, which regulation will eventually catch up and cover.

CONCLUSION

The regulatory issues associated with telehealth are varied and are made more complex by the clinical benefits of telehealth and the use of the internet for health services possibly outweighing regulatory concerns in some circumstances. Where they see a patient benefit, many clinicians will continue to use technologies for the benefit of patients even where regulation has yet to catch up with clinical realities on the ground. Clinicians, regulators, funding bodies and patients should expect to see further advances in regulation either through legislation or rebates/incentives coverage in telehealth in the widest sense of the word across data jurisdiction and use, as well as across the implications of internet usage for healthcare – bandwidth requirements, payments and patient identification, as well as funding and insurance coverage.

REFERENCES

American Academy of Child and Adolescent Psychiatry (AACAP) Committee on Telepsychiatry and AACAP Committee on Quality Issues. (2017). Clinical Update: Telepsychiatry With Children and Adolescents. *Journal of the American Academy of Child and Adolescent Psychiatry*, *56*(10), 875–893. doi:10.1016/j.jaac.2017.07.008 PMID:28942810

Cockburn, A. (2012). *When half a million Americans died and nobody noticed.* Retrieved October 1, 2018, from http://www.theweek.co.uk/us/46535/when-half-million-americans-died-and-nobody-noticed

Department of Human Services. (2017). *Prioritising Mental Health — improving telehealth for psychological services in regional, rural and remote Australia.* Retrieved October 1, 2018, from. https://www.humanservices.gov.au/organisations/about-us/budget/budget-2017-18/health/prioritising-mental-health-improving-telehealth-psychological-services-regional-rural-and-remote

Department of Human Services. (n.d.). *MBS and telehealth.* Retrieved October 1, 2018, from https://www.humanservices.gov.au/organisations/health-professionals/services/medicare/mbs-and-telehealth

International Organization for Standardization. (2004). *ISO/TR 16056-1:2004.* Retrieved October 1, 2018, from https://www.iso.org/standard/37351.html

Matthews, C. (2012, April 12). The Top Ten Fastest-Growing Industries in America. *Time Magazine*.

Prime Minister's Science, Engineering and Innovation Council Working Group on Data in Science. (2006). *From Data to Wisdom: Pathways to Successful Data Management for Australian Science.* Retrieved October 1, 2018, from https://archive.industry.gov.au/science/PMSEIC/Documents/DataForScience.pdf

Stanley, F. (2010), Privacy or public good? Why not obtaining consent may be best practice. *Significance Magazine*, *7*(2).

U.S. Department of Health & Human Services. (2003). *Research.* Retrieved October 1, 2018, from https://www.hhs.gov/sites/default/files/ocr/privacy/hipaa/understanding/special/research/research.pdf

U.S. Department of Health & Human Services. (n.d.). *Summary of the HIPAA Privacy Rule.* Retrieved October 1, 2018, from https://www.hhs.gov/hipaa/for-professionals/privacy/laws-regulations/index.html?language=en

KEY TERMS AND DEFINITIONS

Australian Privacy Principles: The privacy principles that regulates how personal information is used in Australia.

Data Jurisdiction and Storage: The country/region in which the server on which data is stored is located.

Digital Health: The use of the internet and of electronic means to manage health data, healthcare, and health services.

Health Informatics: Design, development, adoption, and application of IT-based innovations in healthcare services delivery, management, and planning, including data usage and analytics.

HIPAA: Health Insurance Portability and Accountability Act of 1996, and it is United States legislation that provides data privacy and security provisions for safeguarding medical information. It is not applicable in Australia.

Online Consultations: The treatment of patients using video conferencing technologies.

Patient and Practice Management Systems: Software (either installed or online) used by practices and practitioners to manage their appointments and bookings, clinical billing, financial reports, and patient records.

Personal Health Record: A health record where health data and other information related to the care of a patient is maintained and/or accessed by the patient.

Practitioners: Clinicians in private practice (rather than in hospitals or other institutions), specifically general practitioners, medical specialists and allied health practitioners.

Chapter 3
Goldstein and Stephens Revisited and Extended to a Telehealth Model of Hearing Aid Optimization

Elaine Saunders
Blamey Saunders Hears, Australia

Sophie Brice
Blamey Saunders Hears, Australia

Roya Alimoradian
Blamey Saunders Hears, Australia

ABSTRACT

Tele-audiology practice is sometimes portrayed or practiced as an extension of conventional audiology practice, but in reality, it should be considered as a more flexible and innovative way of delivering hearing healthcare. It is likely to continue expanding beyond the bounds of conventional audiology into the future. This has far-reaching implications for clinical utility and client satisfaction. One important consequence is that tele-audiology is changing the way individuals are approaching their hearing health. In a connected economy, people are becoming more empowered in managing their health and are metamorphosing from patients, whose only option is to visit a clinical facility, to consumers with choices. There will still be a need for conventional audiology practices to manage more complex cases where medical

DOI: 10.4018/978-1-5225-8191-8.ch003

diagnosis and intervention are involved, or where clients prefer face-to-face service, but this will be as part of a hearing health ecosystem where the consumer makes the choices drawing on a range of influencing factors. There is now substantial evidence from large-scale studies and clinical data that aspects of tele-audiology are prevalent within different service models and that the outcomes are at least as beneficial to the recipients as the outcomes from delivery of conventional audiology services in conventional audiology clinics. In addition to potential improvements to client outcomes, tele-audiology is already starting to improve access to hearing health services, reduce costs, and deliver social and economic benefits to society.

INTRODUCTION

Tele-audiology is a rapidly developing field, particularly as hearing aid manufacturers bring various e-solutions onto the market. A search of the PubMed database for items containing the word "tele-audiology" in any field yielded only seventeen references and one editorial note. A search for "tele-audiology" in Google Scholar yielded 531 results in total and 110 publications since 2016, including one comprehensive book (Rushbrook and Houston, 2016), which received positive reviews. There are also two comprehensive research reviews by Krumm and Syms (2011) and by Swanepoel and Hall (2010), and a more recent review specifically relating to auditory rehabilitation by Tao et al. in 2018. The high ratio of the number of online references in Google Scholar to the listing of peer-reviewed studies in PubMed is symptomatic of the fast-moving fields of tele-audiology, telehealth, and telemedicine, and the fact that peer-reviewed studies are lagging far behind the actual practice of tele-audiology and telemedicine in both public and private healthcare. In this chapter, we have reviewed some of the non-peer reviewed information about tele-audiology from clinical and client perspectives in addition to peer-reviewed research papers, in order to provide an up-to-date and forward-looking perspective of tele-audiology.

Tele-audiology is a subset of telehealth, and developments should be considered in the context of the changes that are sweeping through medicine and healthcare generally. Krupinski (2015) described *telehealth*, the American Medical Association (AMA) has not only promoted the use of telemedicine, but it is also advocating for the formalized training of physicians in telemedicine (The Hearing Review, 2016).

This chapter presents experience with a blended model of care, based on the adaptation of an existing service model of Auditory Enablement.

BACKGROUND

Telehealth is well established in some countries; for example, in Canada, in order to overcome the barriers of physical access, such as remoteness or restricted mobility. Telehealth is having a major impact on access to services, on equity of service provision, on quality of outcomes, and is increasing productivity (Canadian Agency for Drugs and Technologies in Health, 2016). A Canadian report is one of many that show that the benefits arising from telehealth extend far beyond the facilitation of client/clinician communication at a distance. The report includes reference to over forty different medical and allied health disciplines using telehealth (but tele-audiology is not among them). Developments in tele-audiology aim to deliver similar impact and benefits to clients. In Australia, a National strategy is under development and is documented (Australian Digital Health Strategy), and queries the time full uptake will require, assuming that digital health is the path forward. There is a certain tension between the speed of adoption and the relatively conservative approach in medicine towards change. As Silicon Valley physician and tech entrepreneur Jordan Shlain recently put it, *the techie attitude of move fast and break things comes up against the medical attitude of move slowly and don't kill people.* (Vize, 2017). We are at a unique juxtaposition of technology and healthcare, requiring health professionals to extend their skill set and be open to new ways of working: a change that will increase both access to services and consumer empowerment. There is international consensus that telehealth is ready for growth and will deliver widespread benefits to clinicians, clients and national healthcare programs, if formally incorporated into public and private models of health care. This forward thinking also applies to tele-audiology. Much of the technology and infrastructure developed for telehealth applications can be applied directly to tele-audiology.

Coincident with the exciting telehealth developments, there are other social changes and technical developments that are relevant to the development and effectiveness of tele-audiology. It is an ideal framework for client empowerment and truly client centred care, and it is well established in healthcare that engagement of the *patient improves health outcomes.* It can also be an enabler of health empowered communities, based on distributed trust, as evidenced in virtual client communities (Krupinski, 2015) and collaboration communities such as One Million Solutions in Health (2018). Several recently published studies show that hearing aid users can be empowered by fitting their own self-fit hearing aids, when the hearing aids are designed for that purpose using appropriate technology (Blamey, Blamey, and Saunders, 2015; Campos and Ferrari, 2012; Convery, Keidser, Dillon, and Hartley, 2011; Keidser and Convery, 2016) and that digital social networks can be effective adjuncts to clinical management of children with cochlear implants (Aiello and

Ferrari 2015). These are exciting developments that indicate that tele-audiology may be catching up with some of the more advanced telehealth trends.

In Australia, telehealth is ideally placed to support major national programs associated with dementia, mental health, diabetes, dermatology, management of chronic conditions and regional concerns related to rehabilitation, acute waiting list relief and outpatient support. Hearing health is an obvious member of that set of chronic conditions, and hearing aids are part of the solution.

Hearing Aids and the Internet of Things

Hearing devices are the most sophisticated body-worn ultra-low-power personal digital computing devices in the world. They connect directly or indirectly, via wires or wirelessly, with smartphones, computers, other digital devices, and with the internet. The most common connection between a hearing aid and a computer is for programming or fitting the device to the user's hearing aid preferences. With the computer also connected to the internet, the situation is tailor-made for tele-audiology applications and enhancements. For example, the client may fit the hearing aid themselves and transmit the data securely to a remote database, (Blamey et al., 2015) or the clinician may program the device from a remote location. (Wesarg et al., 2010; Kuzovkov, Yanov, Levin, Bovo, and Rosignoli, 2014).

Tele-audiology, used with hearing aids, can be seen as part of The Internet of Things (IoT). This is a system of interconnected computing devices, built on cloud computing. It is mobile and provides instantaneous connection. The first Internet of Things hearing aid was announced in 2016. (PR Newswire, 2016). The hearing aid was differentiated by being able to potentially connect to other IoT devices. The continuous or regular connection of hearing devices to smartphones or the internet is enabling new tele-audiology applications, and changes to the delivery of audiology services. For example, daily monitoring of the hours of hearing aid use may be a useful non-invasive measure of activity and alertness for aged care and treatment of mental or physical illness (Molini-Avejonas, Rondon-Melo, de la Higuera Amato, and Samelli, 2015). Additionally, other monitoring applications may be integrated, which has already given rise to the term "hearables". A recent systematic review of the use of telehealth in the areas of speech, language and hearing reported internet speed and other technical barriers needed to be overcome for widespread adoption of telehealth. Thus, studies of outcomes in tele-audiology and other areas of telehealth are important in informing both health and infrastructure policy.

Tele-Audiology and Big Data

One of the consequences of telehealth practices is that health and medical data are being accumulated and stored in very large data sets that are then potentially available for large scale data studies giving new insights into health from diverse perspectives including the incidence of various health problems, the delivery of health services, and perhaps most importantly the economic burden of disease and disability (Andreu-Perez et al., 2015). The availability of large quantities of audiological data for analysis is one of the major benefits of tele-audiology that is accelerating audiological research and its translation into practice. For example, there are already large scale tele-audiology studies on practical applications of remote audiology (e.g., Brennan-Jones, Eikelboom, Swanepoel, Friedland, and Atlas, 2016; Jacobs and Saunders, 2014).

DEMOGRAPHICS OF HEARING DIFFICULTIES

The World Health Organization (WHO) estimates that over 466 million people (over 5% of the world population) have hearing loss that is disabling and this is accentuated by the ageing of the world's population (World Health Organization, 2018). Hearing loss as a public health burden has often been ignored, even though it is considered by some authorities to be the prevalent disabling condition globally. The WHO estimates of hearing loss is based on a criterion for disability that most scholars would regard as quite conservative; that is hearing loss greater than 40 decibels (dB) in the better hearing ear in adults, and a hearing loss greater than 30 dB in the better hearing ear in children, measured over a four frequency average. Current production of hearing aids meets less than 10% of the global need even with this criterion, and even though production could be accelerated, face-to-face services and audiological facilities are lacking.

Sensorineural hearing damage, which occurs through loss of hair cell function in the cochlea, is the dominant cause of hearing loss in developed countries. In 2050, it is estimated that the prevalence of hearing loss (better ear) will reach up to 900 million people – 10% of the total population (World Health Organization, 2018).

Hearing impairment left unaddressed can lead to progressive auditory deprivation at the cortical level, leading to reduced speech recognition. This is of particular relevance in difficult environments where the signal to noise ratio is significantly varied (in favor of noise). A reduced ability to detect, identify and localize speech sounds in various environments not only affects the lives of the individual with impaired hearing, but also their significant others, as it can cause a breakdown in communication, or a barrier to accessing education and employment. A breakdown in effective communication may lead to feelings of isolation, reduced social activity, and overall poorer quality of life. Acquired hearing loss is known to increase the likelihood of developing mental health and cognitive problems, including dementia (Lin et al., 2013; Arlinger, 2003).

However, disturbingly, even where hearing aids are readily available, such as in Australia, fewer than one in five people who would benefit from hearing aids goes on to own and use them (Access Economics, 2006; Deloitte Access Economics, 2017). Whilst the reasons for this are complex, it may be inferred that these statistics imply a need for more accessible and less costly audiology services and hearing aid fitting. Tele-audiology is a potential cost saving solution to this problem, reducing the need for expensive infrastructure at local sites, and addressing the shortage of highly trained professionals that restricts the availability of face-to-face services. The problem is not too few audiologists, the problem is that each audiologist needs to reach and service a larger number of people with significant hearing loss, who are geographically spread over large areas. Service provision is not triaged into people with complex or low needs. From a clinical perspective in developed countries, tele-audiology is a potential means to enable scalable, and less costly hearing services to help more people and achieve greater impact on the hearing health of the population. The proliferation of online hearing screening tests and questionnaires indicates that audiologists and the general community are well aware of this potential. Tele-audiology is also being used to provide services to clients who live in remote areas. There is a need and an opportunity to change the audiology service delivery model to overcome the problem of the shortage of clinicians, restricted access, and high cost of services. Thus, developed and developing countries have a dual need for tele-audiology, to alleviate the issues caused by insufficient numbers of clinicians, as well as providing client-clinician communication and treatment at a distance.

Several investigators have explored the barriers that may discourage those with hearing loss from choosing to obtain and use hearing aids to assist with their communication needs. Noble, in his book, Self-Assessment of Hearing (2013), described the individual's experience of their hearing difficulties, is greatly shaped by whether they attend to general environments or on environments that are of especial importance. The more a hearing difficulty affects the capacity for a person to contribute to a part of their lifestyle they care greatly about, the more likely they are to acknowledge and recognize the hearing difficulty. People who acknowledge or self-report hearing difficulties are more likely to seek help. (Jenstad and Moon, 2011; Knudsen, Öberg, Nielsen, Naylor, and Kramer, 2010). The individual's experience of their hearing difficulties is greatly shaped by whether they consider hearing generally or whether they are focused on environments that matter to the individual. Cost and perception of value and benefit have been found to be a barrier to access. One of Kochkin's MarkeTrak surveys (2007) in the USA showed that 64%

of respondents reported they could not afford hearing aids, and 45% of respondents also indicated that they felt that hearing aids are not worth the expense. Potentially, tele-audiology has a role in reducing hearing aid costs and reducing these adverse perceptions.

The recent Australian Parliamentary Inquiry into the Hearing Health and Wellbeing of Australia (Parliament of the Commonwealth of Australia, 2017) noted that there is an identified need to inform and educate the potential client about hearing health in general, about their personal hearing health, and about the potential solutions that are available. Similarly, a recent report by service firm PwC (Review of Services and Technology Supply in the Hearing Services Program, PwC, 2017) identified a low level of hearing health literacy, and weak understanding of services available.

TELE-AUDIOLOGY AND AUDITORY REHABILITATION

Tele-audiology is an obvious candidate as a way to deliver hearing health education and rehabilitation programs.

There have been studies investigating the validity of appropriately tailored rehabilitation programs (Henshaw and Ferguson, 2013) and development and evaluation of programs that can be delivered online or on a DVD. These authors found that published evidence for the efficacy of individual computer-based auditory training for adults with hearing loss is not robust and therefore cannot be reliably used to guide intervention at this time. The authors identified a need for high-quality evidence to further examine the efficacy of computer-based auditory training for people with hearing loss. This would include newer market entrants, including the well known independent learning program, LACE (Listening and Communication Enhancement), supplied online by Neurotone, and the newer customized learning exercises for aural rehabilitation, clEAR™ (https://www.clearworks4ears.com/) based on the work of Tye-Murray (2016), has strong academic credentials. Current successful practices such as the one described in this chapter provide the evidence for broader service planning, and provides strong data upon which service improvements can be built, to further improve services. It is the existing successful models of care which provide scientific evidence for a Government sponsored program,

Successful examples in telehealth indicate that tele-audiology provides opportunities to plan services more efficiently to suit the different types of prospective hearing aid users. The remainder of this chapter describes one such service and supporting data.

The Blamey Saunders Model of Client Centred Care

The Blamey Saunders Model of client centred care is a blended model. The Model incorporates tele-audiology, a light touch, face-to-face model (Link clinics) and a full clinical service model. Clients may experience one or more of these models of care, moving between them. The question then is posed: who should use which pathway and when in developing this model of care? Blamey and Saunders drew on the work, initially described by Goldstein and Stephens (1981) and their clinical model of auditory enablement. This model describes a comprehensive methodology towards auditory enablement, without presuming who or how it is administered. For Blamey and Saunders, the model also provided a means to assist clients in choosing their preferred or most suitable path. Goldstein and Stephen's Model implicitly addresses a situation of optimizing resource allocation, where people who need or want more help get it, and those who are able to help themselves pass through the Model quickly, with limited resource utilization. Blamey and Saunders saw this as a methodology that could be applied to a blended model of care that incorporates tele-audiology. Put more simply, non-complex audiology cases can be helped very effectively by a tele-audiology professional, who has sufficient knowledge to work with non-complex cases and to identify clients who need greater technical, audiological and perhaps psychological care. Goldstein and Stephens developed four Types of Client Attitude, to assist in planning time and strategy for successful auditory enablement outcomes, in an economically efficient manner. Since the original publication, there have been 25 years of clinical experience validating this approach (Stephens and Kramer, 2009). The initial study was completed before the availability of tele-audiology as a service platform for auditory rehabilitation. It does, however, provide a robust, validated framework for developing a strong client centered, and cost-effective auditory rehabilitation model.

The Blamey Saunders adaptation of the Goldstein and Stephens Model incorporates tele-audiology, by ensuring a comprehensive systematic evaluation and a practical guide to the interaction of client attitude and audiological complexity, irrespective of the channel of delivery. The tele-audiologist will likely be the first contact point with the system. Their initial role is to help the client identify their most suitable or preferred path forward, with a focus on empowerment and enablement. At this point the Model has aspects of the traditional in that a brief client history is taken, which is sufficient to identify any medical red flags, and to assist the client in making a choice between full face-to-face service, a digital experience, or a blended model. The tele-audiologist is more of a consumer coach than a patient manager, to facilitate a true client centred approach, but needs to be able to act in a triage role and provide strong influence if medical investigation seems advisable. The client's choice of path balances the need for cost efficiency, the achievement of good outcomes and their own preferences. The Goldstein and Stephens Model identifies client *Attitude* as a key differentiator in guiding and advising clients (work that was expanded upon by Knudsen et al., 2010). The use of *Attitude*, as described by Goldstein and Stephen, has been adopted by Blamey and Saunders. Goldstein and Stephens described four rehabilitation Types to guide both clinicians and clients:

Type 1: People who are positively motivated without complicating audiological factors. They are likely to accept relevant hearing aid recommendations and will require little extra help. Their hearing loss is likely to be of gradual onset, bilateral and fairly symmetrical; they have identified that they have hearing difficulties, probably in background noise.

From a tele-audiology perspective, these people are motivated, self-sufficient and will be keen to control their own healthcare. Any tools, systems and processes in an eHealth model should provide ease of access for these people to self-help. This demands a consultative approach that is unfamiliar to many health professionals as they fold into the coaching role, giving up the leading or "telling" position.

Type 2: People who are positively motivated but have complicating audiological factors, including greater severity of loss and personal or environmental factors. They will require more attention with regard to specific hearing aid set up and handling, communication skills and hearing and communication tactics.

In an eHealth model, these people require a blended service approach. They need to build trust and confidence in their own decision-making ability – along with the role of the clinician as coach. A mixed model should enable these clients to drop in and out of moderate to low service needs as their confidence peaks – tools should focus on online help in tandem with verbal confidence boosting via phone or low-touch face-to-face.

Type 3: People who want help but reject the idea of hearing aids, lacking the effort or understanding and persistence that sometimes is needed to cope with hearing loss. This could be termed the sceptical client. People in this category will require careful handling with counselling and will probably benefit from the involvement of their significant others. This group may have wildly inappropriate expectations of hearing aids, thinking they will solve all their problems, instantly. They are sometimes identified early as "serial hearing aid shoppers". They may also have previously had poor experiences in the hearing aid retail industry.

Tele-audiology offers interesting prospects for this group– on one hand, you could argue that this client needs the assistance and assurance of a clinician face-to-face. On the other hand, this client could do very well with a circuit breaker approach that shifts attitudes from the old tried and not trusted to a new approach, and can potentially more easily involve the family, eradicating the phone scripts that are common to ensure people bring a loved one to their appointment, Type 3 provides an interesting challenge for clinicians but one well worth tackling through an innovative service model that respects their viewpoint.

People falling into the Type 4_category are the biggest challenge, as this group denies any personal problem. These people have probably been persuaded to seek help by significant others and will deny any disability even though they patently have marked hearing difficulties. They probably attribute hearing difficulties to other people ("Other people mumble, or don't talk clearly"). They will probably never wear a hearing aid, and will probably reject all other aspects of the auditory enablement process.

Type 4: People may be guided to a different avenue until they are ready to commit to a path of action. Little can be gained via a tele-audiology intervention.

According to Stephens and Kramer (2009) and other authors, 90% of clients will present as Types 1 and 2. This is consistent with the findings of Jenstad and Moon (2011), and is of great assistance in service planning.

When Blamey and Saunders overlaid the Goldstein and Stephens Type categorization onto the different potential approaches to the client interaction, that is; full face-to-face consultation with diagnostic audiology, light touch model, or remote consultation, the following scenario emerged:

Figure 1 shows two intersecting axes of barriers to successfully adopting hearing aids and attitude to getting and using hearing aids. The persona featured as Type 1 is the positively motivated client, and should really enjoy the online, remote interaction and the self-fitting approach.

The persona featured as Type 2 is someone who is positively motivated, but who needs or wants more help with her hearing aids and hearing health. This might involve a full diagnostic assessment.

In between, on the abscissa, is featured a Personna where she needs some help to get started, that is delivered as face-to-face guidance. She might well then migrate to using remote hearing care (tele-audiology), which would be more convenient for her, and she is confident.

Figure 1. Attitude types expressed as a personalized service outcomes model

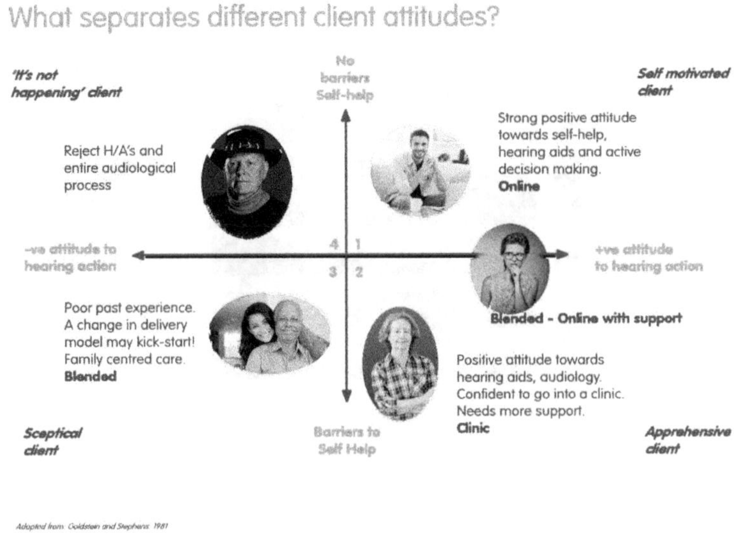

Of note is that Type 3, now called the Sceptical Client. The Goldstein and Stephen's Model suggests that it is a minor percentage of the population that are likely to need a complex level of care, thus freeing up highly qualified and experienced audiologist's time for these more complex cases. This person may enter the Model by any channel, but if disillusioned with the hearing services model due to poor experiences, may find the tele-audiology approach attractive as a start point.

The Clinical Model

The clinical model, inspired by the Goldstein and Stephens Model of care, has the client at the centre. The client may enter the system via referral agencies, or self-referral into any of the available modalities: a full clinic evaluation; a light touch guide, or fully remotely (online, video Link and phone). The goal, however, is an independent and enabled client who won't have to make repeat clinical visits, and who will ideally transition to using self-fit methodologies and interact with the tele-audiology team from home. The tele-audiologist is only a click or a phone call away, and acts as the coach or guide.

Despite the work of Noble (2013), an unpublished study conducted by Blamey & Saunders Hearing Pty Ltd (BSH), identified that potential hearing aid users like to confirm their self evaluation with a test of hearing.

Figure 2. The Blamey Saunders Model: A flexible model of care and empowerment (based on Goldstein and Stephens, 1981)

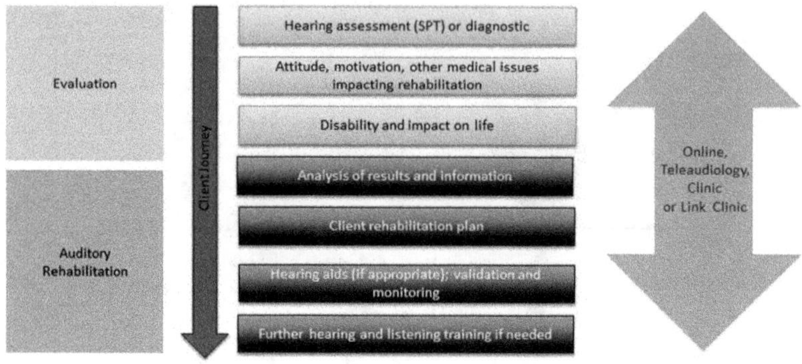

The literature on tele-audiology contains substantial reports of remote audiometry (e.g., Swanepoel et al., 2010; Botasso et al., 2015). Traditionally, the audiogram has held an important position as a way to compare a person's hearing and to predict how well they hear speech. It also has an important differential diagnostic application. This situation has been maintained, despite the high-cost service and technical requirements of a pure tone threshold test. Research has been carried out to compare remotely conducted audiometry with standardized methods. Research studies have reported on the equivalency of results using remote, or less costly devices but have not questioned the need or appropriateness of a hearing threshold test using pure tones. Much of the cost of conventional audiology is incurred in the purchase and maintenance of the expensive sound treated rooms and audiometers required to measure hearing, and there has been scientific debate about whether audiograms can be measured in non-soundproof work environments (Brennan-Jones, 2016). Additionally, there is a high cost of training of personnel to learn and utilize a standardized method, which must be adhered to if audiograms are to be comparable and valid, and in the calibration of instrumentation. Whilst the pure tone audiogram may currently be regarded as a valuable differential diagnostic tool, it has long been known to be a relatively weak tool for assessing receptive speech perception ability, although it is also recognized that speech perception tests in quiet lack predictive ability for hearing aid use in all situations. The point though is that, for post-lingual adults, the audiogram is not an intuitive starting point for the fitting of nonlinear hearing aids or hearing aid validation.

Thus, an alternative approach to accessible hearing assessment is to develop alternatives to the audiogram for hearing aid fitting. Candidate approaches to receptive speech perception hearing assessment are speech perception tests in quiet and in noise, questionnaires, and self-assessment. Carhart (1946) introduced the idea of using speech material as part of hearing aid fitting in the 1940's, and the importance of speech is recognized in the development of the Speech Intelligibility Index (American National Standards Institute, 1997) formally adopted in 1997 and the use of the speech mapping function in modern audiometers for the verification of hearing aid fittings (Moore, 2006). Speech perception measures have the advantage of being more meaningful to the client, and more functionally representative than graphs of hearing thresholds and speech mapping measures. They clearly convey the nature of the hearing difficulty and the effect of hearing aids in overcoming or reducing the difficulty.

The Speech Perception Test (SPT) described by Blamey (Blamey et al., 2015, Blamey and Saunders, 2015) can be used effectively, either within a clinic setting or remotely, to provide an informative self-explanatory measure of hearing difficulty, a means to predict hearing aid first fit, and a verification of hearing aid benefit. The use of speech at conversational levels avoids the need for sound-proof rooms and minimizes remote calibration issues.

The application of a mobile tool, such as the SPT as a replacement for conventional audiometry is an essential component of the Blamey Saunders end-to-end tele-audiology solution.

Speech perception testing and subjective self-report measures are also useful methods of determining real-world hearing difficulties and later real-world benefits of hearing aid performance that do not require extrapolation from the aided and unaided audiogram. According to Cox (2003) there are at least three reasons to use self-report measures of benefit and satisfaction. First, for largely economic reasons, health care is becoming more consumer driven. In this evolving system, the consumer decides what treatment is selected and when it is complete. BSH is trialling an open-ended Consumer Outcomes survey instrument, which is independently managed to tracker user satisfaction. In the first 6 months it has been found that participation rates are about 23%, compared to the norm of 10 to 15%. A Self-report measures of outcome are gaining importance is also related to the fact that many of these real-world experiences simply cannot be measured effectively in laboratory conditions. The traditional hearing aid outcome measures clinicians have used in the past, such as speech recognition in quiet and in noise, do not capture the true experiences of hearing aid use in everyday listening situations. Self-report measures can quantify the true impact on lifestyle that the hearing loss and its associated treatment implementations cause. Even when laboratory conditions are used to simulate real-world listening situations, they do not always resemble the patient's impression of the actual real-life situation.

In the Blamey Saunders Model, the client first carries out a test of hearing for speech (the Speech Perception Test), using their computer or smartphone, at a comfortable listening level. The results are stored in the Blamey Saunders e-health cloud. When a tele-audiologist speaks to the client, it is with some knowledge of the client's hearing difficulties, as seen in the results of the SPT (Beckett et al., 2016). The tele-audiologist's role is to build the relationship and to glean adequate information to assist the client in choosing their path forward. That is, ascertain *Attitude*, and other information that will help the client to decide whether to go forward on the path to auditory enablement through face-to-face contact, or via the digital health channel. This discussion will necessarily include the results of the SPT. From this point on, the tele-audiologist may remain the first point of call, but it may be in a triage type role, resulting in audiologist support, face-to-face or remote support, or in assisting the client's path to auditory enablement. It's an asset in a hearing health ecosystem if the hearing service provider can provide access to assistance remotely, through light touch assistance, to diagnostic and complex care. BSH provide the full spectrum, putting the client and client choices at the centre of the Model.

There are numerous descriptions of the potential role of a tele-audiologist. The tele-audiologists in the BSH team are able to help the client steer a path through audiological triage to informational counselling. They need to be able to interpret audiological data, but not necessarily to be able to carry out the tests. They need to identify when to guide and influence the client, to the most suitable type of care, be it medical or face-to-face audiological, or both. The tele-audiologist needs familiarity with ICT systems so that they are fully comfortable in drawing on the available ICT resources and to be able to confidently switch between available digital tools. They also need to be prepared for many interactions as a tele-audiologist is very easy to contact. The tele-audiologists will have access to an audiologist, and be able to pass on a particular case to an audiologist, whose role draws on a deeper experience and knowledge of audiology and incorporates the expertise to carry out complex and standardized assessments and interpretations.

Complementary Aspects of Audiology and Tele-Audiology

As part of the Auditory Enablement process, and following the collection of adequate information and consultation, BSH send hearing aids to the client, pre-programmed as predicted by the client's SPT. The hearing aids are self-fit, described elsewhere (Keach, 2013), and the client can use a very simple process based on balancing frequency band centred chimes, to shape the frequency spectrum to their needs. The user is guided through further personalization steps as chosen. If help is required,

Figure 3. Audiology and Tele-audiology services overlap

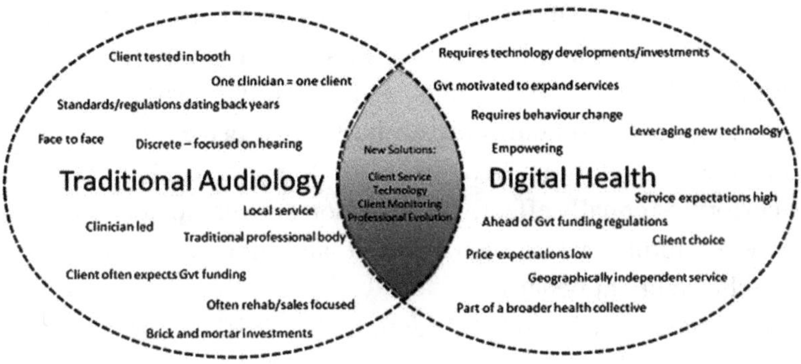
Client tested in booth
One clinician = one client
Standards/regulations dating back years
Face to face
Discrete – focused on hearing
Traditional Audiology
Local service
Clinician led
Traditional professional body
Client often expects Gvt funding
Often rehab/sales focused
Brick and mortar investments
New Solutions:
Client Service
Technology
Client Monitoring
Professional Evolution
Requires technology developments/investments
Gvt motivated to expand services
Requires behaviour change
Leveraging new technology
Empowering
Digital Health
Service expectations high
Ahead of Gvt funding regulations
Client choice
Price expectations low
Geographically independent service
Part of a broader health collective

Figure 4. The Blamey Saunders client journey

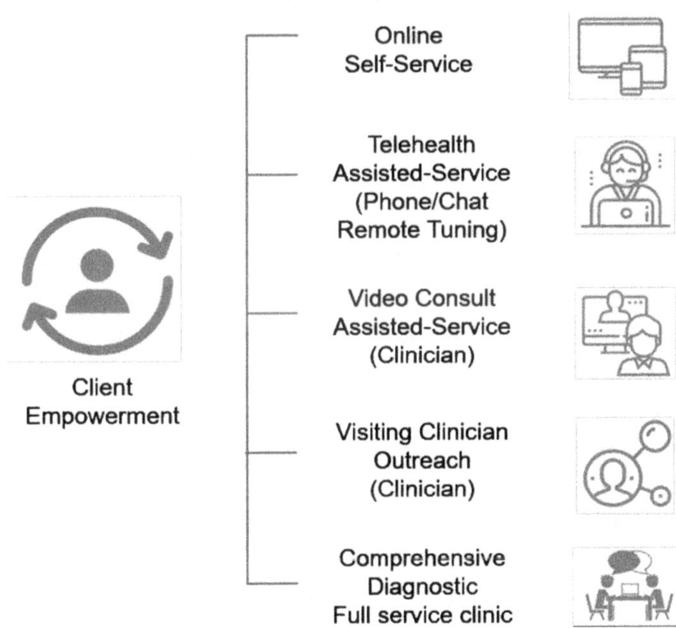

a tele-audiologist can make remote adjustments to the hearing aid, working in partnership with the hearing aid user. The team uses simple outcomes questionnaires, open ended questions, and repetition of the SPT as validation tools.

There are aspects of audiology which cannot currently be done remotely and where someone, be it a remotely supervised assistant or an audiologist, must be in physical proximity to the client. However, this is a dynamic and changing situation where we may expect exciting developments, targeting more accessible and home-based client care. There are other parts of audiology that are relatively easy to perform, such as the online screening of hearing by questionnaires or listening tests, although there is still some scepticism about the accuracy of some of these methods (Bexelius et al., 2008; Sindhusake et al., 2001; Smits et al., 2006; Kimball, 2008).

Between the aspects of audiology that are best performed by face-to-face audiology and those that are easily performed by tele-audiology, there are overlapping aspects that can be performed equally effectively in person or over the internet and is a matter of choice or accessibility by the client. The tele-audiology method will employ new practices to achieve client benefit.

The Blamey Saunders Speech Perception Test (SPT) is an example of a test that has been developed so that a person may get a comprehensible picture of their ability to hear speech at normal levels, and understand their hearing strengths and weaknesses, from the convenience of their home (Blamey and Saunders, 2015). This is important for people who have difficulty accessing diagnostic audiology services due to distance or limited mobility; for people who don't want to face up to a "hearing" test; and for people who get anxious during audiometry testing. The results of this SPT are stored in a central database and the results are used to predict the hearing aid's first fit, fulfilling a suggestion made by Raymond Carhart two generations ago (Carhart, 1946). In order to perform hearing aid fitting via tele-audiology, the once ubiquitous HiPro programmer device (Jelonek, 1994) has been replaced by much cheaper substitutes that are supplied with the hearing aids. Thus, with the BSH system everyone has their own programmer for personal use, or such that they can take it to any independent audiologist who undertakes fee for service work. BSH uses a simple magnetic connection to the programming cable to avoid the necessity of using fiddly connection cables, and rechargeable batteries that connect to the hearing aid Core with a magnetic connector. This modular, self-fit hearing device is called the Facett®.

It's not just hearing aids that can be managed remotely. In another equipment substitution example, a US company, Cellscope, supplies an iPhone attachment for otoscopy that parents can use to send video otoscopy of their child's eardrum for remote evaluation by an otologist (Richards et al., 2015). The iPhone otoscope enables frequent on-demand monitoring of ear health in children that would be prohibitively time consuming and expensive without the device. A similar device is available internationally from British company Cupris. (Mandavia et al., 2017)

It is clear that a complete hearing health solution with adequate clinical utility will need to incorporate both conventional audiology and tele-audiology services, and it is the innovation in the service model that is critical.

Remote, online services are already commonly in use in tinnitus counselling, vestibular therapy, and auditory rehabilitation.

RESEARCH BENEFITS OF LARGE-SCALE DATA IN HEARING HEALTHCARE

The model developed by Blamey and Saunders results in large scale data collection. Until recently, audiological data were siloed in the records of relatively small clinical organizations, with a few exceptions such as the Veterans Administration in the USA and the National Acoustics Laboratories in Australia. This meant that large studies with more than a few hundred participants were rare, and often expensive and difficult to carry out, because of the need to aggregate data from multiple clinics. For example, the widely used NAL-NL2 hearing aid fitting prescription was initially based on only 240 audiograms and fine-tuned on the preferred responses for 187 hearing aid users (Keidser et al., 2011). The largest published studies of cochlear implant outcomes in adults, (Blamey et al., 2013, Lazard et al., 2012) involved the development and use of specialized statistical methods in order to combine and analyze data for 2251 patients from fifteen implant centres in Australia, Europe and North America. Tele-audiology and health informatics are starting to provide much larger datasets collected in a more uniform manner that are easier to analyze. For example, a report entitled "New opportunities and challenges for tele-audiology within Department of Veterans Affairs" indicate that data from 1,170 patients have shown outcomes with remote hearing aid programming to be as good as or better than those from traditional face-to-face encounters. (Donahue et al., 2010)

A similar study (Pross et al. 2016) used the IOI-HA survey to show that out of 42,697 who received hearing aids between January and September 2014, the 1,009 veterans who received tele-audiology care had outcomes that were at least as good as the other 41,688 who received in-person care. These results are consistent with those achieved in a study by Blamey and colleagues (Blamey et al., 2015). The study objectively measured the benefit of hearing aids fitted to 484 people based on information from an online speech perception test, and found the benefit was at least as great as the benefit of hearing aids fitted using face-to-face audiograms to 517 people in a conventional clinic. The large numbers of participants in these studies illustrate the advantages of tele-audiology methods in generating relatively large consistent data sets and the rapid accumulation of strong clinical evidence that may be used to address practical clinical research questions. This is a major advantage over the much smaller University-based or clinic-based audiology studies that dominate the mainstream research methodology.

CHALLENGES TO THE ADOPTION OF TELE-AUDIOLOGY

Implementing any change in healthcare delivery is challenging. The medical model has remained constant for hundreds of years, and initial adoption of telehealth and digital health models are either within current structures or entrepreneurial activities outside of Government structures, with the exception of the work at the Veterans Administration in the USA. The availability of various sensing, digital and robotic technologies allow medicine to move into more personalized practice with much greater consumer empowerment and control (Vogenberg et al., 2010; Agyeman et al., 2015). Not all clinicians are embracing this change despite the positive evidence of the effectiveness of empowerment and client-centered medicine.

A study by Eikelboom (2016) suggests that the lead and initiatives in tele-audiology are likely coming from outside the traditional audiological profession, and are not only client-centered, but client led. In Eikelboom's study, audiologists around the world were surveyed online about their attitudes toward tele-audiology and their willingness to use it. Responses from 269 audiologists from 28 countries indicated limited clinical adoption, which suggests that the products and procedures that they were aware of did not enhance their practice efficiency. The authors concluded that, despite positive attitudes toward telehealth, the low number of audiologists who have used tele-audiology for services indicates limited clinical adoption. Another study (Chien et al., 2011) surveyed 202 hearing healthcare professionals in Canada. The authors concluded that the majority of respondents considered that, apart from improved accessibility to services, tele-audiology was likely to have a minimal effect on the quality of hearing healthcare in audiology and the quality of client-practitioner interactions. A small minority of respondents indicated that tele-audiology would have a negative impact on quality of care in audiology. The study concluded that a willingness to use tele-audiology depended on a combination of the clinical tasks to be performed and the patient populations to be served.

Interestingly, in what might be considered a very advanced and surgically invasive area of auditory rehabilitation, that of cochlear implants, a number of studies indicate satisfaction by both clients and clinicians. For example, Kuzovkov (2014) and his colleagues studying cochlear implant programming in Italy, Sweden and Russia, found that remote cochlear implant programming was both safe and well received by health-care professionals and clients. In this case, we surmise that they have appropriate processes and technologies.

These examples indicate that the majority of practitioners in mainstream audiology see little benefit or need to adopt advanced tele-audiology practices, despite the growing evidence from large studies and specialist services that it can improve productivity and cost-effectiveness of appropriately selected audiology practices by a large factor. Adoption of tele-audiology should herald an era of prompt and personalized care, with a reduced financial footprint.

NEW BUSINESS MODELS FOR TELE-AUDIOLOGY

One of the major potential benefits of tele-audiology is the increase in affordability of hearing health solutions for health agencies and individual users of hearing health services and products, by removing the need for expensive infrastructure. However, it has been recognized that there is a reluctance to provide lower-priced hearing aids (U.S. Food and Drug Administration, 2016) and that insurance companies and other payers are not going to fund telehealth services, including tele-audiology services unless they are convinced that they are proven as effective as those provided face-to-face. Finding a tele-medicine business model that delivers value to the stakeholders, makes operational sense and is economically sustainable, has been reported as problematic (National Academies of Sciences, Engineering, and Medicine, 2016). This is not an insurmountable problem and the Blamey and Saunders Model has been operational in Australia for over seven years (Beckett et al., 2016).

CLIENT PERSPECTIVES

The findings of Lloyd et al. (2001) were that people do not like to be labelled as patients, especially if they have an invisible chronic condition such as sensorineural hearing loss. This label potentially contributes to the perceived stigma of hearing loss. Tele-audiology, coupled with self-fit hearing aids, is a means by which clients can improve their self-image and take control of their hearing and their lives again, within a flexible continuum including tele-audiology care. Table 1 summarizes the authors' interpretation of the advantages to the client of the telehealth and self-fit hearing aid audiology model compared to the traditional audiology clinic model.

The Knowledge Gap

One of the factors that can influence client/clinician communication and the efficacy of tele-audiology is the knowledge gap between the clinician who is familiar with technical terms such as decibel, hearing threshold, sensorineural hearing loss, real-

Table 1.

Tele-audiology model	Traditional clinic model
Client centered	Clinician centered
Wellness/enablement model	Medical/disability model
Personalized sound quality established by client	Clinician chosen sound quality
Cost savings to client and provider	Cost-intensive
Flexible independent or assisted; personal responsibility and "buy-in"	Clinician managed; little personal responsibility; Clinician knows best
Convenient, home-based, no travel costs	Clinician timetable, travel costs

ear gain, and so on, and the client who may not be familiar with the technical terms, but, and importantly, knows about their personal hearing difficulties in quiet and background noise in various real-world situations. Successful direct-to-client tele-audiology requires that communication involves a minimum of technical jargon and does not assume a high level of technical knowledge or competence on the client's part. In a study of 224 clients with a mean age of 67.1 years who had all experienced at least one audiology appointment, 75% were at least moderately willing to use tele-audiology, and those who had a high level of comfort with technology were twice as willing as those with a low level of comfort (Singh et al., 2017).

The use of speech perception tests and self-report methods as alternatives to the audiometer also helps to reduce the knowledge gap. Clients already know about the difficulties they are experiencing with speech perception, and do not need complex explanations about the fact that they may not have scored 100% on the test, and that they can expect an improved score when wearing a hearing aid.

The question of technical knowledge gap for the client needs to be addressed in telehealth, especially in relation to health in the home for older clients. This is not solely a problem in hearing health. Many proposed solutions to the burgeoning problem of chronic care presuppose an increased role for technology. Systems must be designed to suit user needs.

According to the Australian Bureau of Statistics the number of households with access to the internet at home reached 7.85 million in 2016–17, representing 86% of all households (up from 71.8% in 2008-09). In a training and user experience based iterative design study, Kaufman et al., (2006) demonstrated in a study involving 2,000 patients, that the patients were receptive to most aspects of the technology. Collaborative activity in the health space, particularly in a focus on home-based care will be important in large-scale telehealth roll out. In the interim, clients are self-selecting, and in a truly client-centered model, those wishing to see a clinician may be able to access a traditional face-to-face model, depending on distance, or work with a non-specialist facilitator in a clinician to clinician model.

Satisfaction

An important dimension of hearing aid outcomes is satisfaction with the hearing aid experience. Satisfaction differs from benefit in that satisfaction is not necessarily entirely driven by objective performance. For example, a client can experience a significant degree of benefit as measured on aided and unaided tests, but be reporting dissatisfaction as measured on a satisfaction scale, for many reasons including physical discomfort, difficulty with handling, unhelpful peer influence, and loudness dissatisfaction.

Loudness perception, aversion, and satisfaction is a complex topic. Hearing aids differ in the management of loudness and amplification strategy, and many hearing aid studies contribute little to the field of knowledge as different types of hearing aids are bundled together into a single category. Blamey and Martin (2009) showed, in a study using hearing aids which all had the same signal processing features, using the adaptive dynamic range optimization (ADRO®) amplification strategy, that loudness tolerance and loudness satisfaction are related but not equivalent. McKenna and colleagues (2010) drew attention to the prevalence of hyperacusis and the difficulties in distinguishing between hyperacusis and loudness recruitment. It has long been established that hearing aids bring optimal benefit for speech intelligibility where the perceived sound remains in the audible and comfortable range (Valente et al., 1998). Hearing aid technologies and hearing aid delivery mechanisms have been relatively unresponsive to these guidelines that rely on subjective judgements of comfort and satisfaction. Tele-audiology and self-fit methods are controlled by the client who is less likely to select an uncomfortable hearing aid setting than the clinician, and thus likely to have a higher level of satisfaction. This expectation was consistent with the results of Keach (2013) who studied speech perception scores in quiet and noise, and sound quality ratings for fittings a) based on the audiogram with no fine tuning, b) based on the audiogram plus in-situ measures performed by the client, and c) based on the audiogram plus in-situ measures and fine-tuning performed by the researcher. All three fittings improved speech intelligibility in noise and quiet with no significant differences. The results were:

1. Tended to produce greater benefit in quiet than c);
2. Tended to produce greater benefit in quiet than c);
3. Tended to produce better sound quality ratings than (a) or (c); and
4. Tended to produce the greatest improvement in noise.

Motivation

Singh (2012) evaluated 27 factors that might influence the participant's willingness to participate in tele-audiology. The five factors most likely to motivate a client participating in a tele-audiology appointment were access to specialists, flexible appointment times, meeting the practitioner in emergencies, minimizing waiting time, and obtaining appointments quickly. Better access to specialists and meeting the practitioner in emergencies have the potential to provide a better outcome from the tele-audiology appointment than from a conventional audiology appointment. The other three factors are related to convenience for the client. The two most demotivating factors were thought to be that the clinician could not examine the hearing aid, and the clinician could not examine the client. In reality, it has been found in the experience with the Blamey Saunders Model that photography and structured discussion have been effective, and encouraged better self-management.

The study above (Singh, 2012) did not report that cost savings to the client were a motivating factor, although the Canadian telehealth study reported savings of 47 million kilometers of travel and $70 million dollars of travel costs from a total of 187,385 telehealth sessions in 2010. In the case of the Veterans Affairs studies the savings in service provision, apart from client travel costs, were probably retained by Veterans Affairs. Similarly, in the case of privately funded hearing aid provision, the bundling of devices and services works against the savings being passed on to the client. However, if device and service costs are unbundled, and the client pays for clinic visits but not for tele-audiology appointments, there is a significant saving that is passed on to the client. In the private model, this results in a 50% saving by the client who purchases hearing aids, in comparison with purchasing comparable aids through a conventional audiology channel.

IMPLEMENTATION OF A CLIENT-CENTERED TELE-AUDIOLOGY MODEL

The client centered tele-audiology model requires an appropriately trained triage or tele-audiology team that handles client issues at a time convenient to the client, in their own home. As with any triage service, issues may need to be passed on to a specialist: an audiologist, medical person, technician, or scientist, as appropriate. The client will have the option of a conventional clinic appointment or an immediate tele-audiology session. Once a tele-audiology presence is established, the clinical entity is extremely contactable online. The audiology support team is a click or a phone call away. This is important for client confidence. However, the model can and should be set up in a manner that allows for considerable client empowerment. This is an excellent platform for the use of self-fit hearing aids. If the client can fine tune their own hearing aids, and only reaches out for help if they really need it, both client and clinician have multiple benefits. The client benefit may include the ability to fine tune the hearing aids from their mobile phone while experiencing real-world listening conditions. The clinician benefits by being able to help more clients achieve higher levels of satisfaction, whilst adhering to the clinical governance and privacy matters of most jurisdictions.

CONCLUSION

The Goldstein and Stephens Model of Auditory Enablement has provided a strong base for the development of a multi-channel service delivery model that is effective and scalable. Clinical utility will continue to increase through technology changes that further reduce the costs and increase the effectiveness and scope of tele-audiology. Acceptance of tele-audiology by clinicians and clients will grow as regulatory barriers are removed, sustainable business models emerge and are incorporated into broad telehealth funding models, and hearing health professionals become more comfortable with the enabling technologies. The rate of change will accelerate as large datasets are created, demonstrating the benefits of the tele-audiology approach.

ACKNOWLEDGMENT

The authors' research is covered by Ethics Approval from the Royal Victorian Eye and Ear Hospital Human Research and Ethics Committee (project 14/1164H, "Maximising speech perception benefits in hearing aid users". Australian Government and Victorian State Government grants have supported the development of the tele-audiology technologies and services used by Blamey & Saunders Hearing Pty Ltd.

REFERENCES

Agyeman, A. A., & Ofori-Asenso, R. (2015). Perspective: Does personalized medicine hold the future for medicine? *Journal of Pharmacy & Bioallied Sciences*, *7*(3), 239. doi:10.4103/0975-7406.160040 PMID:26229361

Aiello, C. P., & Ferrari, D. V. (2015). Teleaudiology: Efficacy assessment of an online social network as a support tool for parents of children candidates for cochlear implant. *CoDAS*, *27*(5), 411–418. doi:10.1590/2317-1782/20152013061 PMID:26648210

AMA encourages telemedicine as part of "med school of the future." (2016). Available at: http://www.hearingreview.com/2016/06/ama-encourages-telemedicine-as-part-of-med-school-of-the-future

American National Standards Institute. (1997). *Methods for the calculation of the speech intelligibility index*. New York: Author.

Andreu-Perez, J., Poon, C. C. Y., Merrifield, R. D., Wong, S. T. C., & Yang, G.-Z. (2015). Big Data for Health. *IEEE Journal of Biomedical and Health Informatics*, *19*(4), 1193–1206. doi:10.1109/JBHI.2015.2450362 PMID:26173222

Arlinger, S. (2003). Negative consequences of uncorrected hearing loss - a review. *International Journal of Audiology*, *42*(2), S17–S20. doi:10.3109/14992020309074639 PMID:12918624

Australia's National Digital Health Strategy. (n.d.). Retrieved from https://conversation.digitalhealth.gov.au/australias-national-digital-health-strategy

Australian Bureau of Statistics. (n.d.). *8146.0 - Household Use of Information Technology, Australia, 2016-17.* Retrieved June 4, 2018, from http://www.abs.gov.au/ausstats/abs@.nsf/mf/8146.0

Australian Parliament: Inquiry into the Hearing Health and Wellbeing of Australia. (2018). Retrieved from http://www.aph.gov.au/Parliamentary_Business/Committees/House/Health_Aged_Care_and_Sport/HearingHealth

Beckett, R. C., Saunders, E., & Blamey, P. J. (2016). Optimizing Hearing Aid Utilisation using Telemedicine Tools. In I. M. Miranda, R. Martinho, & R. Rijo (Eds.), *Encyclopedia of E-Health and Telemedicine* (pp. 72–85). IGI Global. doi:10.4018/978-1-4666-9978-6.ch007

Bexelius, C., Honeth, L., Ekman, A., Eriksson, M., Sandin, S., Bagger-Sjöbäck, D., & Litton, J.-E. (2015). Evaluation of an internet-based hearing test—comparison with established methods for detection of hearing loss. *Journal of Medical Internet Research, 10*(4), e32. doi:10.2196/jmir.1065 PMID:18940783

Blamey, P., Artieres, F., & Başkent, D. (2013). Factors affecting auditory performance of postlinguistically deaf adults using cochlear implants: An update with 2251 patients. *Audiology & Neuro-Otology, 18*, 36–47. doi:10.1159/000343189 PMID:23095305

Blamey, P. J., Blamey, J. K., & Saunders, E. (2015). Effectiveness of a teleaudiology approach to hearing aid fitting. *J Telemedicine and Telecare, 1*(8), 474-478.

Blamey, P. J., & Saunders, E. (2015). Predicting speech perception from the audiogram and vice versa. *Canadian J Audiology, 2*(2).

Blamey, P. J., & Martin, L. F. A. (2009). Loudness and satisfaction ratings for hearing aid users. *JAAA, 20*(4), 272–282. PMID:19927699

Botasso, M., Sanches, S.G.G., Bento, R.F., & Samelli, A.G. (2015). Teleaudiometry as a screening method in school children. *Clinics SciELO Brasil, 70*(4).

Brennan-Jones, C. G., Eikelboom, R. H., Swanepoel, D. W., Friedland, P. L., & Atlas, M. D. (2016). Clinical validation of automated audiometry with continuous noise-monitoring in a clinically heterogeneous population outside a sound-treated environment. *International Journal of Audiology, 55*(9), 507–513. doi:10.1080/14992027.2016.1178858 PMID:27206551

Campos, P. D., & Ferrari, D. V. (2012). Teleaudiology: Evaluation of teleconsultation efficacy for hearing aid fitting. *Jornal da Sociedade Brasileira de Fonoaudiologia, 24*(4), 301–308. doi:10.1590/S2179-64912012000400003 PMID:23306678

Carhart, R. (1946). Tests for selection of hearing AIDS. *Laryngoscope, 56*(12), 780–794. doi:10.1288/00005537-194612000-00004 PMID:20282107

Chien, E., Geffen, M., & Gordon, D. (2011, May). *Telehealth Benefits and Adoption- Connecting People and Providers Across Canada.* A Study Commissioned by Canada Health Infoway.

Convery, E., Keidser, G., Dillon, H., & Hartley, L. (2011). A self-fitting hearing aid: Need and concept. *Trends in Amplification, 15*(4), 157–166. doi:10.1177/1084713811427707 PMID:22143873

Cox, R. M. (2003). *Assessment of subjective outcome of hearing aid fitting: getting the client's point of view. International Journal of Audiology.*

Deloitte Access Economics. (2017). *The social and economic cost of hearing loss in Australia*. Author.

Donahue, A., Dubno, J. R., & Beck, L. (2010). Accessible and affordable hearing health care for adults with mild to moderate hearing loss. *Ear and Hearing*, *31*(1), 2–6. doi:10.1097/AUD.0b013e3181cbc783 PMID:20040828

Economics, A. (2005). *Listen Hear!* The Economic Impact and Cost of Hearing Loss in Australia.

Eikelboom, R. H., & Swanepoel, D. W. (2016). International survey of audiologists' attitudes toward telehealth. *American Journal of Audiology*, *25*(3S), 295–298. doi:10.1044/2016_AJA-16-0004 PMID:27768191

Goldstein, D. P., & Stephens, S. D. (1981). Audiological rehabilitation: Management model I. *Audiology*, *20*(5), 432–452. doi:10.3109/00206098109072713 PMID:7271594

Henshaw, H., & Ferguson, M. A. (2013). Efficacy of Individual Computer-Based Auditory Training for People with Hearing Loss: A Systematic Review of the Evidence. *PLoS One*, 10. PMID:23675431

Jacobs, P. G., Saunders, G. H., Jacobs, P. G., & Saunders, G. H. (2014). New opportunities and challenges for teleaudiology within Department of Veterans Affairs. *Journal of Rehabilitation Research and Development*, *51*(5), vii–xii. doi:10.1682/JRRD.2014.04.0093 PMID:25334005

Jelonek, S. (1994). NOAH/HI-PRO system offers industrywide standard for fitting programmables. *The Hearing Journal*, *47*, 21–21.

Jenstad, L., & Moon, J. (2011). Systematic review of barriers and facilitators to hearing aid uptake in older adults. *Audiology Research*, *1*(1), 91–95. PMID:26557310

Kaufman, D. R., Pevzner, J., Hilliman, C., Weinstock, R. S., Teresi, J., Shea, S., & Starren, J. (2006). Redesigning a Telehealth Diabetes Management Program for a Digital Divide Seniors Population. *Home Health Care Management & Practice*, *18*(3), 223–234. doi:10.1177/1084822305281949

Keach, E. E. (2013). *Investigation of hearing aid provision via the first-fit efficacy of three adaptive dynamic range optimisation (ADRO) fitting methods* (Master thesis). University of Auckland.

Keidser, G., & Convery, E. (2016). Self-Fitting Hearing Aids: Status Quo and Future Predictions. *Trends in Hearing*, *2016*, 20. PMID:27072929

Keidser, G., Dillon, H. R., Flax, M., Ching, T., & Brewer, S. (2011). The NAL-NL2 prescription procedure. *Audiology Research*, *1*(1), 24. PMID:26557309

Kimball, S. H. (2008). Inquiry into online hearing test raises doubts about its validity. *The Hearing Journal*, *61*(3), 38–46. doi:10.1097/01.HJ.0000314717.42321.4a

Knudsen, V., Öberg, M., Nielsen, C., Naylor, G., & Kramer, S. E. (2010). Factors Influencing Help Seeking, Hearing Aid Uptake, Hearing Aid Use and Satisfaction With Hearing Aids: A Review of the Literature. *Trends in Amplification*, *14*(3), 127–154. doi:10.1177/1084713810385712 PMID:21109549

Kochkin, S. (2007). MarkeTrak VII: Obstacles to adult non-user adoption of hearing aids. *The Hearing Journal*, *60*(4), 24–51. doi:10.1097/01.HJ.0000285745.08599.7f

Krupinski, E.A. (2015). Innovations and possibilities in connected health. *Journal American Academy Audiology*, *26*, 761-767.

Kuzovkov, V., Yanov, Y., & Levin, S. (2014). Remote programming of MED-EL cochlear implants: users' and professionals' evaluation of the remote programming experience. *J. Acta Oto-Laryngologica*.

LACE. (2018). Retrieved from https://www.neurotone.com/lace-interactive-listening-program

Lazard, D. S., Vincent, C., Venail, F., Van de Heyning, P., Truy, E., Sterkers, O., ... Blamey, P. J. (2012). Pre-, per-and postoperative factors affecting performance of postlinguistically deaf adults using cochlear implants: A new conceptual model over time. *PLoS One*, *7*(11). doi:10.1371/journal.pone.0048739 PMID:23152797

Lin,, F.R., Yaffe,, K., & Xia,, J., Lie, X., Satterfield, S., Ayonayon, H.N., ... Simonsick, E.M. (2013). Hearing Loss and Cognitive Decline in Older Adults. *American Medical Association Internal Medicine.*, *173*(4), 293–299.

Lloyd, C., King, R., Bassett, H., Sandland, S., & Savige, G. (2001). Patient, Client or Consumer? A Survey of Preferred Terms. *Australasian Psychiatry*, *9*(4), 321–324. doi:10.1046/j.1440-1665.2001.00358.x

Mandavia, R., Lapa, T., Smith, M., & Bhutta, M. F. (2017). A cross-sectional evaluation of the validity of a smartphone otoscopy device in screening for ear disease in Nepal. *Clinical Otolaryngology*, *43*(1), 31–38. doi:10.1111/coa.12898 PMID:28485038

McKenna, L., Baguley, D., & McFerran, D. (2010). *Living with Tinnitus and Hyperacusis*. Sheldon Press.

Molini-Avejonas, D. R., Rondon-Melo, S., de la Higuera Amato, C. A., & Samelli, A. G. (2015). A systematic review of the use of telehealth in speech, language and hearing sciences. *Journal of Telemedicine and Telecare*, *21*(7), 367–376. doi:10.1177/1357633X15583215 PMID:26026181

Moore, B.C. (2006). Speech mapping is a valuable tool for fitting and counseling patients. *Hearing Journal*, *59*(8), 26-8.

National Academies of Sciences, Engineering, and Medicine. (2016). *Hearing Health Care for Adults: priorities for improving access and affordability*. National Academies Press.

Newswire, P. R. (2016). *Oticon Launches World's First Internet of Things Hearing Aid*. Retrieved from https://www.prnewswire.com/news-releases/oticon-launches-worlds-first-internet-of-things-hearing-aid-584077291.html

Noble, W. (2013). *Self-Assessment of Hearing* (2nd ed.). San Diego, CA: Plural Publishing.

One Million Solutions in Health. (2018). Retrieved from http://www.onemillionsolutionsinhealth.org/

Pross, S. E., Bourne, A. L., & Cheung, S. W. (2016). TeleAudiology in the Veterans Health Administration. *Otology & Neurotology*, *37*(7), 847–850. doi:10.1097/MAO.0000000000001058 PMID:27273404

Richards, J. R., Gaylor, K. A., & Pilgrim, A. J. (2015). Comparison of traditional otoscope to iPhone otoscope in the pediatric ED. *The American Journal of Emergency Medicine*, *33*(8), 1089–1092. doi:10.1016/j.ajem.2015.04.063 PMID:25979304

Sindhusake, D., Mitchell, P., Smith, W., Golding, M., Newall, P., Hartley, D., & Rubin, G. (2001). Validation of self-reported hearing loss. The Blue Mountains Hearing Study. *International Journal of Epidemiology*, *30*(6), 1371–1378. doi:10.1093/ije/30.6.1371 PMID:11821349

Singh, G., Pichora-Fuller, M. K., Malkowski, M., Boretzki, M., & Launer, S. (2014). Survey of the attitudes of practitioners toward teleaudiology. *International Journal of Audiology*, *53*(12), 850–860. doi:10.3109/14992027.2014.921736 PMID:25017424

Smits, C., Merkus, P., & Houtgast, T. (2006). How we do it: The Dutch functional hearing–screening tests by telephone and Internet. *Clinical Otolaryngology*, *31*(5), 436–440. doi:10.1111/j.1749-4486.2006.01195.x PMID:17014457

Stephens, D., & Kramer, S. E. (2009). Living with Hearing Difficulties: the process of enablement. Wiley-Blackwell.

Swanepol, D. W., Koekemoer, D., & Clark, J. (2010). Intercontinental hearing assessment – a study in tele-audiology. *Journal of Telemedicine and Telecare*, *16*(5), 248–252. doi:10.1258/jtt.2010.090906 PMID:20457801

Teleaudiology, S. G. (n.d.). *Are patients and practitioners ready for it?* Retrieved from https://www.phonakpro.com/content/dam/phonakpro/gc_hq/en/events/2012/advances_in_audiology_lasvegas/Singh_G_Teleaudiology_Are_patients_and_practitioners_ready.pdf

Tye-Murray, N. (2016). *A clEAR™ Solution to the Changing Climate of Hearing Healthcare*. Retrieved September 18, 2018 from https://www.clearworks4ears.com/static/media_relations/Audiology%20practices%20proofs.pdf

U.S. Food and Drug Administration. (2016, December 7). *FDA takes steps to improve hearing aid accessibility*. Author.

Valente, M., Bentler, R., Seewald, R., Trine, T., & Van Vliet, D. (1998). Guidelines for hearing aid fitting for adults. *American Journal of Audiology*, *7*(1), 5–13. doi:10.1044/1059-0889.0701.05 PMID:26649513

Vieira Esteves, T., & Pacheco de Oliveira, S. (2015). Telehealth in Brazil: Contemporary Tool for Access to Health. *Studies in Health Technology and Informatics*, *216*, 995. PMID:26262297

VizeR. (2017). Retrieved from https://www.theguardian.com/healthcare-network/2017/sep/08/nhs-embrace-digital-services-risk-left-behin

Vogenberg, F. R., Barash, C. I., & Pursel, M. (2010). Personalized medicine: part 1: evolution and development into theranostics. *P&T*, *35*(10), 560.

Wesarg, T., Wasowski, A., & Skarzynski, H. (2010). Remote fitting in Nucleus cochlear implant recipients. [PubMed]. *J. Acta Oto-Laryngologica*, *130*(12), 1379–1388.

World Health Organization. (2018). *Deafness and hearing loss*. Retrieved August 22, 2018, from http://www.who.int/mediacentre/factsheets/fs300/en/

KEY TERMS AND DEFINITIONS

ADRO: Adaptive dynamic range optimization amplification. The ADRO patent and trade mark is owned by Wolfson Dynamic Hearing Pty Ltd.

Audiology: The study of hearing, balance, and related disorders. Its practitioners assess hearing and balance disorders, assess degree of hearing handicap, implement auditory rehabilitation strategies to overcome hearing difficulties, and refer to appropriate medical specialties.

Cost-Benefit Relationship: Describes the comparison of the benefits and the costs of a course of action in a given situation. In healthcare this defines the cost of providing a treatment or service to a population and the quantified benefits to the population.

Hearing Aid: An approved medical device designed to improve hearing by making sounds both audible and comfortable to a person with hearing loss. The output characteristics are personalized for the user.

Hearing Loss: Term used to quantify someone's hearing difficulties, usually measured in dB in comparison with audiometric zero. Alternative measures include a measure of ability to hear speech sounds.

Chapter 4
The Expected Benefit of Hearing Aids in Quiet as a Function of Hearing Thresholds

Peter J. Blamey
Blamey Saunders Hears, Australia

ABSTRACT

This chapter aimed to estimate speech perception benefits in quiet for clients with different degrees of hearing loss. The difference between aided and unaided scores on a monosyllabic word test presented binaurally was used as the measure of benefit. Retrospective data for 492 hearing aid users with four-frequency pure-tone average hearing losses (PTA) ranging from 5 dB HL to 76 dB HL in the better ear were analyzed using nonlinear regression. The mean benefit for the perception of monosyllabic words in this group of clients was 22.3% and the maximum expected benefit was 33.6% for a PTA of 52 dB HL. The expected benefit can be expressed as a reduction of the error rate by about half for isolated words and about one quarter for sentences across the full range of PTA.

DOI: 10.4018/978-1-5225-8191-8.ch004

INTRODUCTION

Hearing difficulties are common but inconsistently or often not treated in developed countries including Australia, USA, and European countries. Approximately 20% of the Australian population have a significant hearing loss and this percentage rises to 50% for people aged 60 years and over (Access Economics, 2006, Page 5; Deloitte Access Economics for the Hearing Care Industry Association, 2017). Although there is little doubt that modern hearing aids can alleviate hearing difficulties for most people, less than 25% of people who would benefit from hearing aids actually own them and a high proportion of hearing aids end up "in-the-drawer" instead of "in-the-ear" or "behind-the-ear" (Kochkin, 2000; McCormack & Fortnum, 2013). The barriers to improved hearing health in Australia and elsewhere include:

- The high cost of hearing aids purchased through the conventional audiological business model (Australian Competition and Consumer Commission, 2017),
- The inconvenience of the audiological model including distance to the nearest audiologist (Grenness, Hickson, Laplante-Lévesque, and Davidson, 2014),
- The high return rates of hearing aids experienced by conventional audiology clinics (Kochkin, et al., 2010),
- The low usage of hearing aids by hearing aid owners (Kochkin, 2000),
- The perceived stigma of wearing hearing aids (Wallhagen, 2009),
- The reluctance of over 75% of people with hearing difficulty to seek help (Access Economics, 2006), and
- The low expectations of a large proportion of non-hearing aid wearers whose only relevant experience may have been listening to an elderly relative complaining about their hearing aids (Cox and Alexander, 2000; Meister, Walger, Brehmer, von Wedel, and von Wedel, 2008).

Other chapters in this book have addressed the first six dot points above, and this chapter will focus on the last one.

When a potential hearing aid user visits an audiology clinic they are often advised that they should not have unrealistic expectations of the benefit of hearing aids (Dillon, 2008) but there is very little evidence available about what level of expected benefit is realistic for an individual. Furthermore, the evidence that is available is often couched in audiological or scientific jargon that is not easily understood or explained to the layman. Despite this lack of easily understood data, there is widespread consensus among professionals that hearing aids are of benefit to the population of hearing impaired people in general.

A recent systematic review of randomised controlled trials of hearing aids for mild to moderate hearing loss in adults (Ferguson, et al., 2017) found there was a large beneficial effect of hearing aids on hearing-specific health-related quality of life, associated with participation in daily life as measured using the Hearing Handicap Inventory for the Elderly (HHIE, scale range 1 to 100) compared to the unaided/placebo condition (mean difference (MD) -26.47, 95% confidence interval (CI) -42.16 to -10.77; 722 participants; three studies) (moderate-quality evidence). The authors concluded that:

The available evidence concurs that hearing aids are effective at improving hearing-specific health-related quality of life, general health-related quality of life and listening ability in adults with mild to moderate hearing loss. The evidence is compatible with the widespread provision of hearing aids as the first-line clinical management in those who seek help for hearing difficulties. Greater consistency is needed in the choice of outcome measures used to assess benefits from hearing aids.

Purpose

The purpose of conducting the research described in this chapter was to address the need for a quantitative objective measure of hearing aid benefit that could be used to provide realistic expectations of benefit for individual prospective clients. The specific objectives were to analyse existing clinical data to estimate the speech perception benefits in quiet of hearing aid fitting for clients with different degrees of hearing loss and to express them in language accessible to laypersons in order to give them a reasonable expectation of the potential benefit to them personally. A greater depth of information and explanation is provided for hearing care professionals for use in counselling.

BACKGROUND

The literature includes several studies that found that expectations have a significant effect on hearing aid outcomes. For example, Jerram and Purdy (2001) found that higher hearing aid use time and greater benefit in easy and difficult listening situations were predicted by higher pre-fitting expectations. Similarly, Saunders, Lewis, & Forsline (2009) found that positive expectations resulted in more positive outcomes. Cox and Alexander (2000) found that novice hearing aid users had stable pre-fitting expectations about hearing aids, and these expectations were unrealistically high for the typical individual. These studies used the Abbreviated Profile of Hearing

Aid Benefit (APHAB) and other questionnaires to evaluate hearing aid benefit. Blamey, Martin, and Saunders (2010) used the Profile of Hearing Aid Performance (PHAP) which is closely related to the APHAB to show that hearing aid benefit for communication in quiet increased by 0.79% per dB of pure-tone-average hearing loss (PTA). The same study showed consistent average benefits in background noise and in difficult listening conditions independent of PTA. Thus, it is likely that realistic expectations may be different in quiet and in noisy conditions.

A fairly recent review by Knudsen, Öberg, Nielsen, Naylor, & Kramer (2010) considered 39 papers that evaluated the effects of 31 factors influencing help seeking, hearing aid uptake, hearing aid use, and satisfaction with hearing aids. Expectations were considered as a factor in six of these studies, and three of the six studies found that expectations had a statistically significant association with hearing aid use and/or hearing aid satisfaction. Sixteen of the reviewed studies considered hearing sensitivity (degree of hearing loss, PTA) as a factor and nine of these found a significant association with at least one of the four outcome measures.

Meister et al., (2008) found that three predictor variables (expectations towards improvement of quality of life, stigmatization, and self-rated hearing ability) accounted for about 55% of the variability in the data for willingness to wear hearing aids.

In the light of these studies, the question of how to provide a realistic expectation of the benefit of hearing aids to individuals has high clinical significance. If the expectation is unrealistically low, the individual may not be motivated sufficiently to wear the hearing aid, and therefore the potential benefit will not be realised by the individual. If the expected benefit is unrealistically high, the individual is likely to be dissatisfied and may reject the hearing aid as providing insufficient benefit, and therefore the potential benefit will not be realised by this individual either. Between these two extremes lies a happy medium of realistic expectations which increase the probability of delivering realistic benefits to individuals.

In the author's opinion, individuals tend to be torn between the unrealistically optimistic statements in the manufacturers' and retail chains' marketing materials, and the old-fashioned but fairly pervasive view that hearing aids don't work. Neither of these two sources of information is very useful to individuals because they miss the point entirely that hearing aid benefit does not just depend on the hearing aid, it also depends on the individual using it and the sounds they are listening to. Blamey, Martin, and Saunders (2010) found that in quiet, some people benefit a lot and some people don't benefit much at all, while in noisy and difficult listening situations most people benefit a moderate amount.

Traditionally, it has been the responsibility of the clinician to assess the hearing and other circumstances of the individual, estimate the need for hearing aids, the type of hearing aids best suited to the individual, and the likely benefit to the individual. The primary basis for this assessment has been the audiogram, which is meaningful to the clinician, but largely meaningless to the untrained individual. Thus, there is an unmet need for a measure of hearing that is meaningful to untrained individuals and that leads easily and directly to a realistic expectation for the benefit provided by hearing aids to individuals.

METHODS: ANALYSIS OF SPEECH PERCEPTION BENEFITS

Speech audiometry offers a measure of hearing that is meaningful to untrained individuals, but has not been applied to the assessment of hearing aid benefit until relatively recently. Since the early work of Harvey Fletcher (1929), Raymond Carhart (1951), Arthur Boothroyd (1968) and others, speech audiometry has gained acceptance and is routinely used in a variety of ways including speech mapping for hearing aid verification (Moore, 2006) and speech testing to assess suprathreshold hearing function (Plomp, 1978; Glasberg and Moore, 1988). With the advent of nonlinear amplification, noise reduction, and other complex sound processing algorithms, speech and speech-like signals are now more suitable for hearing aid evaluations than the pure-tone signals used in traditional hearing aid test boxes. A recent addition to the speech audiology literature is the Blamey Saunders online Speech Perception Test or SPT (Blamey, Blamey, and Saunders, 2015) which was specifically designed for tele-audiology applications in Australia.

The Speech Perception Test (SPT)

The SPT is a monosyllabic word test with 50 words per list, each having CVC structure (Consonant-Vowel-Consonant). There are 32 different lists of words. The phonemes in each list are phonemically balanced and are representative of the distributions of vowels and consonants in spoken Australian English language as a whole. The list presented in any instance is chosen randomly from the set of 32 and the words within each list are presented in random order to reduce learning effects. The words were recorded by a female native speaker of Australian English and individually normalised to a consistent presentation level. Lists are designed to be presented at a conversational speech level, binaurally or monaurally, depending on the use case, from a computer in a quiet environment. In a clinic environment, the presentation level is set to 60 dBA (Olsen, 1998). Online, the instructions are to set to a normal conversational level, and this is best done by a person known to have good hearing. The responses are ideally typed into the computer by the client to minimise the tester effect. The responses are scored automatically using text to phoneme conversion to avoid spurious errors caused by misspelling or use of alternative spellings for the response word. Each list yields four primary scores – the number of words correct (out of 50), number of words not heard (out of 50), number of consonants correct (out of 100) and number of vowels correct (out of 50). The SPT is similar to CNC word tests that have been used previously for different purposes (Peterson and Lehiste, 1962; Henry, McDermott, McKay, James and Clark, 1998; Blamey and Sarant, 2003), with the innovative addition of an information transmission analysis based on speech features (Miller and Nicely, 1955) that allows estimation of the audiogram from the SPT (Blamey and Saunders, 2015).

Use of the SPT for Tele-Audiology

As the test is hosted on the web at https://apps.blameysaunders.com.au/wordtest/, it can be used by people from home for a variety of purposes:

- **To Detect Hearing Difficulties:** On completion of the online test, the Infogram® is displayed graphically with a full explanation of the results in user-friendly, non-technical language. This includes a clear statement that the listener may have hearing difficulties if the word score is less than 44 words correct, or that the listener has good hearing if the word score is 44 words correct or higher.
- **To Determine Which Speech Sounds They Have Trouble Hearing:** The individual bars of the Infogram show which phoneme contrasts are easy or difficult to hear.
- **To Determine Whether They Would Benefit From a Hearing Aid:** The shaded regions in the Infogram show whether a hearing aid would be of benefit and for which sounds. The bluish shaded region at the top of the Infogram indicates that a hearing aid is not needed for sounds in this region; the gold region indicates that an open-fit Speaker-In-The-Ear hearing aid would be of benefit; and the white region at the bottom indicates that a visit to an audiologist is recommended.
- **To Provide Information in Order to Buy and Fit Hearing Aids Online:** The SPT result provides enough information for Blamey Saunders to produce a good initial fit for a hearing aid, as shown by the phase three validation result in Blamey, Blamey and Saunders (2015).
- **To Measure the Benefit of Hearing Aids:** The difference between an aided score and an unaided score on the SPT under the same conditions shows the benefit of hearing aids. This technique was used in the study described in this chapter.

- **To Track Changes in Hearing Over Time:** The SPT data are recorded in emails and in an online database, and so can be used to document hearing performance at different times.

The online SPT is used to enhance the Tele-audiology services that Blamey & Saunders Hearing (Blamey Saunders hears) delivers to thousands of clients each year. Each time a person completes the SPT online or in a clinic, the data (stimulus-response pairs for 50 words) are recorded in a central database which includes over 50,000 SPT results collected since June 2013 and may be evaluated to answer research questions such as those posed in this chapter.

Study Participants

In the current retrospective data analysis, the Blamey Saunders hears clinical database was searched for all clients who had:

- At least one SPT result in the unaided condition,
- At least one SPT result in the aided condition, and
- At least one audiogram.

There were 492 participants in total who met these criteria in 2016 when the search was conducted. In the cases where there was more than one measure, the highest SPT was selected and the most recent audiogram was selected. The 4-frequency pure-tone-average (PTA) hearing loss was calculated from the most recent audiogram in the better ear. The frequencies used were 500 Hz, 1 kHz, 2 kHz and 4 kHz. The PTA hearing loss varied between 5 dB HL and 76 dB HL within the group. According to audiological convention, hearing loss with PTA between 25 and 40 dB HL is referred to as "mild"; 40 to 70 dB HL as "moderate"; and 70 to 90 dB HL as "severe" hearing impairment. On the basis of their PTA there were 65 participants with "normal hearing", 201 with "mild hearing loss", 223 with "moderate hearing loss" and 3 with "severe hearing loss" in this study.

The participants used their own hearing aids purchased from Blamey Saunders hears for the SPT in the aided condition. They were tested either in a Blamey Saunders hears clinic or online. It is assumed that the online testing occurred at a conversational presentation level in reasonably quiet conditions with no difference between conditions for the aided and unaided SPT but there are no acoustic measures available for the online data. The audiograms were either supplied by the client or tested in a Blamey Saunders hears audiology clinic.

RESULTS

The data below are presented graphically and summarized with the help of curve fitting techniques, sometimes with a smoothing algorithm that makes no assumptions, sometimes using a sigmoid function, and sometimes with a linear regression line. For specific data sets, either the linear regression or sigmoid curve is more appropriate over the whole or part of the range of hearing thresholds. The smoothed data line is shown together with the other curves where appropriate, so the reader has a better feel for how well they fit the specific datasets and why curve fitting is preferred for some graphs and linear regression for others. This is explained in detail for Figures 1, 3, and 4 below and the explanation for other Figures has been reduced for clarity.

Unaided SPT Results vs. PTA

For each participant in the study, a dot is plotted on Figure 1. The selected SPT word score out of 50 in the unaided condition determines the vertical position of the dot and the PTA value for the participant's hearing loss determines the horizontal position of the dot.

A sigmoid-shaped curve was fitted to the data (solid line in Figure 1) using two adjustable parameters. It provides a good representation of the data, accounting for 67% of the total variance. The smoothed average data curve (dashed line in Figure 1) lies close to the fitted curve across the full PTA range, indicating that the sigmoid

Figure 1. Unaided SPT score as a function of hearing loss

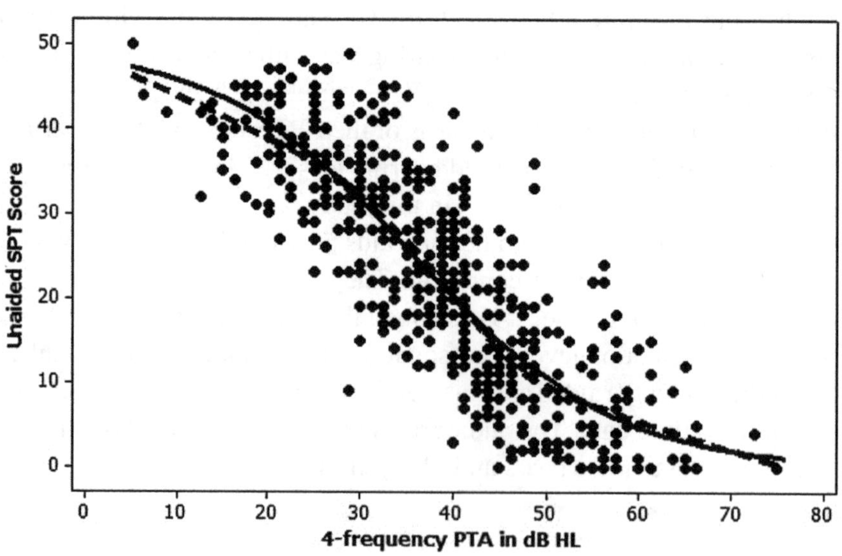

shape is appropriate. The 50% point on the curve is at 35.9 dB HL and the "width" of the curve is 11 dB HL so that the fitted equation is:

Unaided SPT score = 50 / (1+e^{-x}) where x = (35.9 - PTA) / 11

For simplicity, the second adjustable parameter is referred to as "width" because it is a measure of how wide a PTA range is spanned by the curve from approximately 75% correct to 50% correct. The 50% point on the curve at 35.9 dB indicates that a mild hearing loss is enough to reduce the SPT word score to 25 out of 50. It often surprises people who do the SPT that they do not score 100% even though they do not consider that they have a hearing loss at all. This occurs because the high redundancy of the speech signal and the English language make it possible for people to function very well without hearing every phoneme – they literally fill in the gaps without noticing (Assmann and Summerfield, 2004).

Aided SPT Results vs. PTA

Figure 2 shows data for the same participants as Figure 1, while wearing hearing aids.

The sigmoid-shaped curve accounted for 49% of the total variance. The 50% point on the curve is at 53.4 dB HL and the width of the curve is ± 18 dB HL. The 50% point at 53.4 dB lies in the middle of the moderate hearing loss range. Comparison of this result with the 50% point for Figure 1 means that when they are wearing hearing aids, people with moderate hearing loss perform on the SPT like people with mild hearing loss who are not wearing hearing aids.

Figure 2. Aided SPT score as a function of hearing loss

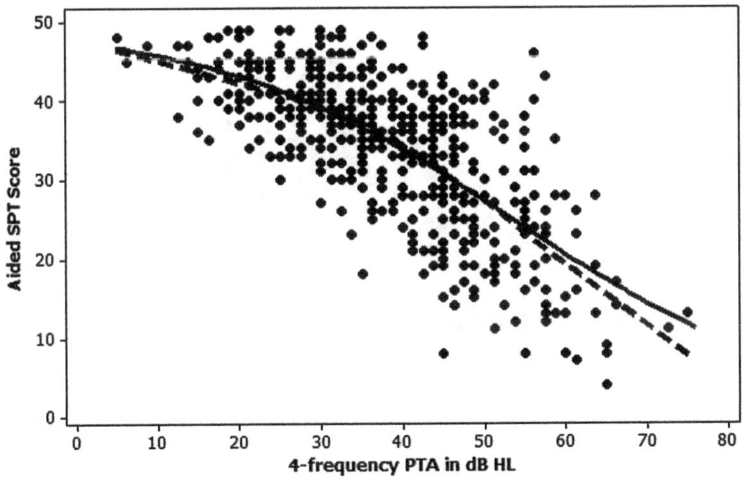

Speech Perception Benefit vs. PTA

Figure 3 shows the difference between the selected SPT word scores in the aided and unaided conditions. The solid line in Figure 3 is the difference between the fitted sigmoid curves in Figures 2 and 1. It accounts for 29% of the total variance. The maximum point on the curve corresponds to 16.8 words or 33.6% improvement between unaided and aided scores at a PTA of 52 dB HL in the moderate hearing loss range.

The dot-dashed line in Figure 3 is the regression line for SPT benefit against PTA. It has a slope of 0.72% per dB. The regression line is a reasonable fit to the data up to a PTA of 60 dB HL but should not be extrapolated to higher PTA.

DISCUSSION: EXPRESSING BENEFIT IN EVERYDAY LANGUAGE

The specific goal of this chapter includes presenting the results in a form that is easily understood by a layperson and establishes a reasonable expectation expressed in everyday language. The results above do not meet this goal, in part because of the use of the expression of hearing loss as PTA in the units of dB HL. In order to overcome this difficulty the results have been replotted in Figure 4. The selected SPT word score out of 50 in the aided condition determines the vertical position of the dot (as in Figure 2) and the selected SPT word score out of 50 in the unaided

Figure 3. SPT benefit as a function of hearing loss

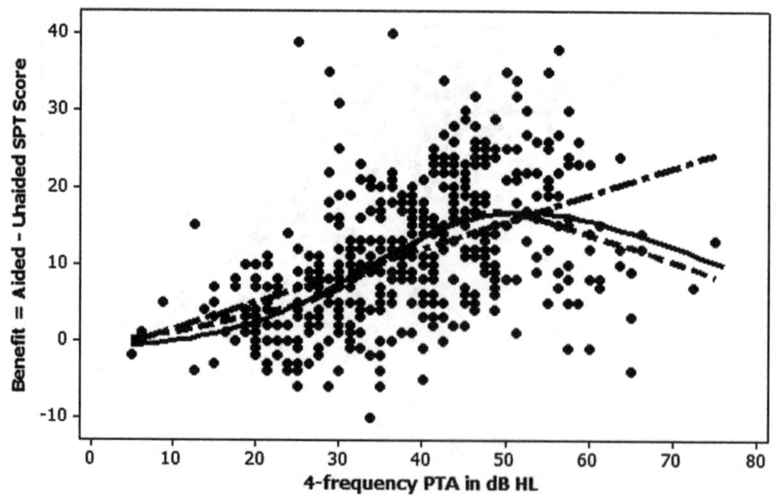

condition determines the horizontal position of the dot (as in the vertical axis of Figure 1). In Figure 4, the unaided SPT score is used as a surrogate measure of hearing loss, with good hearing on the right and poor hearing on the left, in contrast to Figures 1 and 2 where good hearing is on the left and poor hearing is on the right.

As in Figure 3, the solid line is derived from the sigmoid curves for unaided and aided hearing, the dashed line is the smoothed data, and the dot-dashed line is the linear regression fit to the data. The solid curve does not lie close to the smoothed curve for unaided scores less than about 5 out of 50 when the data are plotted in this way. The hearing aid still provided non-zero benefit even though the unaided score was zero for some of the participants. When plotted this way, the linear regression line is a better representation of the trends in the data. The linear regression line has equation:

Aided score = 0.56 X Unaided Score + 22

This can be re-written in terms of error rates as

Aided error rate = 50 – (0.56 X (50 – unaided error rate) + 22)

= 0.56 X unaided error rate

Thus, it is a realistic expectation that the number of errors made in the aided SPT will be about half (56%) of the number of errors made in the unaided condition.

Figure 4. Aided SPT score as a function of unaided SPT score

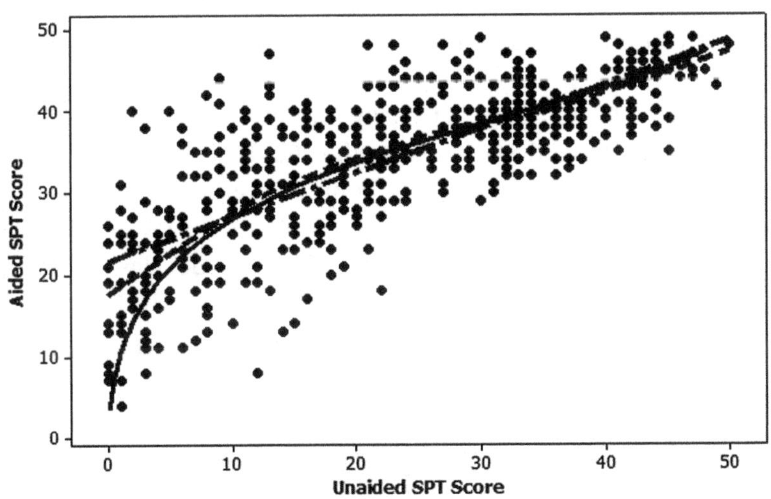

DISCUSSION: HEARING AID BENEFIT FOR RUNNING SPEECH

As mentioned above, people are often surprised at how low they score on the SPT. One of the reasons for this is that the monosyllabic words were purposely constructed to have low phonetic redundancy and no context so that it is necessary to hear every phoneme in order to get the word correct. By contrast, running speech typically has both high phonetic redundancy and high context so that it is not necessary to hear every sound in the utterance to be able to recognize all the words in the sentence (Assmann and Summerfield, 2004). For example it is well known that a sentence with all the vowels omitted is reasonably easy to understand, or if you miss a whole word in a sentence, then it can often be filled in if the context is known.

It is therefore of interest to estimate the effects of hearing aids on the perception of running speech in order to give potential clients a realistic expectation of the real-world benefit. In this paper, we use the known relationship between word recognition and sentence recognition to estimate individual scores on a hypothetical sentence test in aided and unaided conditions. There are several published graphs showing the well-accepted relationship between word and sentence perception scores, including Figure 124 of Fletcher (1929) and Figure 6 of Killion (1985). The former graph was used to transform the words correct data in Figures 1 to 4 and produce the estimated sentence scores in Figures 5 to 8.

Figure 5 is equivalent to Figure 1, showing the estimated unaided sentence perception scores as a function of hearing thresholds. The sigmoid-shaped curve provides a good representation of the data (except for PTA greater than 65 dB HL), accounting for 56% of the total variance. The 50% point on the sigmoid curve is at 48.7 dB HL and the width of the curve is 8.5 dB HL.

Figure 6 is the equivalent of Figure 2, showing the estimated aided sentence perception scores as a function of hearing thresholds. The sigmoid-shaped curve accounts for 33% of the total variance with 50% point at 76.5 dB HL and width of 15.3 dB HL.

Figure 7 is equivalent to Figure 3 and shows the estimated benefit of hearing aids for running speech as a function of hearing thresholds. The solid line accounts for 50% of the total variance. The maximum point on the solid curve corresponds to 55% improvement between unaided and aided scores at a PTA of 60 dB HL in the moderate hearing loss range. The linear regression line (dot-dashed line in Figure 7) is not a good fit to the data either above or below 60 dB HL PTA and is shown only for completeness of the comparison with Figure 3.

Figure 5. Estimated unaided sentence score as a function of hearing loss

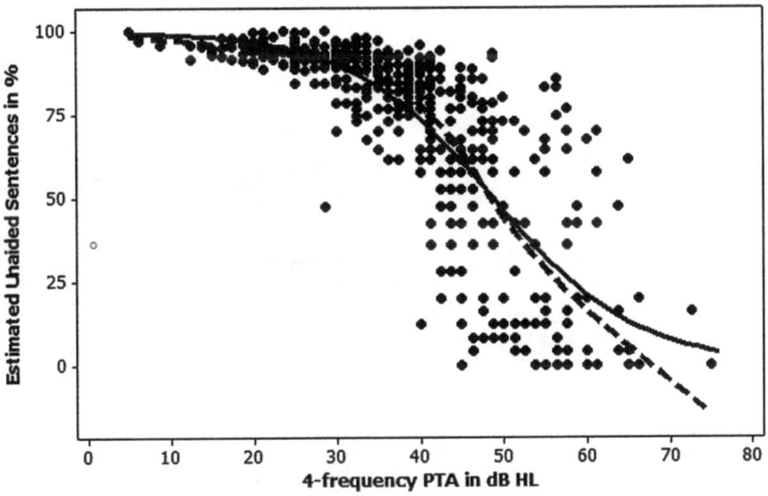

Figure 6. Estimated aided sentence score as a function of hearing loss

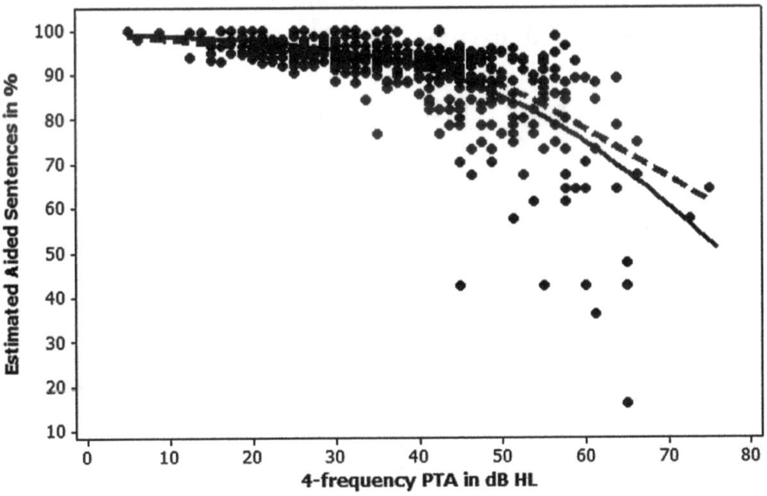

Figure 7. Estimated sentence benefit as a function of hearing loss

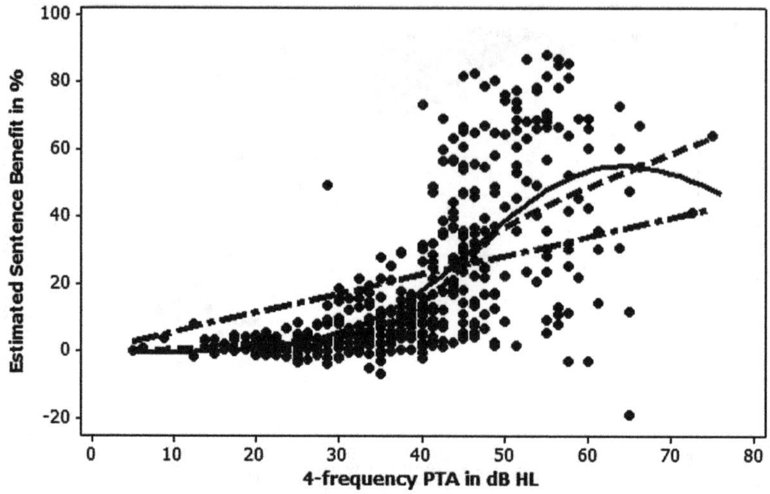

Figure 8 is analogous to Figure 4 and combines the data from Figures 5 and 6. When plotted this way, the linear regression line is a better representation of the trends in the data than the solid curvilinear fit. The linear regression line has equation:

Estimated aided sentence score = 0.28 X Estimated unaided sentence score + 72

Figure 8. Estimated aided sentence score as a function of estmated unaided sentence score

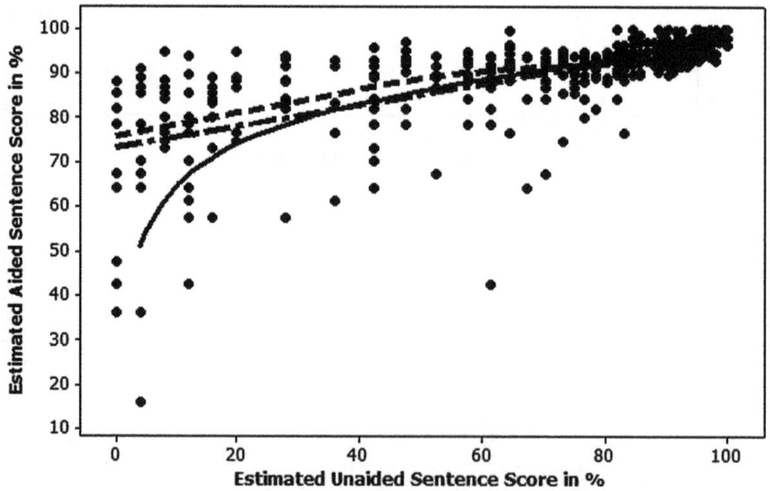

This can be re-written in terms of error rates as

Estimated aided error rate = 0.28 X estimated unaided sentence error rate

Thus, it is a realistic expectation that the number of errors made in aided sentence perception will be about one quarter (28%) of the number of errors made in the unaided condition.

DISCUSSION: SOLUTIONS AND RECOMMENDATIONS

The data and analyses presented in the sections above illustrate one method of objectively measuring hearing aid benefit, together with mathematical formulae for predicting the expected benefit of hearing aids based on these measures. The mathematical formulae use either audiological input data (PTA) or unaided speech perception data as input for the prediction. If these or similar methods are used, it becomes relatively easy for a clinician to calculate the expected performance or benefit on the SPT or in running speech for an individual prospective client from their audiogram. Similarly, it becomes relatively easy for a prospective hearing aid user to self-assess their speech perception performance and expected benefit from hearing aids in quiet conditions.

A less detailed way of looking at the data is to consider that the solid line in Figure 2 is further to the right and has a shallower slope than the solid line in Figure 1. The 50% point has moved from 35.9 to 53.4 dB HL suggesting that the hearing aids on average are equivalent to an improvement of 17.5 dB in PTA. This is enough to move a person from the "mild hearing loss" range into the "good hearing range" or from the middle of the "moderate hearing loss" range to the "mild hearing loss" range. Similar consideration of Figures 5 and 6 shows that the 50% point for sentences moves from 48.7 dB HL unaided to 76.5 dB HL when wearing hearing aids. This improvement of 27.8 dB is enough to move from "severe" to "moderate", "moderate" to "mild hearing loss" and from "mild hearing loss" to "good hearing".

The results of this analysis are in qualitative agreement with the results of other studies of hearing aid benefit. It is reasonably well-known that the benefit of hearing aids in quiet increases as hearing loss becomes greater. The fact that the benefit of hearing aids reaches a maximum for moderate hearing loss (52 dB HL for words and 64 dB HL for sentences) is less well-known although it is accepted that cochlear implant technology provides greater benefit than hearing aids for people with severe-to-profound hearing loss.

The sensitivity of monosyllabic words to clinically significant differences in hearing is well-known. For this reason, monosyllabic words are recommended for cochlear implant candidacy assessment and for post-operative performance evaluation (e.g. Roland, Gantz, Waltzman and Parkinson, 2016; Sladen et al., 2017) and excellent cochlear implant users are reported to achieve scores of 80% correct for monosyllabic word tests.

Limitations

There are some limitations that the reader should be aware of when applying these specific methods. The test/retest reliability of the word score on a 50-word test is relatively poor, with an estimated 95% confidence interval of ±7 words correct (±14%) at the 50% point based on the binomial theorem. Visual inspection of Figure 1 shows that the actual spread of SPT scores near the 50% point is greater than ±7 words. This extra variability is likely to come from multiple sources apart from test-retest reliability. For example, the level at which the SPT is presented is not well controlled when it is performed online with unknown computer and unknown speakers in an unknown acoustic environment. The instructions for the test are to set it to a normal conversational level, and this is best done by a person known to have good hearing. Even so, conversational levels may vary by ±5 dB depending on the voice characteristics of the speaker and the distance between the speaker and the listener (e.g. Olsen, 1998). A variation of ±5 dB in presentation level is approximately equivalent to a change of ±5 dB in PTA and would be expected to produce an additional ±5 words difference in the word scores, estimated from the slope of the curve in Figure 1 at its steepest point.

The linguistic knowledge and experience of the listener is also known to affect the SPT word score. For example, Blamey et al. (2001) shows the relationship between speech perception scores, equivalent language age and hearing loss in children. Children with language equivalent to a 7-year-old child with normal hearing should perform similarly to an adult on the SPT. For similar reasons, people for whom English is not their first language may score lower on the SPT than for people with English as their native language. Linguistic knowledge and hearing loss have different effects on speech perception and thus the expected benefits of hearing aids for people who are not fluent in English should not be estimated using the data or analyses in this chapter. A different type of analysis should be used in this case as illustrated in Blamey and Sarant (2002) for example.

The present analysis is based on a simplified attenuation model of hearing loss and does not take into account distortions in hearing mechanisms that are not perfectly correlated with the 4-frequency average hearing thresholds (PTA). The extent to which these distortions were present in the studied population is unknown, and it is likely that they contribute to the high degree of variability observed. It has been pointed out by Plomp (1978) and others that this distortion component of hearing loss accounts for the limited benefit of hearing aids to some extent.

FUTURE RESEARCH DIRECTIONS

Although the SPT has been thoroughly validated for Australian English (Blamey, Blamey and Saunders, 2015) and has been used clinically by Blamey Saunders hears as part of its Australian tele-audiology practice for many years, it can still be extended. Planned improvements include the development of versions of the SPT for languages other than English. These developments may be especially important in regions where there is no well-established audiology profession.

There is also a need to investigate the application of the information transmission techniques to accents other than Australian. For example, it is known that there are significant phonetic differences between Australian, American, British, and New Zealand accented English that may affect the information transmission analyses. However, these differences are unlikely to affect the word scores and expected benefits as a function of PTA in a very significant way.

It should be noted that the current study is based on retrospective data for 492 individuals using the ADRO® sound processing (Blamey, 2005) in Blamey Saunders hearing aids. It is possible that the benefits of other hearing aids fitted in different ways may lead to different conclusions and this should be evaluated before these results are applied to other devices

Future research should also include the development and validation of an objective evaluation that can be used to establish realistic expectations of the benefit of hearing aids in background noise for individuals. This is an important adjunct to realistic expectations of benefit in quiet because it is often the case that people become aware of their hearing difficulties in noisy and difficult conditions well before they are aware of their difficulties in quiet. It is likely that speech perception measures will provide a suitable basis for realistic expectations in noise, although this is a significantly more complex problem than establishing realistic expectations in quiet. The added complexity arises from the fact that even people who have excellent hearing have difficulty in background noise at levels that are not unusual in everyday life, and performance on speech perception tests depends on the noise level, direction, and type. It is also true that the benefit of hearing aids will depend critically on microphone characteristics such as directionality and adaptivity in noise and is unlikely to be constant across different brands and types of hearing aids. There is also evidence that hearing in noise is affected differently by hearing loss than hearing in quiet. For example Plomp (1978) postulated a “distortion” component of hearing loss that was distinct from the "attenuation" component of hearing loss and primarily affected perception of speech in noise. A promising approach to address this problem has been taken by Killion, Niquette, Gudmundsen, Revit, and Banerjee (2004) who have measured signal-to-noise-ratio (SNR) loss in normal and impaired ears.

CONCLUSION

This chapter shows that it is possible to provide realistic expectations of benefits to potential hearing aid users across a wide range of hearing loss by using a speech perception test as the measure of benefit. The speech perception test score is easily understood by laypersons and is the basis of the expected benefit calculation. It also has the advantage that the layperson can perform the test themselves and indeed measure the benefit of hearing aids for themselves with little or no assistance from professional audiologists.

It is recommended that the SPT results be used to set realistic expectations of hearing aid benefit and that the limitations are clearly stated. The recommended wording for expected benefit is that the number of errors on the SPT would be reduced by about half and the number of errors in running speech would be reduced to about a quarter of the number that occur without hearing aids.

ACKNOWLEDGMENT

Ethics approval for the research was provided by the Royal Victorian Eye and Ear Hospital Research and Ethics Committee, Project 14/1164H, "Maximising speech perception benefits in hearing aid users."

The author wishes to acknowledge the long-term contributions of others in achieving the outcomes described here, including colleagues at Blamey & Saunders Hearing Pty Ltd (Blamey Saunders hears), The University of Melbourne, the Bionics Institute, Dynamic Hearing Pty Ltd (now part of Cirrus Logic), Swinburne University of Technology, the audiologists, audiometrists, and tele-audiologists who worked with the participants in these studies, and the hearing aid users themselves.

The research was funded by Blamey & Saunders Hearing Pty Ltd with government assistance from a Commercialisation Australia grant, a Victorian Technology Voucher, and the R&D tax incentive. Blamey & Saunders Hearing Pty Ltd is a "profit for purpose" company whose purpose is to improve the hearing health of Australians using a sustainable business model. The Bionics Institute acknowledges the support it receives from the Victorian Government through its Operational Infrastructure Support Program.

REFERENCES

Access Economics. (2006). *Listen Hear! The economic impact and cost of hearing loss in Australia.* Retrieved from http://www.expression.com.au/files/editor_upload/File/Research%20Reports/listenhearreport.pdf

Assmann, P., & Summerfield, Q. (2004). The perception of speech under adverse conditions. In *Speech processing in the auditory system* (pp. 231–308). New York, NY: Springer. doi:10.1007/0-387-21575-1_5

Australian Competition and Consumer Commission. (2017). *Issues around the sale of hearing aids.* Retrieved 4 September, 2018 from https://www.accc.gov.au/publications/issues-around-the-sale-of-hearing-aids

Blamey, P., Martin, L. F., & Saunders, E. (2010). *Hearing aid benefit as a function of hearing loss.* Paper presented at the Australasian International Conference on Speech Science and Technology, Melbourne, Australia.

Blamey, P., & Sarant, J. (2002). Speech perception and language criteria for paediatric cochlear implant candidature. *Audiology & Neuro-Otology*, *7*(2), 114–121. doi:10.1159/000057659 PMID:12006739

Blamey, P., & Saunders, E. (2015). Predicting Speech Perception from the Audiogram and Vice Versa. *Canadian Audiologist, 2*(1).

Blamey, P. J. (2005). Adaptive dynamic range optimization (ADRO): A digital amplification strategy for hearing aids and cochlear implants. *Trends in Amplification*, *9*(2), 77–98. doi:10.1177/108471380500900203 PMID:16012705

Blamey, P. J., Blamey, J. K., & Saunders, E. (2015). Effectiveness of a tele-audiology approach to hearing aid fitting. *Journal of Telemedicine and Telecare*, *21*(8), 474–478. doi:10.1177/1357633X15611568 PMID:26556060

Blamey, P. J., & Sarant, J. Z. (2003). Development of spoken language by deaf children. Oxford handbook of deaf studies, language, and education, 232-246.

Blamey, P. J., Sarant, J. Z., Paatsch, L. E., Barry, J. G., Bow, C. P., Wales, R. J., ... Tooher, R. (2001). Relationships among speech perception, production, language, hearing loss, and age in children with impaired hearing. *Journal of Speech, Language, and Hearing Research: JSLHR*, *44*(2), 264–285. doi:10.1044/1092-4388(2001/022) PMID:11324650

Boothroyd, A. (1968). Statistical theory of the speech discrimination score. *The Journal of the Acoustical Society of America*, *43*(2), 362–367. doi:10.1121/1.1910787 PMID:5636798

Carhart, R. (1951). Basic principles of speech audiometry. *Acta Oto-Laryngologica, 40*(1-2), 62–71. doi:10.3109/00016485109138908 PMID:14914512

Cox, R. M., & Alexander, G. C. (2000). Expectations about hearing aids and their relationship to fitting outcome. *Journal of the American Academy of Audiology, 11*(7). PMID:10976498

Deloitte Access Economics for the Hearing Care Industry Association. (2017). *The Social and Economic Cost of Hearing Loss in Australia.* Retrieved June 4, 2018 from http://www.hcia.com.au/hcia-wp/wp-content/uploads/2015/05/Social-and-Economic-Cost-of-Hearing-Health-in-Australia_June-2017.pdf

Dillon, H. (2008). *Hearing aids*. London, UK: Hodder Arnold. doi:10.1201/b15118-293

Ferguson, M. A., Kitterick, P. T., Chong, L. Y., Edmondson-Jones, M., Barker, F., & Hoare, D. J. (2017). *Hearing aids for mild to moderate hearing loss in adults.* Retrieved 5 June, 2018 from https://www.cochrane.org/CD012023/ENT_hearing-aids-mild-moderate-hearing-loss-adults

Fletcher, H. (1929). *Speech and Hearing*. New York: Van Nostrand.

Glasberg, B. R., & Moore, B. C. (1988). Psychoacoustic abilities of subjects with unilateral and bilateral cochlear hearing impairments and their relationship to the ability to understand speech. *Scandinavian Audiology, 1989*(32), 1–25. PMID:2711118

Grenness, C., Hickson, L., Laplante-Lévesque, A., & Davidson, B. (2014). Patient-centred audiological rehabilitation: Perspectives of older adults who own hearing aids. *International Journal of Audiology, 53*(sup1), S68-S75.

Henry, B. A., McDermott, H. J., McKay, C. M., James, C. J., & Clark, G. M. (1998). A frequency importance function for a new monosyllabic word test. Australian Journal of Audiology, November, 20(2), 79-86.

Jerram, J. C., & Purdy, S. C. (2001). Technology, expectations, and adjustment to hearing loss: Predictors of hearing aid outcome. *Journal of the American Academy of Audiology, 12*(2), 64–79. PMID:11261460

Killion, M. (1985). The noise problem: There's hope. *Hearing Instruments, 36*(11), 26–32.

Killion, M. C., Niquette, P. A., Gudmundsen, G. I., Revit, L. J., & Banerjee, S. (2004). Development of a quick speech-in-noise test for measuring signal-to-noise ratio loss in normal-hearing and hearing-impaired listeners. *The Journal of the Acoustical Society of America, 116*(4), 2395–2405. doi:10.1121/1.1784440 PMID:15532670

Knudsen, L. V., Öberg, M., Nielsen, C., Naylor, G., & Kramer, S. E. (2010). Factors influencing help seeking, hearing aid uptake, hearing aid use and satisfaction with hearing aids: A review of the literature. *Trends in Amplification, 14*(3), 127–154. doi:10.1177/1084713810385712 PMID:21109549

Kochkin, S. (2000). MarkeTrak V: "Why my hearing aids are in the drawer" The consumers' perspective. *The Hearing Journal, 53*(2), 34–36. doi:10.1097/00025572-200002000-00004

Kochkin, S., Beck, D. L., Christensen, L. A., Compton-Conley, C., Fligor, B. J., Kricos, P. B., & Turner, R. G. (2010). MarkeTrak VIII: The impact of the hearing healthcare professional on hearing aid user success. *Hearing Review, 17*(4), 12–34.

McCormack, A., & Fortnum, H. (2013). Why do people fitted with hearing aids not wear them? *International Journal of Audiology, 52*(5), 360–368. doi:10.3109/14992027.2013.769066 PMID:23473329

Meister, H., Walger, M., Brehmer, D., von Wedel, U. C., & von Wedel, H. (2008). The relationship between pre-fitting expectations and willingness to use hearing aids. *International Journal of Audiology, 47*(4), 153–159. doi:10.1080/14992020701843111 PMID:18389410

Miller, G. A., & Nicely, P. E. (1955). An analysis of perceptual confusions among some English consonants. *The Journal of the Acoustical Society of America, 27*(2), 338–352. doi:10.1121/1.1907526

Moore, B. C. (2006). Speech mapping is a valuable tool for fitting and counseling patients. *The Hearing Journal, 59*(8), 26–28. doi:10.1097/01.HJ.0000286371.07550.5b

Olsen, W. O. (1998). Average speech levels and spectra in various speaking/listening conditions: A summary of the Pearson, Bennett, & Fidell (1977) report. *American Journal of Audiology, 7*(2), 21–25. doi:10.1044/1059-0889(1998/012) PMID:26649514

Peterson, G. E., & Lehiste, I. (1962). Revised CNC lists for auditory tests. *The Journal of Speech and Hearing Disorders, 27*(1), 62–70. doi:10.1044/jshd.2701.62 PMID:14485785

Plomp, R. (1978). Auditory handicap of hearing impairment and the limited benefit of hearing aids. *The Journal of the Acoustical Society of America*, *63*(2), 533–549. doi:10.1121/1.381753 PMID:670550

Roland, J. T. Jr, Gantz, B. J., Waltzman, S. B., & Parkinson, A. J. (2016). United States multicenter clinical trial of the cochlear nucleus hybrid implant system. *The Laryngoscope*, *126*(1), 175–181. doi:10.1002/lary.25451 PMID:26152811

Saunders, G. H., Lewis, M. S., & Forsline, A. (2009). Expectations, prefitting counseling, and hearing aid outcome. *Journal of the American Academy of Audiology*, *20*(5), 320–334. doi:10.3766/jaaa.20.5.6 PMID:19585963

Sladen, D. P., Gifford, R. H., Haynes, D., Kelsall, D., Benson, A., Lewis, K., ... Westerberg, B. (2017). Evaluation of a revised indication for determining adult cochlear implant candidacy. *The Laryngoscope*, *127*(10), 2368–2374. doi:10.1002/lary.26513 PMID:28233910

Wallhagen, M. I. (2009). The stigma of hearing loss. *The Gerontologist*, *50*(1), 66–75. doi:10.1093/geront/gnp107 PMID:19592638

ADDITIONAL READING

Chisolm, T. H., Johnson, C. E., Danhauer, J. L., Portz, L. J., Abrams, H. B., Lesner, S., ... Newman, C. W. (2007). A systematic review of health-related quality of life and hearing aids: Final report of the American Academy of Audiology Task Force on the Health-Related Quality of Life Benefits of Amplification in Adults. *Journal of the American Academy of Audiology*, *18*(2), 151–183. doi:10.3766/jaaa.18.2.7 PMID:17402301

KEY TERMS AND DEFINITIONS

4-Frequency PTA: The abbreviation for 4-frequency Pure-Tone-Average Threshold, the average hearing thresholds for frequencies of 500, 1000, 2000, and 4000 Hz.

Benefit: The difference in performance when wearing hearing aid(s) compared to performance on the same task under the same conditions when not wearing a hearing aid(s).

dB HL: The abbreviation for "decibels hearing level" relative to the quietest sounds that a young healthy individual ought to be able to hear.

Hearing Aid: A device designed to improve hearing by making sound audible to a person with hearing loss.

Running Speech: The continuous sound of spoken dialogue from which the listener is able to distinguish individual words and sentences.

Signal-to-Noise Ratio (SNR): A measure that compares the level of a desired signal to the level of background noise. SNR is defined as the ratio of signal power to the noise power, often expressed in decibels.

Speech Perception: The process by which the sounds of language are heard, interpreted and understood.

Tele-Audiology: The delivery of hearing health services and products outside of conventional audiology clinic settings, via the internet for example.

Chapter 5
Empowering Cochlear Implant Users in Their Home Environment by eHealth Solutions

Filiep Vanpoucke
Cochlear Technology Centre, Belgium

Birgit Philips
Cochlear Technology Centre, Belgium

Cas Smits
VU University Medical Center, The Netherlands

Paul J. Govaerts
The Eargroup, Belgium

Inge Doorn
Houten, The Netherlands

Thomas Stainsby
Cochlear Technology Centre, Belgium

ABSTRACT

In the chapter, the authors address the prescient need to update accepted care models of cochlear implant (CI) fitting and long-term maintenance to better utilize self-care and tele-medicine possibilities, thus shifting the focus of CI maintenance to the recipient. There is a strong evidence base that such a move will better meet the needs of CI users, giving them greater control of and involvement in their hearing progress. Simultaneously, such an approach can better meet present shortcomings in the market acceptance and delivery of the benefit of cochlear implants, particularly in the elderly segment of the population, where device penetration of the market remains low (c. 7%). Such initiatives make it viable to reach many more users, as the present models are prohibitively expensive for such expansion. A case study of pilot software for CI maintenance based on tele-audiology is described with the inclusion of data collected from initial studies.

DOI: 10.4018/978-1-5225-8191-8.ch005

INTRODUCTION

Cochlear implants (CI) are improving hearing for people with a severe-to-profound bilateral hearing loss, with the personal health and community health-economic benefits being universally accepted after more than three decades of evidence (Vaerenberg et al., 2014). However, with the maturing of the technology beyond a niche specialist discipline to an accepted widespread intervention, it is evident that the delivery and care methods need to evolve to suit this much wider uptake. The case for a wider uptake will only be expanded following the recent adoption by the World Health Authority, in May 2017, of a resolution on the worldwide need to address hearing loss (World Health Organisation (WHO), 2017b). The traditional model of intensive management in specialist (mainly university-based) centres can no longer meet the needs and desires of this wider recipient base, nor is it viable economically for health services to support traditional care structures for so many more users. In addition, society's demographics, expectations and competencies are changing rapidly. The average age of the population is increasing (and the prevalence of hearing loss is correlated with age), while simultaneously people are expecting greater empowerment and involvement in their healthcare decisions. Concurrently, the population as a whole is rapidly getting more literate in the use of ICT (Information and Communication Technology): this is no longer a specialist domain. Considering this combination of societal trends, it is apparent that the widespread increase in technological literacy, coupled with increased personal empowerment for own-healthcare provision, can be harnessed to meet the impending bottleneck in support for the delivery of CI performance monitoring and maintenance.

Since CI involves lifelong management of the technology, and has a large impact on CI users' lives, it is essential that CI users become involved in their treatment and have proper self-care practices. In health-care outcomes, human behaviour is the largest source of variance (Schroeder, 2007). Literature from chronic health domains suggests that an individual's motivation plays a significant role in treatment adherence (Vermeire, Hearnshaw, van Royen, and Denekens, 2001). The self-determination theory health belief framework (Ryan, Patrick, Deci, and Williams, 2008), which is central to the design of proposed model of CI care presented here, is elaborated further later.

In the following chapter, the authors will present a background and outline of the issues with current CI patient care models, consider some theoretical objectives for how this care can evolve along with societal and technological trends, and then present a case study of an implementation of pilot Remote-care and Self-Care CI maintenance software. Results from initial field trials of this software will also be presented.

BACKGROUND

In May 2016, the World Health Organisation,(WHO), unanimously passed Resolution EB139.R1, "Development of a new Health Assembly Resolution and Action Plan for Prevention of Deafness and Hearing Loss" (WHO, 2016). This firmly establishes the need for all healthcare systems to prioritise the prevention, intervention, and treatment of hearing loss. The WHO estimates that over 360 million people – 5% of the world's population – live with disabling hearing loss, 32 million of whom are children. Thus there is a very large need to better address hearing loss for adults, particularly with the population ageing as it is. With prevalence rates rising, the global cost of unaddressed hearing loss has recently been estimated at $750 billion per year (WHO, 2018). Cochlear Implants are a very cost-effective intervention, because they enable people to participate in society and contribute in far more normal ways. This is true if the intervention is during infancy (Barton, Fortnum, Stacey, and Summerfield, 2006), in which case recipients can enjoy a standard education and normal language development, and hence have normal employment prospects, or if the intervention is later in life, because recipients can maintain normal societal participation and employment for longer (National Institute for Health and Care Excellence, 2009; Ear Foundation, 2014). At present, it is estimated that hearing-aid production meets only 10% of the global need for treating hearing loss (WHO, 2013). The benefits of cochlear implantation for adults make it an effective intervention for a much wider group of candidates than had previously been thought, as there are many people for whom hearing aids cannot deliver the benefit required, regardless of a hearing-aid's power (Govaerts, 2016). Note that in the crossover between hearing loss that is treatable by hearing aids alone and that which is treatable by cochlear implants alone, there is a vastly underdeveloped area for combined electrical and acoustic stimulation (EAS), that is, treatment with both hearing-aid and cochlear-implant technology simultaneously (Roland, Gantz, Waltzman, and Parkinson, 2016). Thus, cochlear implants (CI's) will come much more to the fore as a global treatment for hearing loss, and the care and delivery infrastructure surrounding these devices will need to adapt to meet this increased and changing demand.

The established clinical pathway to support CI implantation and habilitation is intense, especially in the first year after implantation. It consists of a number of visits to an implantation centre (Vaerenberg et al., 2014) to decide on candidacy, a surgery to place the implant, and a number of visits in the initial year. In the first session (typically 2-4 weeks after implantation) the sound processor is provided, a first fitting is performed, and the user is counselled on the use of the device. In order to achieve optimal hearing outcomes, the fitting parameters are further fine-tuned in subsequent sessions (typically 6-8) in the first year. In these sessions hearing performance is assessed and additional counselling on device use and communication strategies is provided. In addition, the user typically follows a hearing habilitation programme with a speech and language therapist (depending on the health system of the country). After the first year an annual visit is organized in most countries to follow up on hearing performance and device use. Technical troubleshooting may be required from time to time as well.

In a classic clinical pathway, all aspects of the care are organized in the implantation clinic, typically a university setting, where expert staff are available to provide high quality care. However, this is not a sustainable model. Expert staff are scarce and the cost structure of an expert centre is high. Even without the financial constraints clinics routinely face, there are simply not enough professionals in the training pipeline to meet predicted future demand. For a clinic, over the years, annual check-up visits lead to an ever increasing work load as more implantations occur each year, limiting the time available to care for new CI users. Aftercare for counselling and recipient training is also not well funded in many healthcare systems, so this aspect of habilitation may be under-addressed in a trade-off for greater throughput of new recipients. These issues may contribute to the low penetration of cochlear implants (estimated at 5-7%, e.g. (De Raeve, 2016)).

For the users, the classical pathway care model provides excellent value since they have access to experts. However it may be very inconvenient because of long travel, an obligation to take time off due to the travel, and may be further exacerbated by mobility limitations experienced by some users, e.g. senior users or those with disabilities. Alternative care provision models, where some of the care is moved out of the expert clinic, e.g. to a local clinic or audiological centre, or by connecting remotely to the home of the user, are attractive. This is the direction of development in Health Care Provision outlined by the Eucomed "Contract for a Healthy Future", which envisages the greater role of tele-medicine in the economics of health care for Europe (Pfleger, 2012). Such alternative care provision models have the potential to increase the independence of the end user, with equal or better quality of care, while reducing health-care cost. The authors have characterized some of the models of care into four levels (where Expert Care is the present standard and the others can be considered potential alternatives), shown in Figure 1, which are now described in turn:

1. **Expert Care:** Where the care is delivered in a centre that is specialised in CI support. Such a centre is usually associated with the implanting clinic and/or a University or teaching hospital. This level of care offers direct contact with the implanting team, but requires that service be provided by highly trained and specialised clinicians. It may also require extensive travel by the recipient for every appointment. The extent of the issue of travel depends heavily on the

geography and market structure in each country, and thus some health-care systems will find this level of care harder to support than others.

2. **Local Care:** Where care is dispensed more locally by trained hearing professionals, but these need not be directly connected with the implanting team as such. While the level of training is still specialized for CI (with the exception of that required for some simple tasks, such as the changing of broken cables, etc.) this care can be offered independently of the original surgical centre, so it is more likely that there will be more professionals available closer to the recipient. This level of care still offers excellent support for the CI recipient, but by being more local to the patient, can be more convenient by virtue of the improved accessibility and the decreased need for travel. The health economic benefits are limited however, as specialised CI staff still need to be available, except for the simpler tasks mentioned above. Of course, there will remain some more complicated cases where the surgical team will still be needed to resolve an issue, in which case a referral back to the implanting centre would be necessary.
3. **Remote Care:** Where care is dispensed outside of a specialist CI centre. This could take several forms, but in each incarnation the commonality is that information and guidance are driven remotely from a specialised CI centre, and then implemented by individuals who are more local. In one form of Remote Care, the support may be offered by a more general hearing professional, such as an audiologist or speech therapist (or GP's and nurses with appropriate training in hearing care) in a local clinic, with reference to and guidance from a CI expert. This model has the advantage that the number of hearing professionals with this more-general level of training is greater, and thus it already goes some way to alleviating a potential bottleneck in CI care provision, by obviating the need for personal contact with a CI specialist. This type of care provision has been termed the "hub and spoke" model. Another form of care at this level is Home Care by the recipients themselves via the internet, but still, crucially, under the guidance of a hearing professional. Given the care is physically located in the home, the professional could have a varying degree of specialisation (a less-specialised practitioner would still refer to a CI specialist for guidance, still saving direct recipient interaction). Whether it be remote contact with a CI specialist or other hearing professional, the big saving to the recipient is the removal of the need to travel. From the health economics perspective, the big saving is in the reduction of physical infrastructure required, though it does not remove the need for the presence of a professionally trained individual, and thus it does not fully resolve potential bottlenecks in the provision of care.

4. **Self Care:** Where the CI recipients interact directly with software themselves, without the need for direct personal contact with a hearing professional. Important advantages are the convenience of not having to travel, and the ability to use the software at any time of the day that suits the recipient's routine. This model offers both the greatest increase in convenience to the users, while simultaneously offering the greatest savings in terms of health economics. The greatest challenge of this type of care, however, is in the sophistication of the software that has to be developed to ensure that recipient performance is not compromised. The present standard model of care from a specialist clinic offers the established benchmark of recipient benefit, and to decrease this would be unethical, whatever the collateral advantages. The way forward for this level of care is sophisticated and well-controlled software at the user end, combined with a well-developed 'Cloud' back-end, wherein all the data are collected and accessible to CI specialists and the implanting centre when necessary. 'Smart' data analysis can also monitor performance through knowledge of individual data that is interpreted in the context of the sum of collective expertise. This would represent the use of an 'Intelligent' Expert System and so-called 'Big Data'. Note that there is even potential at this point for outcomes to be improved above the benchmark, as an Intelligent System with access to collective knowledge may offer guidance beyond that which might be intuitive to any individual, regardless of their level of specialisation. Recipients could also participate in open-ended training and automated counselling, limited only by their personal time commitment. This is a luxury not possible with care by appointment at a specialist centre. Another crucial aspect of this level of care is that the feedback loop to the recipient be closed, to ensure that they receive the best guidance possible based on data they input themselves. This would satisfy the requirement that the level of care is not diminished from that deliverable by personal expert care, within a pre-defined 'non inferiority' margin (Walker and Nowacki, 2011). It seems intuitive that some compromise would result in a trade of convenience and cost savings for the intensity of specialist care, but by establishing non-inferiority, one could be confident that care is not being traded detrimentally for other benefits.

Such innovative distributed care models require a common platform for all actors to have access to the latest data. Technological advances, such as low power wireless links, have the potential to enable access to data, and data sharing over the internet, although they are not able to do so on their own within the present technological framework. With the development of the appropriate automated tools and cloud data-sharing support, advances that are available at the point of the user could enable a rapid expansion of the level of care that is possible remotely.

Figure 1. Different care delivery models

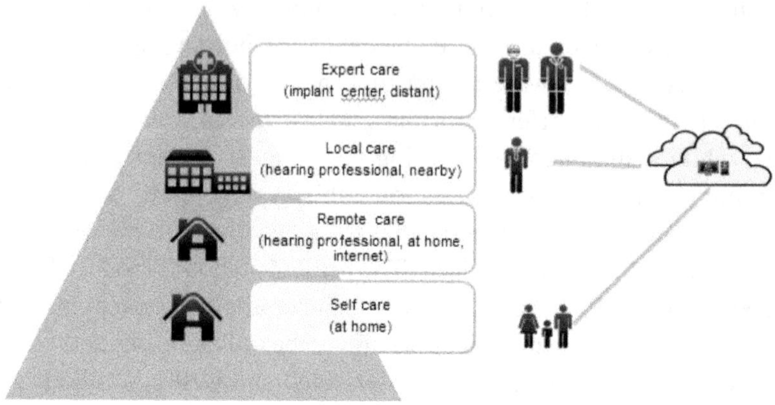

MAIN FOCUS OF THE CHAPTER

An analysis of the present standard model of CI provision and maintenance (i.e., that which is at the "Expert Care" level defined above) reveals a number of fundamental shortcomings:

1. There is a large unmet need for hearing implants. Only 5-7% of candidates that could benefit from a hearing implant have access to one (Athalye, Archbold, Mulla, Lutman, and Nikolopoulous, 2015; De Raeve, 2016). This is most apparent in the elderly portion of society. While major progress has already been achieved in delivering the benefit of CI usage to the paediatric population, largely due to universal hearing screening and standardized care for infants (at least in the most developed countries), similar success has not yet been realised for older citizens, for whom knowledge of, and involvement in, options for dealing with hearing loss are far more varied.
2. The need is growing, as hearing loss is linked to ageing. Demographics are such that there is a wave of elderly people coming in the next decades (WHO, 2004). Also, as CI results continue to improve, candidacy criteria are likely to continue to be loosened. The combination of an increased pool of older citizens needing intervention for hearing loss, wider candidacy criteria, and an increase in the awareness of the option for CI's as an appropriate treatment for those in this age group, will compound this shortcoming.
3. The current care model is not sustainable. Hearing care is a lifelong commitment with the users of an implant. For example, they typically come to the clinic on an annual basis for a check-up visit. Most national health care legislations make such a visit a mandatory step to ensure quality of care. This ever expanding

aftercare is not well funded, and creates capacity issues hampering the provision of care to new users. Under the current health economic models, there is inadequate funding to keep providing the after-care in the expert centre, the implantation clinic. Even maintaining the present rate of uptake (c. 7%) with a growing patient base over time is unsustainable, let alone the demands that would come if uptake rises significantly as a proportion of the population.

4. A shortage of staff is emerging. There are not enough audiologists with sufficient knowledge of hearing implants to provide the care required. For example, in 2016 there were an estimated 2,000 audiologists trained in CI fitting in the USA, whereas it is estimated that around 1,000,000 American hearing-aid users could benefit from having a CI (US Bureau of Labor Statistics, 2017). This shortfall can be somewhat met by making devices that offer more intrinsic support. The device manufacturers can significantly improve this by providing increased cloud/internet service support. These types of solutions come under the "Remote Care" and "Self Care" levels defined above.
5. Many patients demand to be more empowered, expressing a sincere desire to be less dependent on their clinicians (Athalye et al., 2015). This is reflective of a general trend across many areas of healthcare, as information becomes much more freely accessible through online resources (e.g., Medtronic, another manufacturer of medical devices – www.medtronic.com). This desire can be met at the fourth level of care described above: "Self Care".

These issues can be interpreted and analysed in the light of the different models of care explored in the "Background" section above, and are taken up and investigated further during the project reported on later in this chapter.

In 2014 the authors were granted a project, called Supporting Hearing in Elderly Citizens (SHiEC, www.shiec.eu), funded by the Active Ambient Living program (http://www.aal-europe.eu/) of the European Union, to develop an ICT solution to support new users of a hearing implant, mainly during the first year of living with an implant. This project thus explores solutions to the 3rd and 4th levels of care expounded above, namely "Remote Care", and "Self Care". The project consortium consisted of a mix of companies (Cochlear and Otoconsult), clinical centres (VU University Medical Center, Amsterdam, and Eargroup, Antwerp) and the Dutch society of users of a cochlear implant (Onafhankelijk Platform Cochleaire Implantatie - OPCI). The "Issues, Controversies, and Problems" section of this chapter will explore the knowledge gathering and problem definitions that resulted from research within this project, while the "Solutions and Recommendations" section will describe the pilot Tele-Audiometry software solution that was produced as a result, and present the results of initial studies related to this work. The final sections of the chapter will consider where this leads for future technology development in this field.

Issues, Controversies, and Problems

Given that the SHiEC project examines a recipient-driven software tool, the first question that needed to be addressed was the establishment of the technological abilities of the target CI recipient base; namely, older users. To this end, an initial study was run by the Dutch CI Users' group, OPCI. A summary of the results is presented below, and elaborated later in the section describing 'Study 2'.

From workshops that were conducted with patient groups, within the SHiEC project, but also outside of the project, the patient's perspective was constructed. It was found that patients want to hear the best they can, while spending the least amount of time and effort in rehabilitation activities. During the first few months, they are happy to invest in their hearing. After this period, essentially most people want to get on with their life, and be distracted as little as possible because of their hearing loss.

Through user groups, several key needs were identified early on in the project, as summarized diagrammatically in above:

- Need for information and counselling about device use
- Insight into personal device use
- Assurance that the device is functioning properly
- Access to hearing exercises, and
- Performance assessment in the home environment.

The needs identified above will ultimately lead to a radical change of the model in which care is delivered. The fundamental trend in medicine is to put the patient in the centre with all actors in the care model, from the early phase to the chronic lifelong phase, delivering their health care services to the patient.

Later, Figure 2 considers how the identified needs are addressed in traditional care models, and how the My Hearing Application (MHA), which was developed in SHiEC project, offers an alternative approach. The design of the MHA followed the principles of the self-determination theory health belief framework (Ryan et al., 2008). This theory postulates that in order to empower end-users and increase their self-efficacy, it is crucial to build up the users' competence in hearing with, and living with, an implant (e.g. taking care of their device(s)), to increase their autonomy such that they can make their own choices, and to provide them with meaningful relations, such as fluent access to peers and care providers.

The SHiEC project envisioned a solution that consists of a software environment which aimed to deliver continued Self Care for Cochlear-Implant (CI) Recipients through an interaction of three components: 1) Cloud infrastructure to communicate between the Recipient, Clinician and central Company support; 2) A Tablet-based

App ("MyHearing App") for the Recipient to use at home; and 3) A Clinician PC-based Application allowing the tracking of the Recipient's progress in greater detail than is available to the Recipient in the MyHearing App (MHA).

To enable such a model, a crucial enabler is a platform in which the different parties, including first and foremost the patient, can exchange information. This idea has been central to the development of the My Hearing App. All data is securely stored in the Cloud, and the information is available, e.g. to the audiologist in the clinic, who can remotely track the evolution of the user's hearing performance. But the information can also be of use in a conversation with the speech and language therapist, or to discuss with the people in the support network surrounding the patient.

SOLUTIONS AND RECOMMENDATIONS

The preceding sections outlined the identified user needs and fundamental approach taken in the SHiEC project. This section will break down that solution by describing the different software components in detail, and present evidence gained from pilot trials of this technology. Four studies will be reported on: 1) An initial questionnaire regarding ICT use in the target elderly population conducted by OPCI; 2) A usability study of the MyCochlear recipient support portal from Cochlear; 3) A study in experienced CI recipients using the software (Validation, and Testing in the Home) and a study in new users, conducted by the VU University Medical Center in Amsterdam; and 4) A study of software usability in experienced users, conducted by OPCI. The lessons thus learned enable the authors to outline proposed avenues for further development at the end of the chapter.

As already described, five main areas of recipient requirements were identified through consultation with the OPCI CI user group. The five requirements are listed in Figure 2, along with a description of how each need is already met by the traditional care path, and how the new SHiEC pilot described in this chapter would alternatively address the same needs. It is evident that the new model of care better answers the contemporary need for patient-centric care, while simultaneously offering a way to address the impending bottleneck in the amount of support that can be provided by the conventional CI treatment model.

The architecture of the MyHearing App (MHA) was specifically designed to meet each of the identified patient requirements in turn. While the supporting Clinician Application could be more versatile in the ways in which patients' data were processed, it was felt that the user interface for the MHA should directly follow the user requirements in order to gain maximum acceptance and provide optimum support.

Figure 2. Comparison of the conventional and SHiEC (My Hearing App) Hearing Care Journey for CI

User needs	Conventional Hearing Care Journey	SHiEC Hearing Care Journey
Hearing Behavior	-Sound Processor keeps track of hearing behavior, environment and device use -Only accessible by the clinician during a clinic visit	-Richer and faster data logging -Accessible by the user at home -Accessible by the speech therapist and audiologist
Device Functioning	-Some device status information available on a remote assistant: Rather complex to access and to understand	-MyHearing App Dashboard will show information on Program Use and Events since the last fitting: easy accessible and straightforward to understand
Counseling Information	-Counseling provided by clinicians (audiologists, speech and language pathologists) -Self-help limited to paper manuals -Access to clinic limited to clinic working hours	-Provide self-help tools empowering the user by means of a personalized Recipinet Portal, tailored to the needs of the CI recipient -Accessible 24/7
Speech Performance Tracking	-Testing requires expensive specialized equipment: Sound booths, audiometers -Only available in clinic -Due to clinic time constraints not all relevant speech tests can be performed during one visit	-CI user can also track his performance at home or in the waiting room -Tests that should be performed are listed by the clinician
Hearing Rehabilitation	-CI user follows sessions with the Speech and Language Pathologist: limited number of sessions at the clinic	-Computer-Based Auditory Training: CI user can perform hearing rehab at home

Each of these five modules is now described in detail.

1. Hearing Behaviour

The datalogging features of the sound processor in the Nucleus system are ideally suited to presenting the implant user with an automated analysis of their device usage, and hence their hearing behaviour. This information could be conveniently relayed in a dedicated panel of the App's main page, entitled "Datalogging". With this feedback, the recipient can adjust their usage according to their own targets. For example, one can set a goal of progressively increasing participation in speech, perhaps listening to more music, and seeing how attainment of these goals evolves over time. This information is automatically logged by tracking the performance of

Figure 3. The Master Page of the My Hearing Application (MHA)

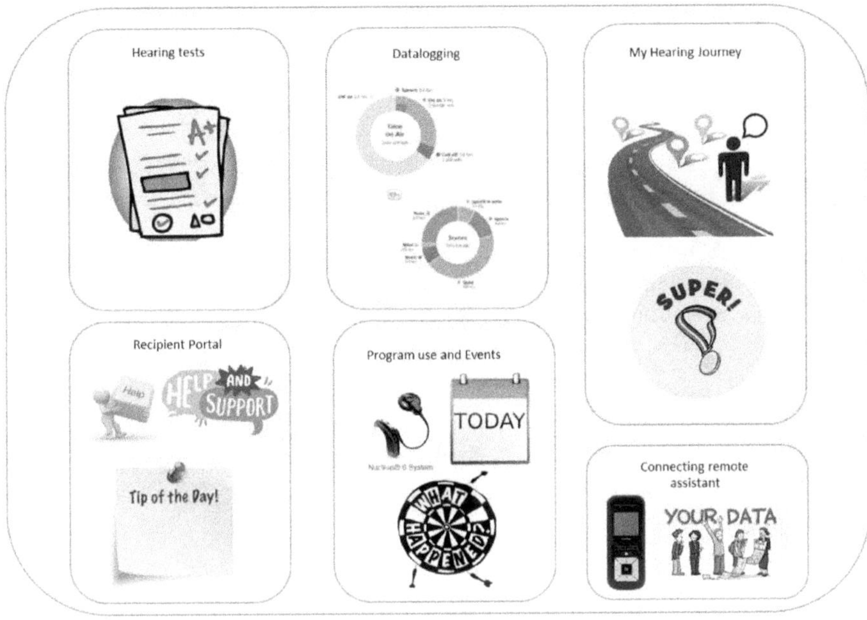

the SCAN (specific to the Nucleus CI System) automated scene classifying algorithm, and can be easily downloaded for display in the MHA. Such a use case fits the type of empowerment that patients already experience in other health domains (e.g. Medtronic). Figure 4 displays the view offered to the user for this feature.

2. Device Functioning

A key concern of both clinicians and recipients is making sure that the CI is functioning optimally for as much time as possible. Time lost due to undetected device deficiencies can be quite detrimental to a patient's habilitation, particularly if it goes undetected for a long time. The processor (Nucleus 6 in this study) already contains data-logging and self-diagnostic capabilities. By providing timely feedback of this information to the user, and also centrally to the clinic and manufacturer via the Cloud infrastructure of the application, any shortcomings can be rectified as quickly as possible. In the past, problems may have gone undetected until the next scheduled clinic visit (e.g. the need to change a microphone cover, or incorrect device configuration), but by using the tele-audiology paradigm, such problems can be automatically flagged, and an additional clinic visit can be scheduled to remedy the problem. The view offered to the user for this functionality is shown in Figure 5.

Figure 4. The Datalogging view of the MHA. This functionality addresses the concern of users to track their hearing behaviour, identified as User Need 1

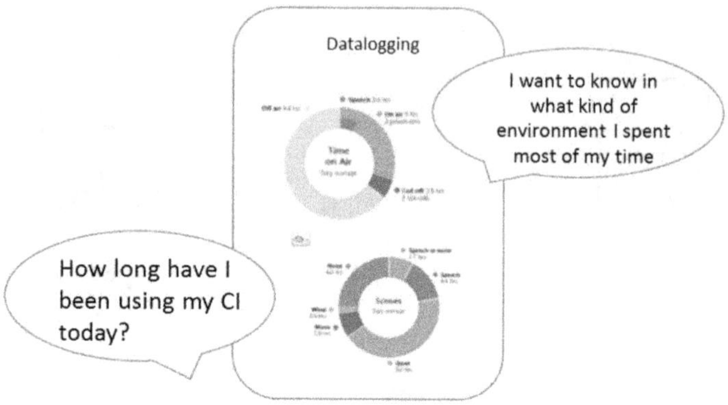

Figure 5. The view of the MHA that addresses User Need 2: Knowledge of correct device functioning

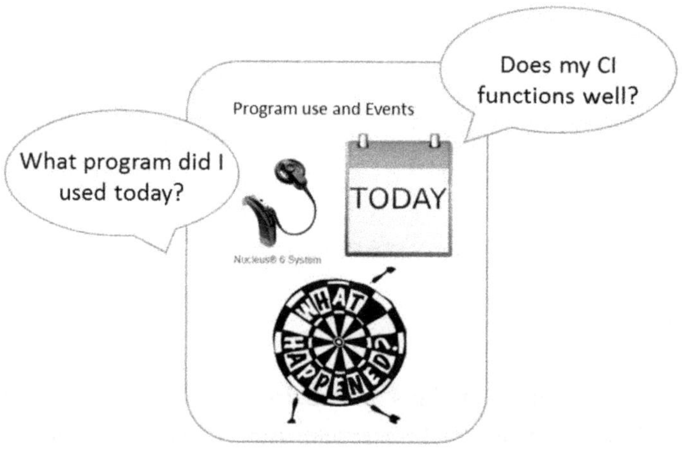

3. Counselling Information

The counselling module offers the opportunity for guidance materials to be incorporated into the App in a progressive way, where they can be accessed on demand, 24 hours a day, at a pace set by the user's personal requirements. Such material can also be structured in a progressive manner, obviating the need for much work that may have previously occupied a sequenced schedule of clinic visits, which required one-on-one contact with the specialist clinician. The relevant view is shown in Figure 6.

Figure 6. The view of the MHA that offers counselling and guidance materials with access to the MyCochlear web Portal

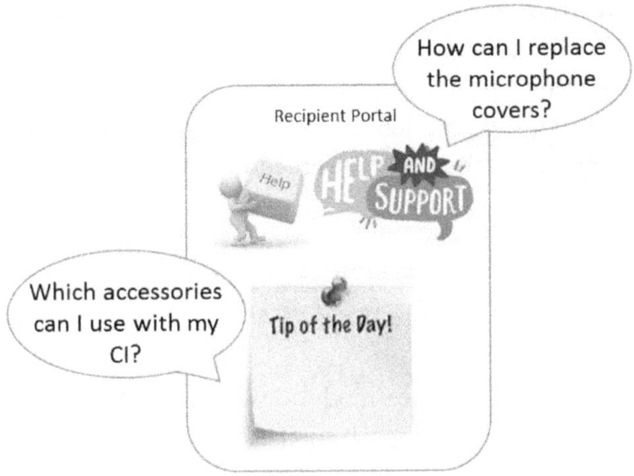

4. Speech Performance Tracking

The possibility for in-built speech testing is particularly exciting. Similar to the move away from clinician-focussed counselling, the ability to self-administer speech testing can potentially free up a lot of clinical resources. It can also automatically flag when additional intervention is required. In the MHA, Speech-in-Noise testing is implemented using the digit-in-noise test (a digit-triplet test), and Speech-In-Quiet testing is implemented using a CVC (consonant-vowel-consonant) word test. The summary of these test results is shown in Figure 7.

Figure 7. The view showing a summary of the recipient's progress on the various speech tests available via the MHA

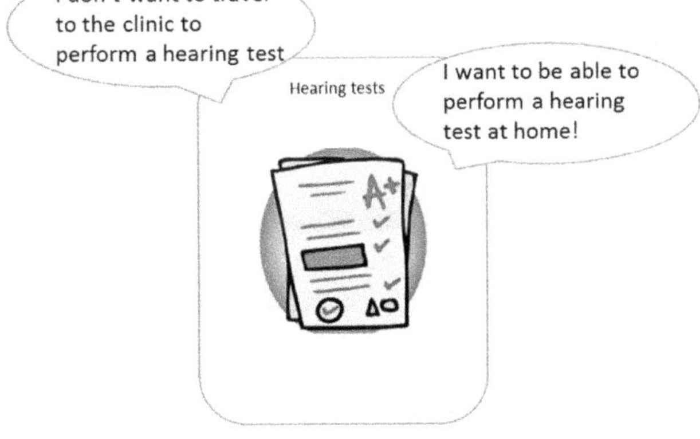

5. Hearing Rehabilitation

In keeping with the Application's established philosophy of motivating the recipient through personal empowerment and ownership of their own care, a view is provided representing the recipient's progress "My Hearing Journey". During the habilitation process, the recipient collects 'badges' to represent Milestones in performance as they are reached. This scorecard is represented in Figure 8.

ARCHITECTURE OF THE WHOLE MYHEARING APPLICATION SYSTEM

As introduced above, the Self-Care model described in this chapter is embodied in a collection of Cloud-based support, a CI Recipient App based on a Windows Tablet (MHA), and an Application for use by the Clinician on a PC. The relationship between these three components is shown in Figure 9.

Figure 8. The My Hearing Journey View displays a record of the recipient's habilitation progress, shown as a scorecard such as the one above

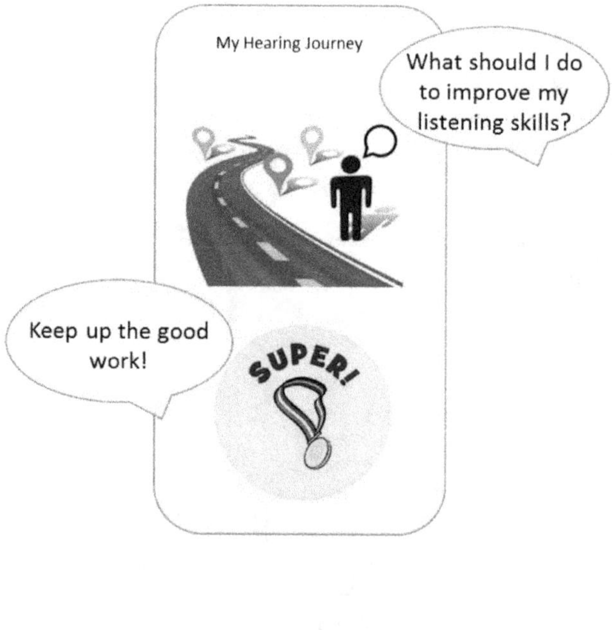
My Hearing Journey
What should I do to improve my listening skills?
Keep up the good work!
SUPER!

Figure 9. The MyHearing App environment, showing the connection of the different software components. The MHA recipient App just described is only one of the three main components of the system.

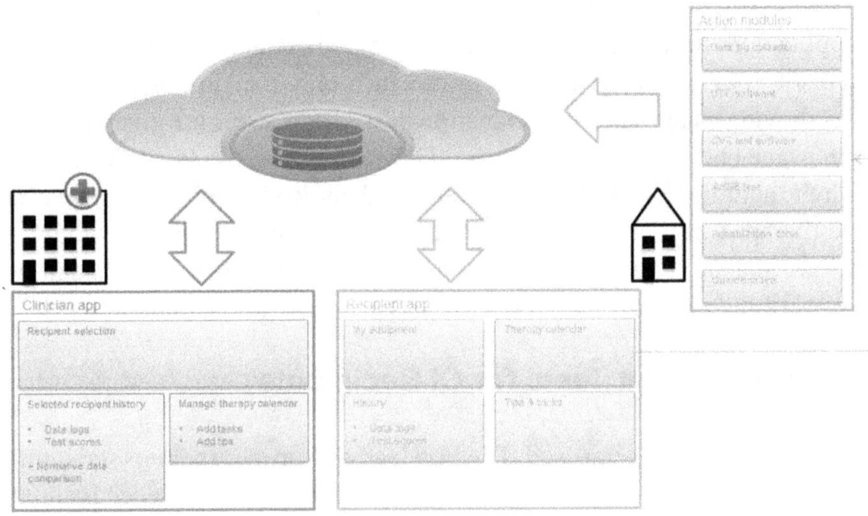

THE NEED FOR INFORMATION AND COUNSELLING ABOUT DEVICE USE

To address the need for information, an information portal was developed with personalized counselling material. CI recipients can find specific information about their CI system via the personalized Recipient Portal, named the MyCochlear Portal. In a first evaluation with 28 users (described below), senior CI users gave a high rating on its usability, (the System Usability Score (Brooke, 1996, as cited in Jordan, Thomas, Weerdmeester, and McClelland, 1996) average score = 73% (SD 7.53 and range 58-85)) and considered such a portal as a reliable source of information to the extent that they would first look up the answer to a question in the portal instead of contacting their audiologist. This study is described in detail below in the section "Study 2", so nominated because it was the second study of the SHiEC project.

The MyCochlear Portal offers a variety of support for the user, such as the pages providing guidance on device usage and maintenance.

CI RECIPIENT INSIGHT IN PERSONAL DEVICE USE

To increase insight in how users were using their own devices, the data logging feature available in the Nucleus 6 sound processor generation was incorporated in the MHA application. In the standard clinical setting, the feature of how long a user is wearing his/her device and in which environment, is only available in the audiological clinic. By moving usage pattern information into an app, users are given insight into their own usage patterns on a daily basis. They can then share this information not only with the audiologist, but other interested stakeholders, such as their speech and language therapist or their significant others. This increases their autonomy, their competence, and strengthens their relations with hearing professionals and peers. A summary of the more detailed usage logs is available to the clinician.

Hearing Assessment Tests for CI Recipients

At present, four tests have been used. The MyHearingApp incorporates standard tests for listening in quiet and in noise, and the A§E (Auditory Sound Speech Evaluation) test battery (Govaerts et al., 2006) is used for testing Phoneme Discrimination and Loudness Scaling. The assessment of hearing performance is a key element of the clinical pathway. To enable reliable testing in the home environment, we opted for the digit-in-noise test (DIN) (Smits, Goverts, and Festen, 2013). The DIN test is a feasible, reliable and valid test for the assessment of speech recognition in noise in listeners with cochlear implants. (Kaandorp, Smits, Merkus, Goverts, and Festen, 2015). This DIN speech-in-noise test was developed as a diagnostic test (Smits, Goverts, and Festen, 2013), while an earlier digit-triplet test was developed for screening of hearing loss in the general population (Smits, Kapteyn, and Houtgast, 2004). The test is an adaptive speech in noise test using triplets of digits as the speech material. The noise is adaptively adjusted until the 50% recognition point (at triplet level) is reliably determined. The user interface for this test is shown below in Figure 10. Due to its small and well known vocabulary and the ease of its user interface, this test is highly suitable for a home test. To solve the problem of calibration and background noise in the home environment, the audio signal was injected into the sound processor through the aux input port of the Nucleus 6 sound processor. Substantial attention was given to careful calibration (de Graaff et al., 2016).

In addition to the DIN test described above, speech perception in quiet was also assessed with the standard Dutch test with CVC words. The user interface for this test is shown below in Figure 11. Initial studies (de Graaff et al., 2016), comparing

Figure 10. DIN test user interface

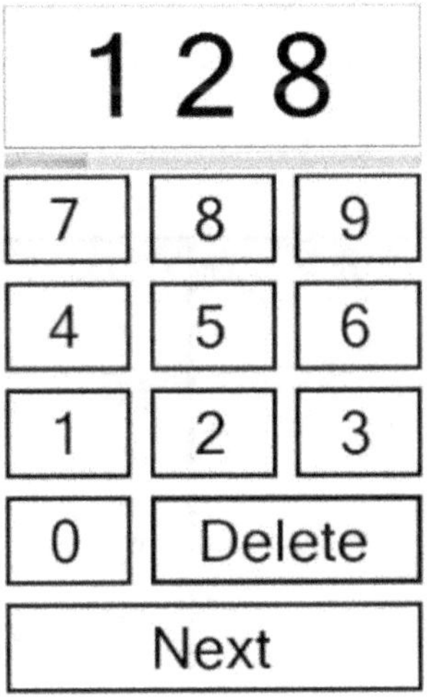

Figure 11. CVC Test User Interface

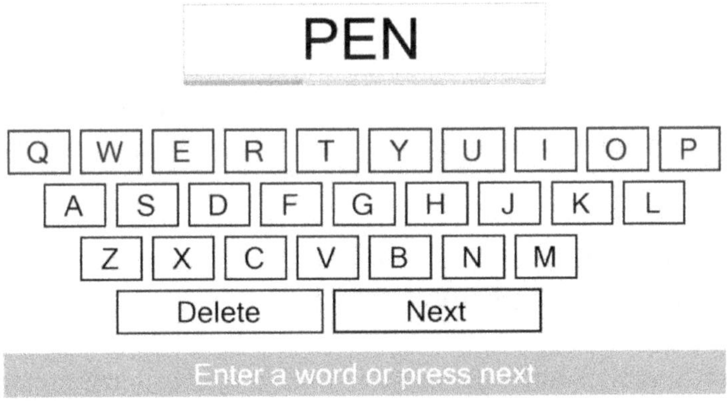

performance in the clinic using the standard audiological equipment, proved equivalence between home testing and clinic testing, both for speech in noise and speech in quiet CVC tests. A richer set of speech evaluations, based on the A§E test suite (Govaerts et al., 2006), is under development.

User speech tests are performed in quiet for the CVC material, and in noise for the DIN material. An example of the user feedback provided for these tests is shown below in Figure 12. With this style of feedback, users can track variation in their

Figure 12. Example of speech testing results displayed to the user, for both speech in quiet and speech in noise

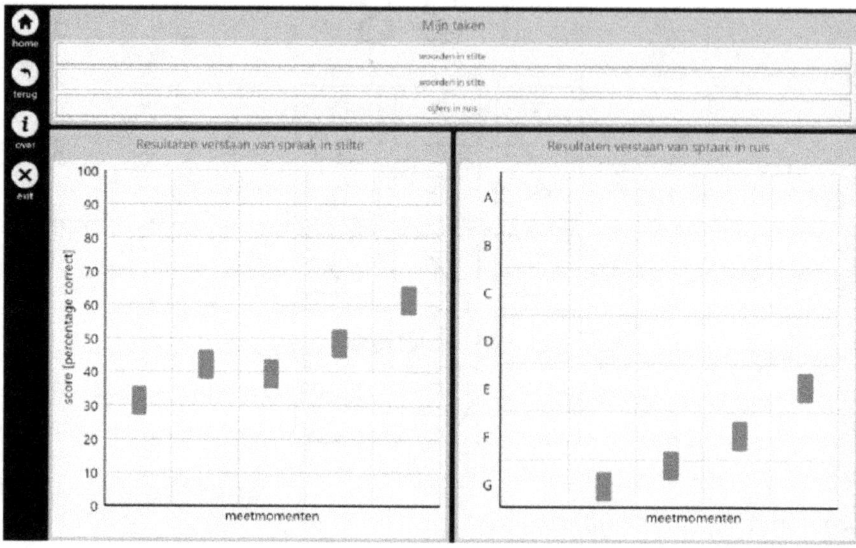

performance over time, normally showing improvement during the course of CI habilitation, particularly during the first 12-18 months. Decrements in performance can be flagged remotely to the clinician to signal that a clinical visit and intervention may be required.

Using The A§E Test Battery to Assess Phoneme Discrimination and Loudness Scaling

The Auditory Speech Sounds Evaluation (A§E) Testing environment has been developed over the last decade by Otoconsult and the Eargroup, both based in Antwerp, Belgium (Govaerts et al., 2006). This environment is highly developed and validated, and provides a range of tests for monitoring the performance of aided hearing-impaired listeners. In the SHiEC project, the Phoneme Discrimination and Loudness Scaling tests from the A§E environment were employed, though not all of the tests available were used. Note that within the SHiEC project, these existing tests, which were previously administered by an audiologist in a clinic, were re-developed on an Android/Windows platform so that they could be performed by the users themselves, outside the clinic.

The discrimination test displayed in Figure 13 shows 14 background sounds and 14 stimulus sounds. The user clicks a button to select one background and one stimulus phoneme. The stimulus phoneme will be presented at random in a series

Figure 13. The screen for testing phoneme discrimination in A§E

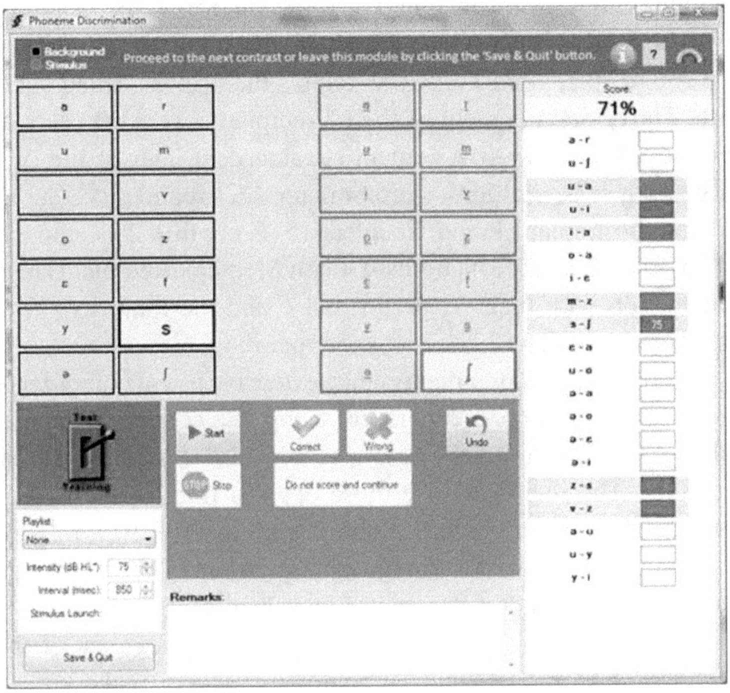

of repetitive background phonemes. The time intervals between the phonemes can be modified in the range 500-3000 milliseconds (msec) and is set at a default value of 850 msec.

The scores are 'correct' in the case of good discrimination, 'false' in the case of absence of discrimination.

The Loudness Scaling Test aims to assess the patient's intensity coding, because this may assist in the tailored programming of hearing devices. It consists of a typical loudness scaling task at 250, 1000 and 4000 Hz, assessing the loudness growth function of the (aided) cochlea. These noises are used in an identification task to scale the subjective loudness. The results may provide useful feedback for the programming of the hearing device (hearing aid or cochlear implant), in ways specific to each patient's requirements, using the discretion of the audiologist.

Study 1: Experienced Users: Survey on Cochlear Implants and Technology Within Senior CI Recipients

Computer technological developments are increasing the opportunities for remote cochlear implant (CI) care and rehabilitation. What types of mobile technology are CI recipients currently using and do they see remote CI-care as useful? To get answers to these questions the Onafhankelijk Platform Cochleaire Implantatie (OPCI), developed the questionnaire "CI and Technology".

A total of 266 people, almost all CI recipients themselves, filled out the on-line questionnaire. Thirty-eight percent of the CI recipients were 60 years or older, as shown in Figure 14. Seventy-five percent became deaf later in life or were born with severe hearing loss, and 86% were unilateral CI recipients. The majority of recipients chose the implant brand Cochlear (57%), while 29% chose Advanced Bionics, 11% MED-EL and 2% Neurelec/Oticon Medical. Recipients reported high levels of satisfaction with their CI performance and the majority, 79%, reported wearing their processors for 12 hours or more per day.

The survey showed that CI recipients make extensive use of computer technology in their personal lives. The recipients report using one or more computers devices for personal use 71% use a laptop, 61% a tablet, 52% a smartphone, and 40% a desktop computer. The recipients use these devices frequently, 42% use for 1-3 hours per day and 46% use more than 3 hours per day. Over 91% of recipients use the internet regularly. A small percentage of respondents (9%) report they already use their devices to monitor some aspect of their health.

The results of this study show that the target elderly segment of the hearing-impaired population have sufficient computer literacy to make an eHealth app viable, although it must be remembered that the methods used to reach users (via the internet) would not be able to target those elderly users who are uncomfortable with such technology. Other avenues, and more traditional support models, would need to ensure that such users are not excluded. Even so, an eHealth App is clearly

Figure 14. Recipient age distribution

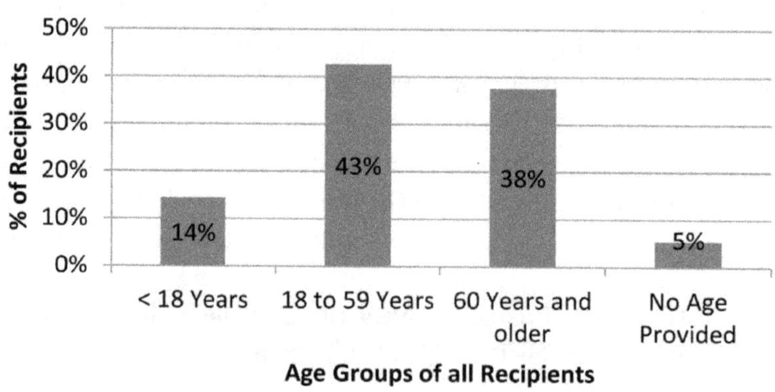

a good direction to follow, given several big evolutions in medicine in general and in the management of chronic conditions in principle. An eHealth app empowers the end user, enabling them to take more control and to reduce their dependence on external care-givers. The principle also applies to the field of audiology in general, and the field of hearing implants in particular.

Study 2: Evaluation of the Recipient Portal by Elderly Cochlear Implant Recipients

As mentioned above, the Recipient Portal was evaluated in its study, which is now described in more detail in this section. Usability of this "MyCochlear" Portal was assessed using 28 experienced CI users, of whom 20 provided completed questionnaires. This group was evenly split between 10 males and 10 females. A range of socio-demographic data were collected with an initial questionnaire. The average age of this cohort was 65.7 years (range 45-71). Of these, 60% stated that they lived with a partner, while 30% stated that they lived alone. 40% of this group stated that they were working, 25% stated that they were volunteering, while 25% described themselves as retired. Most were unilaterally implanted (80%), while 20% were bimodal users (CI in one ear and a hearing aid in the other ear).

The general protocol of the study is shown in Figure 15. Note that there was an initial visit with the audiologist during which baseline questionnaires were administered. Following this, recipients were asked to use the MyCochlear Portal at home for 6 weeks. During this time, recipients were able to give feedback via the

Figure 15. Summary of the protocol for Study 2

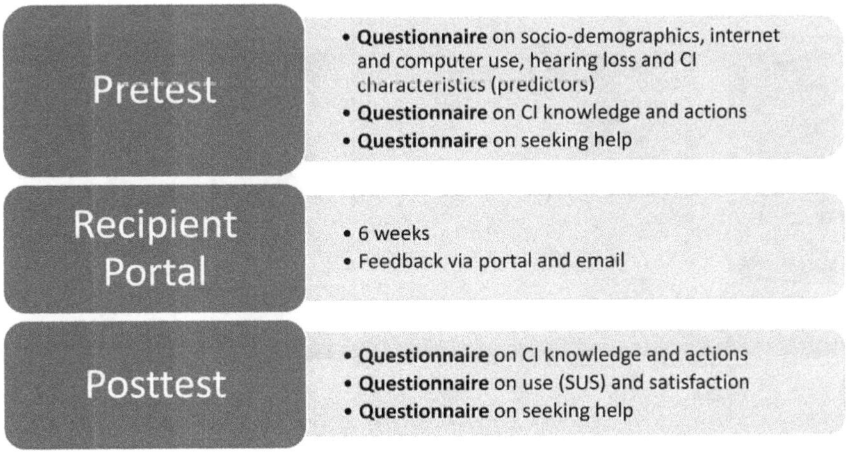

Portal and by email. After this period, they returned for a session to answer three post-test questionnaires. The initial session not only captured the socio-demographics just described, but also investigated further details of hearing loss, ICT use, and CI knowledge. A separate questionnaire investigated the methods the recipients used to get help with their CI's.

In the second visit, three questionnaires were administered. The first consisted of seven questions concerning actions (e.g. "*Do you know how to replace the microphone covers of your sound processor*") and seven questions concerning knowledge about the CI system (e.g. "*Do you know whether you can have an MRI scan with your sound processor*"). The results from this questionnaire are provided in the left panels of Figure 16 (7 questions about knowledge), and Figure 17 (7 questions about actions), showing how recipient knowledge changed before and after using the portal. The results indicate that useful learning was gained by recipient use of the portal, though the change was not large. Both prior to, and after, receiving access to the portal, participants were asked through which methods they would use to find help/information with respect to the 14 questions posed concerning CI actions and CI knowledge. Possible response options prior to having access to the portal were: 1."I would surf on the internet", 2."I would contact my audiologist/speech and language pathologist", 3."I would ask a friend or family member", 4."I would post my question on an internet forum", 5."I would read the paper manual of my sound

Figure 16. Results showing how user proficiency and attitudes changed following use of the MyCochlear Portal

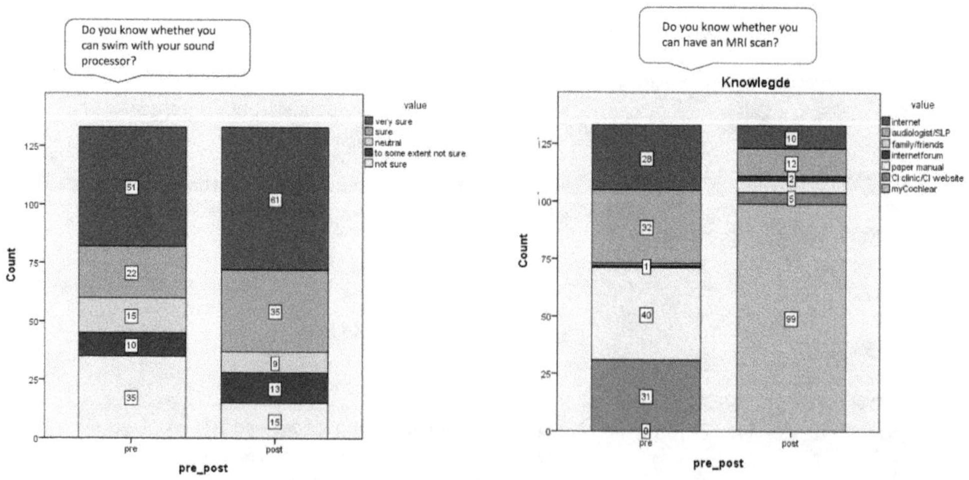

Figure 17. Similar to Figure 26, answers are displayed from the first and third questionnaires, again before and after use of the Portal

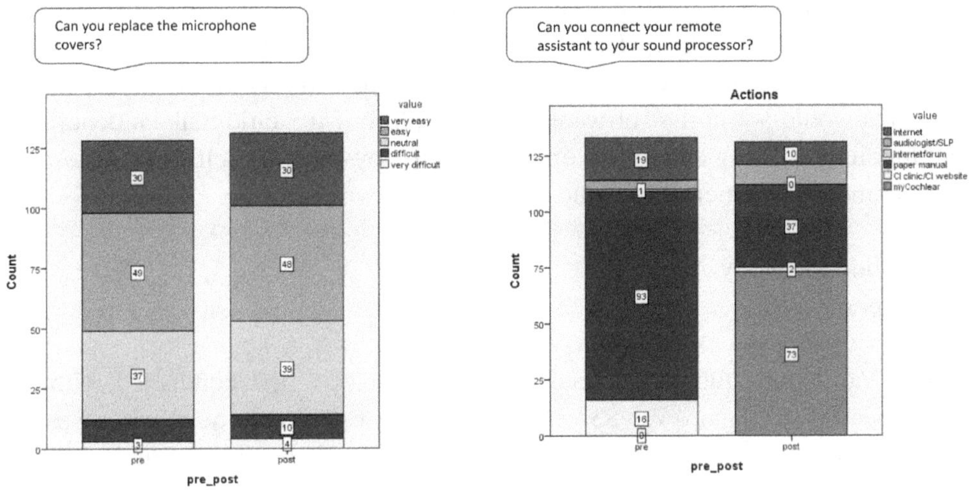

processor", 6."I would surf to the website of my CI team or CI manufacturer". The same response options were shown at the post questionnaire, with an additional 7th, namely "I would surf to my recipient portal" (Right panels of Figure 16 and Figure 17). Prior to having access to the recipient portal, resources of where to find help are diverse among the participants. After having access to the portal, results indicate that both for CI actions (58.9%) and CI knowledge items (72.6%), the participants will visit the recipient portal in order to find an answer. It can be seen that the major channel of information that recipients would use by the end of the trial had become the MyCochlear Portal.

The second questionnaire was a standardized test of system usability to assess the design of the Portal, called the System Usability Scale (Bangor, Kortun, and Miller, 2008). This consisted of 10 questions measured with a Likert Scale, (5 questions in each direction) about standard universal aspects of how easy a system is to use. The results were quite favourable, with the group mean producing an SUS score of 73% (SD 7.53 and range 58-85).

In summary, this study represented a high acceptance of the portal. It was rated as highly usable, and it had some effect on recipients' knowledge of use and maintenance of their device, and a much more significant effect on their preference to use the Portal as the primary channel for gaining information. This is very encouraging for the likely acceptance of Remote Care software.

Study 3: Validation Study in Experienced and New Users at VUmc

The next study of the SHiEC project was conducted at the VU University Medical Center, Amsterdam (VUmc). The aim was to see if equivalent or better results could be obtained in the home setting instead of in the clinic, assess how newly implanted recipients would adopt the software, and to explore if it would make a beneficial path for clinical fitting and follow up at the centre, by enabling self-directed testing in the home environment. This study consisted of two parts:

1. Validation study
2. User Study

The Validation study (de Graaff et al., 2018) was first conducted with 16 experienced users (ages 44 to 83 years). Speech recognition in quiet was assessed with CVC-word lists in four test condition. CVC words were presented at 65 dB and 55 dB, and marked according to the number of phonemes correct. Figure 18 (reprinted from de Graaff et al., 2018) summarises the comparison between testing at home and in the clinic, and it demonstrates that there were no significant differences between data from the home and the clinic.

Speech recognition in noise was assessed using the Digits-in-Noise test developed at the VUmc. Performance was measured in terms of the Speech Reception Threshold (SRT), which shows a Speech-to-Noise Ratio (SNR), at which 50% of digit triplets can be correctly repeated. Where there were differences, namely between the free-field and Audio Cable results for the Speech-in-Noise SRT tests, similar differences existed between the modalities in the home or clinic, supporting the claim that there is no change in performance by testing at home. The results suggest that even in a soundbooth, free-field testing is not the perfect test environment. This was probably because of an interaction between room acoustics, the sound from the patient who is responding, head movements and processor features.

Another important finding of this study was that recipients did not have difficulty performing the testing at home. They were able to connect the audio cable, launch the application, and perform the tests themselves. Thus, there was no penalty for performing the testing at home versus the clinic. It is also important to note that the recipients liked testing themselves. This increased involvement and self-motivation is consistent with the self-determination continuum described by Ryan and Deci (2000), and the findings of Athalye et al. (2015) that recipients want to be less dependent on clinicians for their care.

Once the software was validated in this manner, a follow-up study (de Graaff et al., in preparation) was conducted with 10 newly implanted CI recipients (ages 33 to 78 years). Speech testing was then conducted only in the home, as the software

Figure 18 (reprinted from de Graaff et al., 2018). Speech recognition in quiet measured in four different conditions across the three test sessions of the Validation Study conducted at the VUmc. The symbols represent individual scores and the horizontal lines represent mean and ±1 standard deviations.

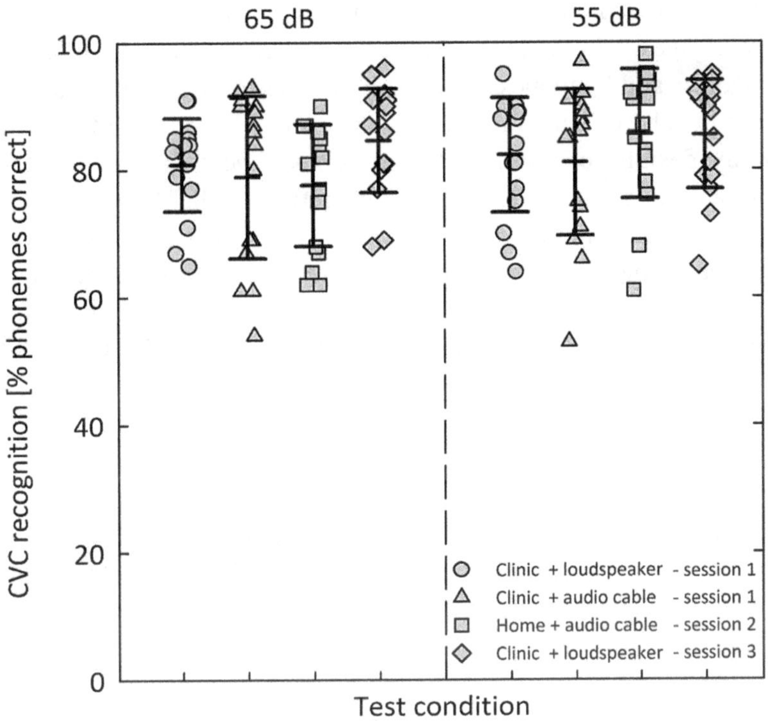

had already been validated. The protocol called for subjects to test themselves twice a week for the first three months after the initial activation of the speech processor. Each testing session consisted of Speech-in-Quiet testing using two CVC sentences, and one SRT determination using the Digits-in-Noise test. A general pattern can be seen whereby performance increases over the first month or so, and then plateaus.

When assessing Speech Perception in Noise, again a plateau of best performance seems to be reached after about a month. In at least one subject, a slightly different pattern of results for the Speech-in-Noise testing was observed, where a plateau was not clearly reached, principally because the data showed only slow, yet pronounced improvement over the whole 12 weeks of testing.

In summary, the results show that recipients are capable of administering speech tests themselves in the home, and that improvement is apparent over the 12 weeks of testing that data were collected. This is very encouraging for the viability of administering speech tests using the Self Care model.

Study 4: Validation Study II via OPCI

After the initial survey of general device usage and ICT competence, and the study of the usability of the MyHearing Portal were conducted, as described above, a more structured and focussed study was conducted with a smaller group of 18 experienced CI users (mean age 68.7 years, SD = 5.2) The full study is reported in Philips, Smits, Govaerts, Doorn, and Vanpoucke (2018), while a description and some preliminary data are provided here. This was conducted by OPCI, The Dutch CI Users' group.

The study design consisted of two sessions. The first session consisted of counselling and an explanation and demonstration of the App, conducted by an audiologist. A pre-questionnaire was administered at this point, to assess the starting situation of each subject prior to adopting the App. Subjects were then sent home to have two weeks of free use with the App, structured according to their desires. The second session, two weeks later, consisted of the subject returning to the audiologist. At this point, a second questionnaire was administered to provide an assessment of how the subjects had experienced the App, and these experiences were discussed with the audiologist.

The results of the Post-Test questionnaire in the second session, using the same SUS scale as previously, showed that general usability of the App was rated at 75.7% ("good"). The subjects also ranked the six functionalities of the App, and the highest preference by a sizeable margin was for the "My Hearing Test", as shown in Figure 19.

Figure 19. Ranking of the six functionalities of the My Hearing App by the 18 recipients in the OPCI study of experienced users

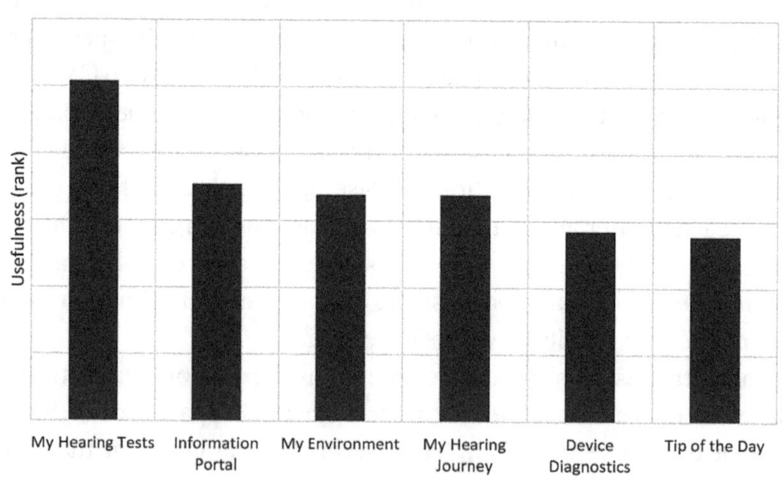

Users' opinions of the App were also examined in the Post-Test Questionnaire using the Intrinsic Motivation Inventory (IMI) (Ryan, 1982), which consisted of seven subscales:

- **Interest/Enjoyment:** "This was fun to do"
- **Perceived Competence:** "I think I am pretty good at this".
- **Effort/Importance:** "I put a lot of effort in this"
- **Pressure/Tension:** "I felt pressured while doing these."
- **Perceived Choice:** "I did this because I wanted to."
- **Value/Usefulness:** "I think this is an important activity."
- **Relatedness:** "I felt like I could really trust this person."

Note that the questions regarding the final category, 'relatedness', were not the standard ones from the IMI, as it was more relevant to ask custom questions regarding family and friends. These are the answers reflected in the 'relatedness' dimension shown in Figure 20, which summarises the results for all seven dimensions.

To summarise the various aspects of Participants' responses to the components of the Post-Test Questionnaire, it can be said that Participants 1) want to continue to use the app in the future, 2) would recommend its use to others, 3) believe it improves their CI care, and 4) want their health insurance to cover any costs. The last point is relevant to the consideration of the types of business models that might be used to implement such Self-Care.

Figure 20. Results of the Intrinsic Motivation Inventory from the 18 Users in the OPCI study

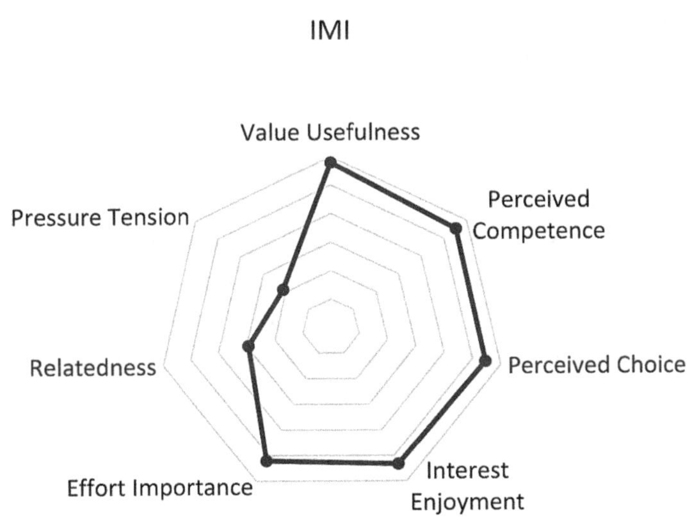

Finally, the results of the IMI allow us to relate the results from the experienced users back to the Self-Determination Theory expounded in Figure 4 from the earlier section "Issues, Controversies, Problems". In general, the participants found the MyHearing App to be valuable and important, perceived autonomy and competence were high, and relatedness to the Health Professional (i.e., dependence upon) is weak. We can conclude that the study supported the belief that users' intrinsic motivation for Self-Care is high, and that the perceived 'good' usability of the MyHearing App suggests this would be a worthwhile model to follow.

FUTURE RESEARCH DIRECTIONS

The preceding sections have outlined the present status of the MHA and the hearing tests presently available. This of course represents only a beginning, especially as this was a pilot App designed for testing on a small number of closely monitored subjects. The next step is to translate the application to a more scalable platform, both in terms of a more advanced server back-end, and a user App that is available on a more widely supported platform.

In terms of functionality, the authors see the need to further develop four main areas:

1. **Rehabilitation:** The application needs a more structured and developed habilitation pathway, where progress is actively encouraged and managed in a staged manner. Exercises could be presented that focus on specific abilities in a managed way. Greater intelligence in the back-end support could systematically set goals based on the interpretation of self-administered hearing tests.
2. **Self Fitting:** A great increase in the potential of the Home-Care paradigm could be realised if recipients could adjust their actual MAP parameters themselves. Apart from the health-economic benefits of such decentralisation, fitting in the home instead of a sound booth in the clinic would provide added buy-in for the recipient through greater self-empowerment, which could lead to striving for better hearing performance.
3. **The Local Care Network/ Inclusion of Significant Others:** A supportive local care network, such as family and significant others, has the potential to greatly increase self-motivation and adherence to habilitation programmes and the extended training that is empirically known to be necessary to reach full hearing potential. This could both raise individual performance and further relieve the clinical bottleneck.

4. **Extended Self-Assessment:** While the present App already contains multiple tests to monitor hearing performance, it may be desirable to increase the number of tests to obtain a more detailed picture of the listener's hearing progress. Aside from refining the algorithms that are used in the present tests, there are a number of potential new tests that could assess different aspects of hearing performance.

The move to a more decentralized model of recipient care needs to be accompanied by a supportive change in the established reimbursement models. Many health systems are currently structured around reimbursing a certain number of clinic visits. This would clearly need to change when habilitation and even basic MAP fitting takes place in the home environment. The authors have outlined how performance can be raised in parallel with a development of more cost-effective and scalable treatment models. It is by redirecting reimbursement appropriately that the greatest health-economic benefits can be realized, as this would encourage the use of the full potential that is offered by these new technologies. Reimbursement could take into account measures of progress that are captured remotely in the Cloud, if the emphasis moves from the time spent in face-to-face clinician interaction. Such new paradigms would obviously necessitate the involvement of the CI manufacturers, thus supporting an increased development of a more service-based business model of patient-centerd development of CI use.

CONCLUSION

This chapter has considered an approach that could be taken to developing a more decentralized, recipient-driven model of CI support that can be implemented outside of the specialized clinic, presumably in the home environment. It began with a consideration of the future requirements of the CI care system, and then offered an analysis of how the present model of care works. It was shown that, at present, care predominantly takes place in specialized, implanting centres in large hospitals, which are often centrally located and not convenient to the user. The authors then considered different care models, and provided evidence that a more patient-oriented approach has the benefit of both 1) motivating and empowering the recipient to strive for better performance, and 2) offering a way around the impending bottlenecks that will inhibit the scalability and wider delivery to a larger CI population, thus delivering much needed health economic benefits in the process.

A pilot application was then described; the MyHearing App. This consisted of a recipient App for self-directed use, a clinician application with additional functionality, and a Cloud-server back-end to record and communicate data on recipient performance, and thereby guide future improvements in fitting. The results of user input were also presented, offering insight into what recipients themselves require from their CI's.

This led to a clearer definition of which future developments are needed. Greater functionality will need to be incorporated into the recipient App to enable self-fitting and greater rehabilitation. Significant potential exists for centralized expert systems to guide ways in which individual performance can be improved, probably in conjunction with enhanced assessment tools that provide more detailed information of existing hearing performance. Functionality could also be extended to harness the power of the Immediate Local Care Network, thus offering greater support and increasing intrinsic motivation.

Finally, consideration was given to how reimbursement models would need to adapt to increasing decentralization of care, thus incentivizing users and manufacturers to pursue this option. The authors view this route as an obvious future path that will be scalable and able to meet the challenge of a future hearing landscape which involves a much higher uptake of cochlear implants across all segments of the population, particularly those that are presently under-represented. This can only result in greater recipient satisfaction and performance, via a more affordable route, which ultimately increases the accessibility to many of the abundant advantages of hearing that would otherwise be unavailable to them.

ACKNOWLEDGMENT

AAL –European Programme to assist Active Ambient Living (ongoing programme now renamed AAL- Active and Assisted Living), which funded the SHiEC (Supported Hearing in Elderly Citizens) project on which this chapter was based.

REFERENCES

Athalye, S., Archbold, S., Mulla, I., Lutman, M., & Nikolopoulous, T. (2015). Exploring views on current and future cochlear implant service delivery: The perspectives of users, parents and professionals at cochlear implant centres and in the community. *Cochlear Implants International, 16*(5), 241–253. doi:10.1179/1754762815Y.0000000003 PMID:25780991

Bangor, A., Kortum, P. T., & Miller, J. T. (2008). An Empirical Evaluation of the System Usability Scale. *International Journal of Human-Computer Interaction, 24*(6), 574–594. doi:10.1080/10447310802205776

Barton, G. R., Fortnum, H. M., Stacey, P. C., & Summerfield, A. Q. (2006). Hearing-impaired children in the UK IV: Cost-effectiveness of paediatric cochlear implantation. *Ear and Hearing, 27*(5), 575–588. doi:10.1097/01.aud.0000233967.11072.24 PMID:16957506

Brooke, J. (1996). SUS: "A quick and dirty" usability scale. In P. W. Jordan, B. Thomas, & B. A. Weerdmeester (Eds.), *Usability Evaluation in Industry*. London: Taylor and Francis.

de Graaff, F. I., Huysmans, E., Merkus, P., Goverts, S. T., & Smits, C. (2018). Assessment of speech recognition abilities in quiet and in noise: A comparison between self-administered home testing and testing in the clinic for adult cochlear implant users. *International Journal of Audiology*, 1–9. doi:10.1080/14992027.2018.1506168 PMID:30261772

de Graaff, F. I., Huysmans, E., Qazi, O. U., Vanpoucke, F. J., Merkus, P., Goverts, S. T., & Smits, C. (2016). The Development of Remote Speech Recognition Tests for Adult Cochlear Implant Users: The Effect of Presentation Mode of the Noise and a Reliable Method to Deliver Sound in Home Environments. *Audiology & Neuro-Otology, 21*(1Suppl.), 48–54. doi:10.1159/000448355 PMID:27806354

De Raeve, L. (2016). Cochlear implants in Belgium: Prevalence in paediatric and adult cochlear implantation. *European Annals of Otorhinolaryngology, Head and Neck Diseases, 133*(Suppl 1), S57–S60. doi:10.1016/j.anorl.2016.04.018 PMID:27246742

Ear Foundation. (2014). *The real cost of adult hearing loss.* Retrieved October 1, 2018, from http://www.earfoundation.org.uk/research/current-research/the-real-cost-of-adult-hearing-loss

European Patient Forum. (n.d.). Retrieved from http://www.eu-patient.eu/campaign/PatientsprescribE/

Govaerts, P. J. (2016). Expert opinion: Time to ban formal CI selection criteria? *Cochlear Implants Intl.*, *17*(S1), 74-77.

Govaerts, P. J., Daemers, K., Yperman, M., De Beukelaer, C., De Saegher, G., & De Ceulaer, G. (2006). Auditory speech sounds evaluation (ASSE): A new test to assess detection, discrimination and identification in hearing impairment. *Cochlear Implants International*, *7*(2), 92–106. doi:10.1179/146701006807508106 PMID:18792377

Kaandorp, M. W., Smits, C., Merkus, P., Goverts, S. T., & Festen, J. M. (2015). Assessing speech recognition abilities with digits in noise in cochlear implant and hearing aid users. *International Journal of Audiology*, *54*(1), 48–57. doi:10.3109/14992027.2014.945623 PMID:25156097

Medtronic plc. (2011). *Medtronic CareLink® Network Remote Monitoring Helps Improve Patient Care and Reduce Healthcare Costs*. Retrieved October 1, 2018 from http://newsroom.medtronic.com/phoenix.zhtml?c=251324&p=irol-newsArticle&ID=1771836

National Institute for Health and Care Excellent (NICE). (2009). *Cochlear implants for children and adults with severe to profound deafness*. Retrieved October 1, 2018, from https://www.nice.org.uk/guidance/ta166/chapter/4-evidence-and-interpretation

Pfleger, R. (2012). *Contract for a Healthy Future*. Presented at Innovation in Healthcare without borders, Brussels, Belgium. Retrieved October 1, 2018, from http://ec.europa.eu/research/health/pdf/event13/roland-pfleger_en.pdf

Philips, B., Smits, C., Govaerts, P. J., Doorn, I., & Vanpoucke, F. (in press). Empowering senior cochlear implant users at home via a tablet-computer application. *Journal of American Audiology.*

Roland, J. T. Jr, Gantz, B. J., Waltzman, S. B., & Parkinson, A. J. (2016). United States multicenter clinical trial of the cochlear nucleus hybrid implant system. *Laryngoscope*, *126*(1), 175–181. doi:10.1002/lary.25451 PMID:26152811

Ryan, R. M. (1982). Control and information in the intrapersonal sphere: An extension of cognitive evaluation theory. *Journal of Personality and Social Psychology*, *43*(3), 450–461. doi:10.1037/0022-3514.43.3.450

Ryan, R. M., & Deci, E. L. (2000). Self-Determination Theory and the Facilitation of Intrinsic Motivation, Social Development, and Well-Being. *The American Psychologist*, *55*(1), 68–78. doi:10.1037/0003-066X.55.1.68 PMID:11392867

Ryan, R. M., Patrick, H., Deci, E. L., & Williams, G. C. (2008). Facilitating health behavior change and its maintenance: Interventions based on Self- Determination Theory. *Eur. Health Psychology*, *10*, 2–5.

Schroeder, S. A. (2007). Shattuck lecture. We can do better–improving the health of the American people. *The New England Journal of Medicine*, *357*(12), 1221–1228. doi:10.1056/NEJMsa073350 PMID:17881753

Smits, C., Goverts, S. T., & Festen, J. M. (2013). The digits-in-noise test: Assessing auditory speech recognition abilities in noise. *The Journal of the Acoustical Society of America*, *133*(3), 1693–1706. doi:10.1121/1.4789933 PMID:23464039

Smits, C., Kapteyn, T. S., & Houtgast, T. (2004). Development and validation of an automatic speech-in-noise screening test by telephone. *International Journal of Audiology*, *43*(1), 15–28. doi:10.1080/14992020400050004 PMID:14974624

United States Department of Labor, Bureau of Labor Statistics. (2017). *Occupational Outlook Handbook*. Retrieved October 1, 2018, from http://www.bls.gov/ooh/healthcare/audiologists.htm

Vaerenberg, B., Smits, C., De Ceulaer, G., Zir, E., Harman, S., & Jaspers, N. (2014, February 4). …Cochlear implant programming: A global survey on the state of the art. *The Scientific World Journal*. PMID:24688394

Vermeire, E., Hearnshaw, H., van Royen, P., & Denekens, J. (2001). Patient adherence to treatment: Three decades of research. A comprehensive review. *Journal of Clinical Pharmacy and Therapeutics*, *26*(5), 331–342. doi:10.1046/j.1365-2710.2001.00363.x PMID:11679023

Walker, E., & Nowacki, A. (2011). Understanding Equivalence and Noninferiority Testing. *Journal of General Internal Medicine*, *26*(2), 192–196. doi:10.100711606-010-1513-8 PMID:20857339

World Health Organization (WHO). (2004). *Global Burden of Disease Report*. Retrieved October 1, 2018, from http://www.who.int/healthinfo/global_burden_disease/GBD_report_2004update_part4.pdf

World Health Organization (WHO). (2013). *Millions of People in the World have Hearing Loss that can be Treated or Prevented*. Retrieved October 1, 2018, http://www.who.int/pbd/deafness

World Health Organization (WHO). (2016). *Executive Board 139th Session: Resolutions and Decisions Annex.* Retrieved October 1, 2018. From http://apps.who.int/gb/ebwha/pdf_files/EB139-REC1/B139_REC1-en.pdf

World Health Organization (WHO). (2018). *Deafness and Hearing Loss.* Retrieved October 1, 2018, from: http://www.who.int/mediacentre/factsheets/fs300/en/

Chapter 6
A Framework for Designing and Evaluating Internet Interventions to Improve Tinnitus Care

Eldré W. Beukes
Anglia Ruskin University, UK

Vinaya Manchaiah
Lamar University, USA

Gerhard Andersson
Linköping University, Sweden

Peter M. Allen
Anglia Ruskin University, UK

David M. Baguley
University of Nottingham, UK

ABSTRACT

Tinnitus can be a debilitating hearing-related symptom. Access to evidence-based tinnitus interventions remain limited. Tele-audiology can assist by providing a clinically and cost-effective tinnitus management route. This chapter highlights how this is made possible by focusing on one form of tele-audiology, namely an internet-based intervention. Guidelines are provided for the development of such interventions. A framework outlining the various processes involved in evaluating newly developed interventions is also provided. The chapter closes by discussing factors that may facilitate or hamper the dissemination of new interventions into existing service delivery models. This well-defined outline for intervention development and evaluation can be applied and used to guide innovative intervention models by stakeholders.

DOI: 10.4018/978-1-5225-8191-8.ch006

INTRODUCTION

Technological advances can assist with the provision of healthcare interventions aimed at improving the health of individuals. Utilising these developments should be explored, especially when a chronic condition or symptom exists which may require multiple complex interventions and place a substantial burden on health organisations (West, 2012). Implementing novel interventions without a systematic process of careful development and evaluation may result in them failing to reach their full potential or produce the desired outcomes (Craig et. al., 2008). The aim of this chapter is to encourage utilisation of digital healthcare in the context of an auditory-related condition known as tinnitus. It provides a comprehensive and systematic framework for the design and evaluation of these interventions. The examples and well-defined guidelines can be applied by those interested in improving service delivery models such as clinicians, scientists, researchers, students, and government based workers.

This chapter was written by a diverse range of professionals, including a clinical psychologist, audiologist, a tinnitus expert, and academic-researchers, with a common interest in helping those with tinnitus. While working in clinical settings, each noticed some recurring themes surrounding barriers to providing the quality care patients required. Many stories of unmet needs and people desperate for help were heard. The authors, therefore, pioneered models to improve interventions, which will be shared in this chapter.

The objectives of this chapter are:

1. To outline the barriers to accessing tinnitus care in current tinnitus care models
2. To highlight how inclusion of tele-audiology can improve access to evidence-based intervention for tinnitus
3. To provide a framework for the development of Internet-based interventions
4. To outline the sequential procedures required for Intervention evaluation
5. To identify key processes that aid implementation of newly developed interventions

BACKGROUND

Tinnitus is often characterised by perceiving sounds such as ringing or buzzing in the absence of an identifiable external sound source (Baguley, Andersson, McFerran, and McKenna, 2013). As one of the most distressing and debilitating hearing-related symptoms, the effects can be devastating (Cima, Vlaeyen, Maes, Joore, and Anteunis, 2011). Whether emerging gradually or suddenly, the onset is frequently a significant life event and often associated with numerous challenges and increased levels of stress (Scott et al., 2016). Those experiencing tinnitus may feel isolated, when in actual fact it is one of the most highly prevalent chronic auditory-related symptoms, affecting an estimated 10–15% of the adult population across the globe (Davis and Rafaie, 2000; Khedr et al., 2010; Michikawa et al., 2010; Shargorodsky, Curhan, and Farwell, 2010). This incidence is likely to continue to rise, due to factors such as an increase in life expectancy and recreational noise exposure (Martinez, Wallenhorst, McFerran, and Hall, 2015). Finding a cure that permanently abolishes tinnitus remains elusive due to the heterogeneous aetiology, varying individual experiences and limited understanding regarding the mechanisms and pathophysiology (Elgoyhen, Langguth, De Ridder, and Vanneste, 2015). This realisation of having to live with hearing these sounds all the time, together with the loss of silence, can result in a range of distressing emotional reactions. For those greatly troubled by tinnitus, associated adverse consequences may include insomnia, reduced concentration, anxiety, and depression which can impact both short and long term functioning (Hall et al., 2018; Langguth, 2011).

Individuals often feel helpless and unsure how to manage their tinnitus. Some withdraw and limit going to places they believe will worsen their tinnitus. This approach is often associated with greater distress and poorer long-term outcomes (Beukes et al., 2017a; Hayes, Wilson, Gifford, Follette, and Strosahl, 1996). Those with tinnitus often do not realise that there are ways to cope, despite having tinnitus. The ultimate goal during tinnitus interventions is to become accustomed to, i.e. habituating, to hearing the sounds. Habituation is the point where perceiving tinnitus no longer results in a negative emotional response and does not affect day-to-day functioning. Tinnitus interventions can aid habituation and help those living with tinnitus to overcome the devastating effects tinnitus can have. Ensuring that interventions are available for those with distressing tinnitus is, therefore, imperative.

RESTRICTIONS IN CURRENT TINNITUS CARE MODELS

Considering the distress often associated with tinnitus, appropriate clinical care pathways are crucial. Unfortunately, these are not always available due to obstacles preventing delivery of appropriate interventions. A clear understanding of these limitations is required prior to considering potential solutions to address them. The main restrictions include provision of evidence-based interventions, access to tinnitus care, and the costs associated with intervention delivery as outlined in the following sections.

Limited Provision of Evidence-Based Interventions

In terms of tinnitus management, a significant barrier is the lack of standardisation in the approaches used (Hoare, Kowalkowski, Lang and Hall, 2011). Moreover, there is a lack of evidence supporting the efficacy of many tinnitus management strategies (Landgrebe et al., 2012). What adds to the complexity of tinnitus is that tinnitus-related distress is not related to the loudness or character of tinnitus experienced, but rather to the psychological complaints thereof (Andersson, 2002). Tinnitus interventions targeting the tinnitus sound itself, are, therefore, often less effective than psychological interventions which focus on improving functionality and minimising the effects tinnitus may have (Hoare et al., 2011). The intervention with the most evidence in reducing tinnitus distress at present is cognitive behavioural therapy (CBT), a type of psychological therapy (Grewal, Spielmann, Jones, and Hussain, 2014; Hesser, Weise, Westin, and Andersson, 2011). Despite this evidence, there is limited provision of CBT in clinical practice, largely due to a shortage of trained professionals to provide CBT for tinnitus (Gander, Hoare, Collins, Smith, and Hall, 2011). Further discrepancies exist, in that the management routes most frequently offered to patients are often those with the least evidence of efficacy. Bhatt, Lin, and Bhattacharyya, (2016) for instance reported that doctors in the USA recommended medications 45% of the time opposed to cognitive behavioural therapy only 0.2% of the time. Hall et al. (2011) reported a similar trend with doctors in the USA, UK and Europe recommending pharmaceutical treatment for acute tinnitus 77% of the time and psychological interventions for chronic tinnitus 35% of the time.

Lack of Access to Speciality Care

Accessing specialised health services largely depends on geographic location, both within countries and in different countries where Audiology as a profession for instance does not exist. This may be related to a shortage of resources, increase in service-demand, lack of trained professionals, poor infrastructure and a focus on basic healthcare (Smith, McKeon, Blunt, and Edwards, 2014). The demand for these services may also lead to an increase in appointment waiting times which has been associated with poorer outcomes for a variety of health issues (Pizer and Prentice, 2011; Smith et al., 2014). Despite psychological treatment modalities having the best evidence base for successful tinnitus management, they may not be available as demonstrated by a survey performed in the UK (McFerran, Hoare, Carr, Ray, and Stockdale, 2018). For patients experiencing significant levels of health-related distress, such as those with chronic tinnitus, overcoming these barriers by maximising access to care and minimizing the waiting time for this care should be prioritised

(Gander et al., 2011). Service delivery models should focus on improving access to evidence-based care.

The Costs Associated With Intervention Delivery

Provision of healthcare cannot be considered without evidence of the cost-effectiveness of these interventions. As no cure has been identified, treating tinnitus remains challenging and costly at an estimated annual healthcare cost of £750 million and resulting societal cost of £2.7 billion per year in the UK (Stockdale et al., 2017). Due to its chronic nature, healthcare services are further pressurised as processes are often extensive and often encompass referrals to various disciplines to address hearing difficulties and possible indirect psychosocial effects (Cima et al., 2009). The incidence of tinnitus is likely to continue to rise, due to factors such as an increase in life expectancy and recreational noise exposure (Martinez et al., 2015) which may place further financial constraints on healthcare systems that are already pressurised. Innovative planning is required develop interventions that are able to meet these additional demands and challenges e.g. poor patient to health professional ratios.

Of importance is ensuring that these services are sustainable and meet the demands and challenges such as the poor patient to health professional ratio.

THE ROLE OF TELE-AUDIOLOGY FOR TINNITUS

The automation and transferability of telehealth provides unique opportunities to overcome barriers and improve healthcare options for numerous health-related difficulties (Polisena, Coyle, Coyle, and McGill, 2009: Totten et al., 2016). Telehealth encompasses a range of alternative formats of healthcare delivery such as use of the Internet, computer-based technologies, videoconferencing and smartphone applications. Due to the versatility of the Internet, many telehealth self-help interventions are Internet-based (Reavley and Jorm, 2011). The Internet has become a means for many people with tinnitus to connect, as is seen with the increasing specific online tinnitus forums and online support groups (Kaplan, Salzer, Solomon, Brusilovskiy, and Cousounis, 2011). Self-help tinnitus management is often advocated as a means of increasing an individual's knowledge of tinnitus (Nyenhuis, Golm, and Kröner-Herwig, 2013) and utilizing the Internet provides a means to enable self-help management. The Internet is also a familiar vehicle used widely by patients who seek information about health-related difficulties they face (Reavley and Jorm, 2011). This chapter will focus on one form of tele-audiology, namely Internet-interventions. Within this field there are various forms of tinnitus Internet-interventions, including educational resources such as the Tinnitus E-Programme (Greenwell, Featherstone, and Hoare, 2015), those based on acceptance and commitment therapy (Hesser et al., 2011) or cognitive behavioural therapy (Andersson, Strömgren, Ström, and Lyttkens, 2002). This chapter will concentrate on cognitive behavioural therapy delivered on the Internet (iCBT) as it is the intervention with the greatest evidence-base and has been used in current healthcare models. These iCBT interventions have been shown to be effective for a range of difficulties, including auditory related problems (Thorén, Öberg, Wänström, Andersson, and Lunner, 2014), anxiety (Tulbure, 2011), mood disorders, depression (Johansson and Andersson, 2012) headache, insomnia, and somatic problems such as chronic pain (Arnberg, Linton, Hultcrantz, Heintz, and Jonsson, 2014; Cuijpers, van Straten, and Andersson, 2008; van Beugen et al., 2014). The principles discussed in this chapter are, however, transferable to other forms of tele-audiology.

When considering the role of any form of tele-audiology for tinnitus, it is important that it is seen as an additional intervention route, and not the only management route. Due to the heterogeneous nature of tinnitus, having a variety of management options to suit different needs is important. By nature of the intervention, those undertaking it need access to a computer, the Internet, and should have the ability to read, write and understand text. There will be people who do not have the available resources or language skills to undertake such interventions, and alternate management formats should be available to them.

The Potential of Tele-Audiology

An Internet-intervention has clear service delivery advantages, including widespread access to tinnitus services particularly in underserved communities, but the application is not restricted to those with reduced clinical access. It can also be accessed easily by those who may find attending hospitals difficult due to mobility issues, needing to take time off work, reliance on others for transport or poor health (Chiang, Chen, Dai, and Ho, 2012). Additional intervention routes ensure that distressed patients can be treated in a more timely manner, which, in turn, can reduce the anxiety and distress often associated with waiting for an intervention. Health professionals can also be freed up to see patients who require urgent care. Service delivery costs are always an important factor. A delivery model including an Internet intervention could be more cost-effective than face-to-face (F2F) interventions, as fewer resources are required (Hedman et al., 2014). The Internet is a viable alternative for people who are unable to access F2F care for reasons such as a long travelling time, the stigma of seeing a therapist, communication difficulties due to hearing impairment or other health-related problems that may make attending an appointment difficult (Cuijpers et al. 2008). Another advantage is the ability to access an intervention at home, at a comfortable pace and when individuals are in the right emotional state to absorb new information (Griffiths and Christensen, 2007; Muñoz, 2010). Learning and retention can be facilitated as the information can be revised at any stage. (Ferguson and Henshaw, 2015), for instance, found improved knowledge of hearing aids for those patients who obtained information online as opposed to those only receiving instructions in a clinical setting. This mode of intervention may also suit those who find it hard speaking to someone F2F about personal problems due to reduced stigma and online anonymity (Griffiths, Lindenmeyer, Powell, Lowe, and Thorogood, 2006). Outcome monitoring can be embedded in the intervention, allowing closer monitoring of progress, easier data management and time-saving capabilities. It can improve efficiency in healthcare as interventions can be standardised regardless of the therapist or clinic attended. Changes in health care behaviours towards more self-management have been evident following the use of self-monitoring fitness and health-related apps and devices (Chiauzzi, Rodarte, and DasMahapatra, 2015). An Internet-based intervention can empower individuals to take responsibility and promote self-efficacy (Bendelin et al., 2011; Williams and Whitfield, 2001). Tele-audiology thus holds real potential for bridging barriers evident in healthcare provision.

A FRAMEWORK FOR DEVELOPING INTERNET-BASED INTERVENTIONS

The potential of tele-audiology will not be realised if interventions are not systematically developed and evaluated. The sections that follow are aimed at providing such a framework specifically for tele-audiology using the principles outlined for developing and evaluating complex interventions (those with a number of interacting components) provided by the medical research council (Craig et al., 2008). The process is lengthy, but all the stages are important. Neglect of any of these steps can make it less probable that the intervention will be implemented successfully. It is likely that the differences reported in efficacy and effectiveness of individual Internet-interventions are due to optimal designs for intervention development and evaluation not always been used (Morrison, Yardley, Powell, and Michie, 2012). This section is intended to highlight the key components that could improve outcomes and minimise barriers. The framework presented has largely been drawn from Andersson, Carlbring, Berger, Almlöv, and Cuijpers (2009) "What makes Internet therapy work?" article. Further insights from (Morrison et al., 2012) outlining design features leading to effective e-Health have also been incorporated. Guidelines for developing Internet-based interventions are presented below.

Suitable Functionality of the Internet-Intervention Platform

Internet interventions should ensure flexibility within the design in order to adapt to technological advances and the progression of new knowledge. At present these include ensuring the page layout is fully responsive, transparently adapting to screen size and ensuring a fully functional experience regardless of whether the platform is accessed using a desktop computer (PC and Mac), smartphone or tablet. This makes the intervention more accessible and improves engagement. One example is the *Iterapi* purpose-built web-based platform (https://www.iterapi.se/), designed at the Department of Behavioural Sciences and Learning at Linköping University, Sweden (Vlaescu, Carlbring, Lunner, and Andersson, 2015; Vlaescu, Alasjö, Miloff, Carlbring, and Andersson, 2016). This platform has undergone continual improvements following experience in providing interventions since 1998 for various difficulties, including auditory-related symptoms. It allows varying levels of access to different aspects of the intervention should be possible by assigning users different roles and privileges. This included what materials, therapeutic contact and discussion forums individuals had access to. Data logging is beneficial to record the frequency of login, modules read, worksheets completed, and the number of messages sent.

Security Considerations

One of the main concerns regarding Internet-interventions is the security of stored personal data. Country specific security regulations need to be followed such as European regulations (Bennett, Bennett, and Griffiths, 2010), the UK Data Protection Act 1998 (UK Parliament, 1998), and The Privacy and Electronic Communications (EC Directive) Regulations of 2003 in the UK (Riach, 2003). These considerations include appropriate technical and organisational measures to safeguard user privacy and confidentiality (Vlaescu et al., 2015; Vlaescu et al., 2016) as outlined below:

- The security of the servers is an imperative consideration to ensure the servers are only accessed by authorised personnel. Multiple backups are required so that data is never lost due to system failure.
- Data storage should be encrypted and the encryption key should only be accessible to two administrators.
- Login should ideally use a two-step process requiring a user code, password and code that is sent to a users' mobile phone. However, a balance between securing data and ensuring login is not too complex, needs to be customised to each intended population. In countries where recipients are familiar with Internet-banking, these processes should be less complex than for countries where users are unaccustomed to these procedures.

- Any intervention related correspondence takes place within the platform so no confidential information is sent unencrypted via email.
- Users need to be informed regarding how collected information may be used and shared. Provided information about Cookie usage and opting out of the programme should be transparent.

A Multidisciplinary Partnership

It is essential to involve a multi-professional team in the process of Internet-based intervention planning. This is particularly important in the context of chronic conditions and symptoms such as tinnitus, which are optimally treated within a multidisciplinary team (Cima et al. 2009). The importance of an experienced webmaster, preferably with expertise in Internet-intervention design and delivery is key. Including a range of professionals ensures that the various aspects of Intervention development are considered. An example of such a team is seen in the development of a UK based Internet-intervention which included clinical psychologists, audiologists, clinical scientists, researchers, a webmaster and a public-patient forum (Beukes et al., 2016).

The Required Infrastructure

Hand-in-hand with this development is ensuring the infrastructure is in place and the associated costs can be supported. Basic requirements include capital costs such as computers, servers and secure storage of these. Employing staff, including a webmaster, those involved in developing and supporting the interventions are, furthermore, required. Ongoing costs such as SSL certificates, Internet connectivity, service maintenance, encryption packages etc. all need to be factored in.

A Strong Theoretical Base

At the heart of intervention design is a secure theoretical base so that the intervention is built on proven conceptual models (Campbell, Fitzpatrick, Haines, and Kinmonth, 2000). The theoretical base of the iCBT self-help programme developed by (Andersson and Kaldo, 2004) combined both a cognitive rationale (Henry and Wilson, 2001) and a learning theory approach (Hallam, Rachman, and Hinchcliffe, 1984) as shown in Table 1. Evidence-based CBT techniques used included negative automatic thought analysis, cognitive restructuring, imagery, applied relaxation, exposure techniques, sleep hygiene and concentration management. Clinically effective audiological principles, such as sound enrichment, hearing tactics and advice for sound sensitivity (e.g. Jastreboff, 2007) were also included. In addition, there were modules based on targeting practical aspects of daily life such as sleep, concentration management and

Table 1. Example modules used in Internet-based cognitive behavioural therapy Interventions

Introduction
• Rationale for the use of cognitive behavioural therapy
• Navigating the website
• Information about tinnitus
• Defining personal goals
• Identifying ways to prioritise spending time on the programme
Tools Provided Within the Intervention
• Applied relaxation
• Positive imagery
• Enhancing focusing
• Exposure to tinnitus
• Sound enrichment
• Reducing sound sensitivity
• Hearing tactics
• Cognitive restructuring
• Sleep management
• Concentration management
Evaluation and Maintenance
• Key point reflection of each intervention tool and evaluation of the effectiveness of each
• Planning how to maintain positive effects
• Relapse prevention planning

future planning. A progressive relaxation programme, together with techniques such as positive imagery, was incorporated to deal with the physical aspects of tinnitus and to promote behavioural change.

To emphasise the theoretical base individual modules should be organised into a clear structure, including an overview, explanation, and rational step-by- step instructions and further help section, covering possible difficulties that may have been experienced.

Providing Support

Internet interventions are either independent of professional support (unguided) or offer some form of support (guided). Guidance is a mechanism whereby individuals can obtain external information about themselves and their progress

(Barak, Klein, and Proudfoot, 2009). Guidance can be synchronous (such as real-time chats), asynchronous (such as emailing) or a blended approach combining various means (Andersson, Carlbring, Ljótsson, and Hedman, 2013). This contact ensures that individuals are supported but require less health professional contact time in comparison to face-to–face interventions (Paxling et al., 2013). The literature consistently shows that guided interventions lead to better outcomes, increased adherence and fewer dropouts, in comparison to unguided programmes (see (Baumeister, Reichler, Munzinger, and Lin, 2014) for a systematic review). Encouragingly, evidence has suggested that therapeutic alliance is important, and that the format thereof (e.g. face-to-face, video, or audio formats) does not lead to substantially different outcomes (Andersson et al., 2012; Day and Schneider, 2002). The Internet-intervention should, therefore, incorporate the flexibility to enable these communication systems. In guided interventions individuals can ask questions about the techniques or difficulties they experience and the health professional can provide further advice, support, motivation, feedback and encouragement as required. To enable appropriate support, the intervention should include notifications to the therapist when individuals have completed worksheets. Feedback can then be provided in a timely manner. A minimum of a weekly check is suggested for reviewing all recipients and providing messages appropriate to the level of engagement.

Overall, to date, evidence indicates that guidance is important and highly rated by individuals undertaking the interventions (Baumeister et al., 2014). Many questions remain regarding the optimal form of this guidance. There is no clear dose-response relationship between support and outcome (Palmqvist, Carlbring, and Andersson, 2007). Furthermore, there is no difference in outcomes when using an experienced or inexperienced therapist (Andersson et al., 2012). Titov et al. (2009; 2010) also found no difference in outcome when guidance was provided by a technician instead of a health professional. It appears as though having the support is the crucial element, rather than who provides the support. In many European based studies providing iCBT, clinical psychologists have provided the support as they are trained in providing CBT. In the UK, tinnitus is largely treated within the audiological community. To follow this approach an audiologist was used to provide iCBT in a UK based study (Beukes, Allen, Manchaiah, Baguley, and Andersson, 2017b; Beukes, Baguley, Allen, Manchaiah, and Andersson, 2017c). As the outcomes were similar to those from previous iCBT interventions using a clinical psychologist for support (e.g. (Jasper et al., 2014; Weise, Kleinstauber, and Andersson, 2016) using an audiologist in this context may be a viable option. Further research is required to directly compare outcomes obtained using different froms of guidance.

As those with tinnitus often feel isolated, peer support in group therapy can facilitate coping with tinnitus (Thompson, Pryce, and Refaie, 2011). Internet-interventions can include many forms of support. As one example, a discussion forum can, therefore, be included and this forum can be closed (allowing recipients to only read about peer experiences) or open (allowing users to communicate to each other, but moderated by the therapist). An example of a discussion forum topics for an iCBT intervention for tinnitus may be examples of how tinnitus can be reinterpreted, examples of where cognitive restructuring has been applied and how to make relaxation part of daily life.

Tailoring the Intervention

Interventions can be fully standardised or tailored by developing specific aspects based on individual characteristics (Kreuter, Strecher, and Glassman, 1999). This may be personalised communication and/or the ability to select certain therapeutic aspects of the intervention. Providing a tailored intervention aligns the intervention with specific difficulties individuals may be experiencing. Andersson and Kaldo (2004) included tailoring aspects in their tinnitus programme, such as personal treatment goals and receiving individualised weekly feedback. Due to the heterogeneous nature of tinnitus, a tailored intervention, with the flexibility to address individual needs and preferences, is more appropriate than a solely standardised approach. The evidence base supporting this is surprisingly inconclusive. In a meta-analysis reviewing 40 studies, (Lustria et al., 2013) found that tailored interventions resulted in significantly greater improvement in health outcomes compared to non-tailored interventions. On the other hand, Păsărelu, Andersson, Bergman Nordgren, and Dobrean (2017), did not find that tailored interventions lead to improved outcomes in a meta-analysis reviewing 19 Internet-based CBT studies for anxiety and depression. Tailored elements incorporated into Internet-delivered tinnitus programmes developed by Andersson and Kaldo, 2004 included aspects such as personal intervention goals and receiving individualised weekly feedback. The programmes included both optional and compulsory modules thereby acknowledging individual preferences by adapting the intervention according to the specific needs and capacity and by providing a choice of intervention modules according to the symptom profile (Andersson, Estling, Jakobsson, Cuijpers, and Carlbring, 2011). An example of tailoring by letting individual's select optional modules that match their symptom profiles is shown in Figure 1.

Figure 1. Example of a tailored intervention showing both fixed and optional modules from the tackling tinnitus internet-intervention

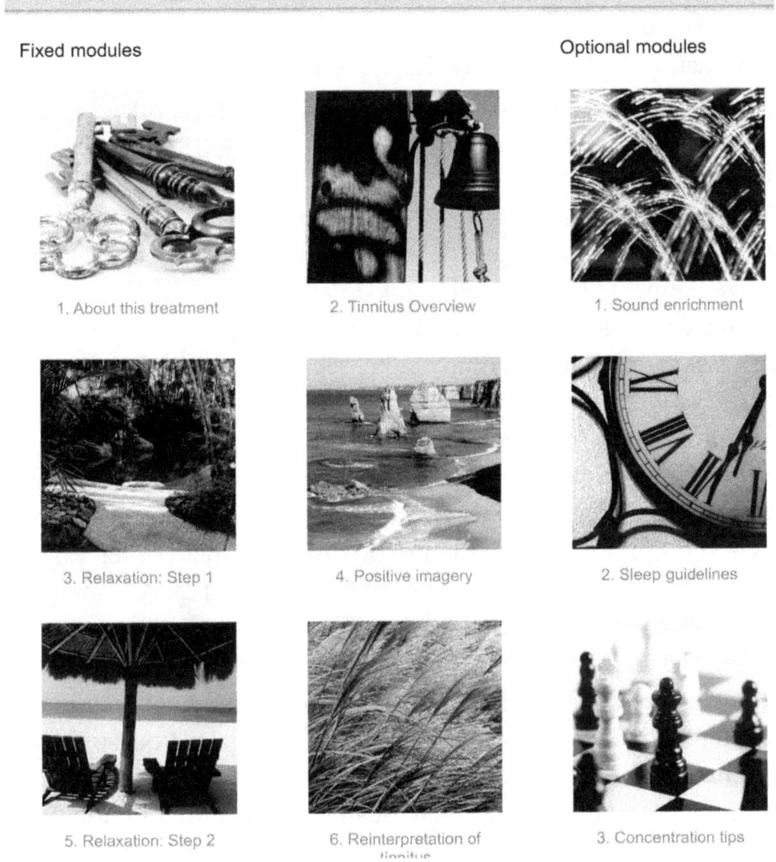
Fixed modules
Optional modules
1. About this treatment
2. Tinnitus Overview
1. Sound enrichment
3. Relaxation: Step 1
4. Positive imagery
2. Sleep guidelines
5. Relaxation: Step 2
6. Reinterpretation of
3. Concentration tips

Facilitating Participation

The intent of Internet-interventions is to maximise positive outcomes. Active involvement is a key component to deriving intervention benefit (James, 2013). Minimising technological barriers is imperative by ensuring information is straightforward to read and easily accessible. During the development of an Internet-based intervention for tinnitus in the UK, Beukes et al. (2016) facilitated participation by incorporating an interactive approach containing a mixture of information, videos, quizzes, diagrams, suggested techniques to apply to daily life, worksheets to keep track of progress, solutions for common problems and downloadable information. Multifunctional tools were used to address a variety of different learning styles. These tools also provided a means to assess and monitor progress which allowed the health professional to provide appropriate feedback. To ensure linguistic appropriateness, the Fletcher reading ease (ease of reading on a scale of 0–100) and Flesch-Kincaid Grade Level (the years of education required to understand the writing) of the intervention was assessed. The target was the generally recommended levels of around 60–70 and seven on each scale, respectively (Laplante-Lévesque, Brännström, Andersson, and Lunner, 2012) to ensure that this is not a barrier to participation.

Monitoring Aspects

In addition to the content for users, an Internet-intervention requires a strong administrative element. This should include data logging of the number of times users login, which modules they access, which worksheets are completed, and the number of messages sent. The administrative section is also required to assign roles to users, such as what therapeutic contact they may have and which discussion forums they have access to (Vlaescu et al. 2016).

The ability of the design to monitor progress over time as well as after completion of an intervention is essential. It has been established that collecting outcome measures online does not compromise the psychometric characteristics (Ritter, Lorig, Laurent, and Matthews, 2004; Thoren, Andersson, and Lunner, 2012). Advantages of online data collection include minimising the risk of missing items and that alerts can be provided when red flag questions, such as indicating possible onward referral, are answered. Responses can be verified where required by telephonic interview as a follow-up to the online questionnaire completion. Integrated questionnaires which can be automatically or manually assigned to users, reminders to complete the questionnaires and graphical progress indicators, are useful additional monitoring features.

A FRAMEWORK FOR EVALUATING INTERNET-BASED INTERVENTIONS

Barriers are often encountered during the translation of health-related research into clinical practice and policies (Grol, 2001; Harvey and Kitson, 2015). These barriers lead to discrepancies in evidence-based practice and to the public failing to benefit optimally from advances in healthcare (Grimshaw, Eccles, Lavis, Hill, and Squires, 2012). Tinnitus studies vary in design and there is significant heterogeneity in the evaluation of tinnitus perception and the questionnaires used (Landgrebe et al., 2012). This jeopardises comparison between trials and precludes meta-analysis of intervention effects. The lack of long-term results in addition to the common use of combined approaches in the management of tinnitus are in part responsible for the lack of conclusive evidence (Landgrebe et al., 2012). It is likely that the differences reported in efficacy and effectiveness of individual Internet-interventions are due to sub-optimal designs during intervention development and evaluation (Morrison et al., 2012). Ensuring that experimental designs include sequential phases of development and evaluation minimise these hurdles (Craig et al., 2008). Suggestions for the evaluation of Internet interventions in a clinical trial format are provided below.

Determining Functionality and Usability of the Intervention

The first step following intervention development is ensuring that no hindrances to its usage exist. In terms of an Internet intervention, the following functionality features should be tested as a minimum:

- Ensuring messages to recipients are delivered and not sent to spam folders is essential. It may be that certain email providers reject emails from providers as a result of certain words used in the messages.
- Checking that recipients are able to login without too much difficulty and providing clear login instructions.
- Testing the navigational aspects, hyperlinks, interactive components, media clips and media links included in the intervention are fully functioning.

In addition, competence associated with computer use can affect engagement with Internet interventions. Cultural differences in the level of computer literacy have previously been reported (Pflug, 2011). Aiming the functionality aspects of the intervention to match the estimated population of cultural computer skills is importance to aid its application.

User Satisfaction and Acceptability of the Intervention

The acceptability of an intervention has always been regarded as one of the key features regarding translating research into practice (Kaltenthaler et al., 2008). Lack of acceptability may influence take-up rates, increase dropout rates and therefore affect the overall effectiveness of an intervention. Acceptability is required by not only individuals undertaking the intervention but also by professionals and non-professionals who have an interest in tinnitus. An effective way is measuring perceived benefit of the actual intervention components in a multidimensional manner. Public patient forums are an ideal channel to enable these evaluations. Beukes et al. (2016) took the approach of letting both tinnitus professionals and users from a tinnitus support group evaluate iCBT adapted for those with tinnitus in the UK. These users were all accustomed to the standard face-to-face tinnitus interventions provided in the UK, so had this as their point of reference. Both groups highly rated the interventions suitability, content, usability, presentation and monitoring aspects. Open-ended questions were also used to identify which aspects of the intervention required improvement.

Nyenhuis, Zastrutzki, Weise, Jäger, and Kröner-Herwig, (2013) investigated the acceptance of iCBT versus that of group-based face-to-face (F2F) CBT for tinnitus by presenting both groups the same CBT manual material. They found that participants were as satisfied with the iCBT as they were with group-based cognitive behavioural therapy (GCBT) and the dropout attrition was similar, at 35% for both groups. However, more people in the iCBT group did not complete the programme at 64% opposed to 55% for the GCBT. They found that satisfaction was affected by the age of participants, confirming findings by Wise and collegues (Wise, Rief and Goebel,1998). Satisfaction with group training increased with age and satisfaction with iCBT decreased with age. Lower levels of initial tinnitus distress were associated with a higher satisfaction for iCBT, a trend not found for the F2F group.

Establishing Intervention Feasibility

Feasibility studies have the purpose of answering the questions regarding whether a study can be done, before the main study is attempted (Eldridge et al., 2016). Establishing the feasibility of a new intervention is crucial prior to more costly and larger scale studies. Various aspects of feasibility may be explored, depending on the nature of the intervention. These are discussed by Thabane et al. (2010) and include:

- Testing the safety of treatment or interventions
- Assessing recruitment potential
- Identifying the standard deviation from the main outcome measure to estimate sample size
- Determining the willingness of participants to be randomised or clinicians to recruit participants
- Retention rates
- Compliance, engagement and adherence rates
- To assess the time and resources required to run the trial
- To determine whether the the eligibility criteria is sufficient or too restrictive

Attrition rates are often a concern of any intervention including iCBT, with varying ranges reported such as 57% by Abbott et al., 2009) versus 5% by Hesser et al. (2011). Initial feasibility studies can help assess attrition rates and adjust protocols to reduce these if required. As iCBT for tinnitus has not been used in the UK before, Beukes et al. (2017b) ran a feasibility study to identify the recruitment potential, retention rates and intervention engagement. In comparison to the recruitment rates in Sweden, the initial take-up rates in the United Kingdom were low and the target population was not reached. This identified that the recruitment strategy was not optimal and strategies were put in place to improve recruitment for subsequent trials. Some participants struggled to engage with the iCBT intervention and the barriers identified included time constraints, work pressures, and poor health.

Kaldo et al. (2008) found that 43% of participants did not complete the full iCBT programme, but explained that this was similar when compared to the number of sessions actually attended by those receiving group-based CBT. Possible reasons have been attributed to (a) a higher intrinsic motivation for those that valued task completion (Donkin and Glozier, 2012), (b) were actively involved and (c) had a positive attitude and hope (Heinrich et al., 2016). By investigating such feasibility issues, they can be addressed before larger scale studies.

Piloting the Intervention

A pilot study is a smaller version study, resembling the design of a further larger scale trial (Eldridge et al., 2016). The importance of running a full pilot study as a proof-of-concept evaluation is often underestimated and omitted. It can assist with preparing and planning larger scaled investigations by examining the reliability and validity of the proposed study design (Thabane et al., 2010). The aim of a pilot study is not to evaluate a treatment effect, but rather to identify shortcomings in both the intervention and the protocol and can help to facilitate the smooth running of subsequent larger trials (Thabane et al., 2010). Pilot studies ensure that efficacy testing has the best chance of success by troubleshooting potential issues early on. They can increase the clinical experience of running a new intervention, generate data for sample size calculations and refine the inclusion and exclusion criteria. They can assess the time required to complete questionnaires and to do the intervention. Pilot studies have different objectives to the main trial and should include an intention for future work.

Assessing Intervention Efficacy

Determining the efficacy of an intervention is an important step during intervention evaluation. The design selected is crucial to ensure sound methodological principles are incorporated and bias is minimised. Efficacy trials prioritise internal validity and therefore include a control group in the study design. They evaluate whether an intervention can work under ideal circumstances (Cochrane, 1972). The use of randomised clinical trials (RCT) is a central component in evaluating new interventions. Participants are randomised into groups with the aim of obtaining an unbiased and reliable comparison these groups. Randomisation is important as it ensures that participants are objectively similar regarding demographic and prognostic factors in the selected groups. Randomisation achieves this as each participant has a known chance of being given the intervention in an allocation that cannot be predicted (Altman and Bland, 1999). Masking participants and researchers to group allocation where possible should be incorporated, as this removes any systematic bias there may be during the assessment and allocation during the trial conduct. To ensure that rigorous methods are selected, the Consolidated Standards of Reporting Trials (CONSORT) guidelines should be followed (Schulz, Altman, and Moher, 2010). These guidelines set standards to adhere to such as ensuring the trial will have enough power to produce statistically valid results.

The assessment measures selected to measure outcome need careful consideration to ensure they are appropriate for the study design. Self-reported assessment measures are generally used in clinical practice to quantify tinnitus distress and identify associated difficulties that may be present. An Internet intervention design has the advantage of enabling data collection of these assessment measures online. This reduces the administrative requirements associated with using hard copies. Algorithms can be used to automatically score responses and results can be easily exported.

Selecting assessment measures that have been psychometrically validated and match the trial design is important. The primary outcome of a tinnitus intervention would be a reduction in tinnitus-related distress after undergoing the intervention. It is of value to know if the intervention is effective at reducing any associated effects. Secondary outcomes may involve tinnitus-related difficulties such as insomnia, anxiety and depression (Hall et al., 2018). As an example Beukes et al. (2017c) included measures for insomnia, anxiety, depression, hyperacusis, hearing disability, cognitive failures, and life satisfaction.

Results of efficacy trials to date have indicated promise that iCBT for tinnitus can reduce tinnitus distress and many of the associated comorbidities as shown in Table 2. The results of early trials had small effect sizes, whereas later trials indicated medium to large effect sizes (by overcoming methodological shortcomings of some of the earlier trials).

Can Intervention Effects Be Maintained?

Evidence that intervention effects are maintained over time is important, especially when outlining the benefits of a new intervention. Measuring the stability of intervention effects at least 1 year post intervention is therefore important. It may be a challenge to obtain results at this time frame, and strategies need to be sought to encourage completion of assessment measures such as telephoning individuals prior to these assessments. Studies have evaluated the results of iCBT up to 1 year

Table 2. Results from iCBT efficacy trials using passive and active controls

Study	Country	Groups	Between group effect size for tinnitus distress post-intervention	Assessment Measures
Andersson, Strömgren, Ström, & Lyttkens, (2002)	Sweden	1. iCBT: n = 26 2. WLC: n = 64 who later undertook the intervention	$d = 0.27$	• Tinnitus distress • Anxiety • Depression • Insomnia
Kaldo et al. (2008)	Sweden	1.iCBT (n = 25) 2. GCBT (n = 26)	1. $d = 0.73$ 2. $d = 0.64$	• Anxiety • Depression • Insomnia • Visual analogue scales for tinnitus loudness, distress and perceived stress
Abbott et al. (2009)	Australia	1. iCBT: n = 32 2. Information only control (IOC): n = 24	$d = 0.25$	• Tinnitus distress • Depression
Hesser et al. (2011)	Sweden	1. iCBT: n = 32 [shorter text of 157 pages divided into 8 modules] 2. Internet based acceptance and commitment therapy (iACT): n = 35 [104 pages] 3. A discussion forum group control (DFC): n = 32	$d = 0.70$ for iCBT versus the control	• Tinnitus distress • Tinnitus acceptance • Anxiety • Depression • Quality of life • Perceived stress
Nyenhuis et al. (2013)	Germany	1. iCBT self-management (n=79) 2. CBT bibliotherapy (n = 77) 3. GCBT (n =71) 4. Information-only control (n = 77)	$d = 0.57$ for iCBT versus the control	• Tinnitus distress • Depression
Jasper et al. (2014)	Germany	1. iCBT (n = 41) 2. GCBT (n = 43) Internet-based discussion forum control (n = 44)	1. $d = 0.56$ for iCBT versus the control	• Tinnitus distress • Depression • Insomnia
Weise et al. (2016)	Germany	1. iCBT (n = 25) 2.GCBT (n = 26)	$d = 0.84$	• Tinnitus distress • Tinnitus • Acceptance • Depression • Anxiety insomnia
Beukes et al., (2017c)	UK	1. iCBT (n=73) 2. A weekly check in control (n=73)	$d = 0.69$	• Tinnitus distress • Anxiety • Depression • Insomnia • Hyperacusis • Hearing Disability • Cognitive failures • Satisfaction with life

post-intervention and have found maintenance of intervention effects. Three of these long-term studies have been in Sweden (Andersson et al., 2002; Kaldo et al. 2008; and Hesser et al. 2011), one in Germany (Weise et al., 2016) and a further one in the UK (Beukes, Allen, Baguey, Manchaiah, and Andersson, 2018a). Further exploration of intervention effects for 2 and 3 years post intervention is required.

Establishing Intervention Effectiveness in Regular Clinical Settings

It is not always clear whether results from efficacy studies can be generalised into normal clinical practice. A limitation of efficacy research is that intervention effects are not contextualised as they are not applicable in typical intervention settings (Glasgow, Lichtenstein, and Marcus, 2003). As a follow-up from these, effectiveness studies examine whether the intervention is effective in real-world clinical settings and in situations that health professions encounter in their daily routine practice (Lutz, 2003). This type of study emphasises the external validity of the research findings.

Effectiveness studies can take various forms. Some compare new interventions to the usual clinical care which is regarded as the gold standard of evaluating new interventions. The aim is generally to show that a new intervention is not inferior when compared to an existing intervention. Consort guidelines should be followed when running non-inferiority and equivalence randomised trials (Piaggio et al., 2012).

Internet interventions delivered in regular clinical services for a range of conditions and symptoms, consistently show sustained effects with moderate to large effect sizes (Andersson and Hedman, 2013). Previous trials comparing iCBT to the usual tinnitus care are summarised in Table 3.

There have been two Swedish studies looking at iCBT for tinnitus in a regular clinical setting (Uppsala Hospital in Sweden), using clinical psychologists and not using advertisements to recruit participants. The first was an open effectiveness trial by Kaldo-Sandström, Larsen, and Andersson (2004) using 77 participants. The within group effect size was Cohen's $d = 0.56$. The second offered two parallel interventions, namely, iCBT (n = 293) and a low-intensity version of iCBT (n = 81) aimed at those with lower tinnitus distress (Kaldo et al., 2013). Results indicated a reduction in tinnitus distress (Cohen's $d = 0.58$), depression, anxiety, and insomnia for those undertaking the full iCBT intervention. Those undertaking the low-intensity version also showed a reduction in tinnitus, although effect sizes were smaller. This may have been related to a lower baseline tinnitus distress levels. The authors concluded that guided iCBT could be successfully used in a regular clinical setting to reduce tinnitus distress. As iCBT has not to date been compared to individualised therapy, Beukes and colleagues (2018) compared iCBT to usual individuated tinnitus therapy

Table 3. Results comparing iCBT to usual clinical care

Study	Location	Groups	Within group effect size
Kaldo-Sandström, Larsen & Andersson (2004)	Sweden	iCBT (n = 77) not randomized from CBT waiting list	*Within group effect size for the iCBT group: d =* 0.66
Kaldo et al. (2013)	Sweden	1. iCBT (n = 293) 2. Low intensity iCBT (n = 81) Not randomised	*Within group effect size for the iCBT group: d =* 0.58 *Low intensity group: d = 0.26*
Beukes et al. (2018)	United Kingdom	3. iCBT (n = 46) 4. F2F individualised tinnitus care (n = 46)	*Between group effect size: d = 0.32* *Within-group iCBT effect size d = 1.28*

Acronyms: F2F: Face-to-Face; **GCBT:** Group-based cognitive behavioural therapy; **iCBT:** Internet-based cognitive behavioural therapy

in England in a non-inferiority randomised control trial and found that results from both interventions were comparable.

IMPLEMENTATION

Implementation of new interventions is complex and may require adaptation of settings and service systems (Andrews and Williams, 2015). Some aspects of guided Internet-Intervention make implementation easier than face-to-face therapies. These include having a highly structured and scripted nature, leaving less room for therapist drift. Outcome monitoring is also embedded in the implementation, thus facilitating the assessment of progress and safety. Rolling out implementation in different settings is also less complex due to the reduced need to duplicate resources, as the same intervention can be used in a centralised manner (Andersson and Titov, 2014). Strategies to aid implementation are discussed in the sections that follow.

Process Evaluation

Presenting the results of assessment outcomes alone do not provide enough information to determine whether new interventions work. A more holistic approach is required to interpret the results and identify factors that facilitate and hamper the application of interventions (Saunders, Evans, and Joshi, 2005). Process evaluation is a means of uncovering various aspects related to implementation and delivery of interventions over time (Manchaiah, Danermark, Ronnberg, and Lunner, 2014). This includes indicating the research context, factors that contribute to positive outcomes and how interventions can be optimised (Moore et al., 2015). Process evaluation provides the opportunity to collect both quantitative and qualitative information that can provide a holistic view of any intervention effects. These models can be used to provide a framework for evaluating an intervention's potential for successful implementation. The models that have been widely used in healthcare interventions include those of Baranowski and Stables (2000) that suggest 11 components, and the Reach, Efficacy, Adoption, Implementation and Maintenance framework (RE-AIM; (Glasgow, Vogt, and Boles, 1999). These models give balanced attention to both internal and external validity elements of research design and evaluation and can be used to estimate the potential public health impact of interventions.

Despite the relevance of process evaluation, there has only been one comprehensive process evaluation to date investigating factors that facilitate or hinder implementation of iCBT for tinnitus (Beukes, Manchaiah, Baguley, Allen, and Andersson, 2017). The parameters they chose are shown in Table 4. Performing a process evaluation indicated barriers that would need to be addressed prior to implementing this intervention. These included improving engagement and motivation, which was found to be variable and encouraging intervention take-up in groups least likely to undertake the intervention such as young adults and those in remote areas.

Establishing Cost-Effectiveness

Where possible cost-effectiveness should be established together with clinical effectiveness in order to be useful for decision makers/budget holders. To date, this aspect has been rarely evaluated (Kaldo et al., 2008) reported that iCBT for tinnitus was 1.7 times more time-effective than seven sessions of group-based CBT in Sweden whereas Beukes and collegues (2018) found iCBT 2.7 times as time-effective compared with individualised tinnitus care. A lexicon of assessment and outcome measures for tele-mental health has been developed as a resource for the evaluation of these services (Shore et al., 2014). Evaluation metrics include treatment utilisation, travel costs, stigma, anxiety, waiting times, training, and motivational readiness. Future research can use these domains to standardise approaches, to determine cost effectiveness and provide a more comprehensive comparison of services.

Key Strategies to Aid Implementation

There are some key strategies to help new intervention translation into routine practice as suggested by Craig et al. (2008). Implementation of new interventions is dependent

Table 4. Process evaluation parameters used by (Beukes et al., 2017)

Process	Description	Assessment measure
Processes related to the research context		
Recruitment	Procedures used to approach and attract participants	Monitoring traffic on the recruitment website via Google analytics
Reach	The extent to which the intervention was received by the targeted population of those with distressing tinnitus who were underserved with previous interventions for tinnitus	Demographic questionnaire
Context	The social, demographic and socio-economic characteristic of the participants that may affect generalisability of the outcomes	Demographic questionnaire and baseline levels on assessment measures
Processes related to the intervention delivery		
Treatment (dose) delivered	Intervention components actually provided to participants	Nature of the guided-intervention
Treatment (dose) received	The extent to which participants engaged in and adhered to the intervention	Data logging
Processes related to the outcomes obtained		
Barriers affecting the outcomes obtained	Barriers that may affect the outcomes obtained	Post-intervention satisfaction questionnaire
Factors facilitating effectiveness	Intervention's effectiveness from the participant's perspective	A benefit questionnaire was used to rate the iCBT modules

on removing known barriers that are likely to prevent implementation. These may include legal, confidentiality, data-security, cost, acceptance and operational barriers (Hill and Powell, 2009).

In addition, intervention credibility is required. Acceptance of new interventions is largely based on health professionals' attitude toward them (Perle et al., 2013). Much work is still required to improve attitudes towards Internet-interventions from both the perspectives of patients and healthcare professionals (Eikelboom, 2016). Unfounded fears, such as concerns that clinical intervention routes will no longer be required need to be addressed. Additional management routes are required to complement existing interventions as many people are unable to access tinnitus interventions at present. Approaching these fears in a culturally sensitive manner is important (Hadjistavropoulos, Thompson, Klein, and Austin, 2012).

Patient's perception of Internet interventions is also important. Musiat, Goldstone, and Tarrier (2014) found that perceptions in the UK of computerised interventions were poor and a greater acceptance was found for face-to-face interventions. In Europe, variable results have been found. Kaldo et al. (2008) compared intervention credibility ratings for those experiencing significant tinnitus. They found that group CBT was rated more credible than iCBT. On the other hand, Kaldo-Sandström et al. (2004) did not find a difference in credibility rating between iCBT and group-based CBT. Much work is still required in this area before Internet-interventions are viewed as credible interventions by patients, health professionals and stakeholders alike.

SOLUTIONS AND RECOMMENDATIONS

This chapter has outlined the potential for Internet-Interventions to improve healthcare for tinnitus. The ultimate health-care goal would be to help implement innovative interventions that demonstrate benefits into clinical practice. In reality there is poor translation of these research findings into practice due to the challenging and multifaceted processes required. This chapter aims to improve rates of success by providing a framework to assist in the design of evidence-based effective interventions that have been appropriately evaluated.

Effectiveness studies are required as a minimum to ensure the intervention works in practice, can be delivered in the intended setting, and be cost effective. Prior to implementation, it is recommended that two efficacy and two effectiveness trials are performed to ensure the intervention can be delivered in the intended settings and within the proposed budget (Tomlinson, Rotheram-Borus, Swartz, and Tsai, 2013)

In terms of Internet interventions for tinnitus, these should be regarded as a complement to other services and by no means a replacement for face-to-face therapies which are beneficial particularly to those with complex needs and those unable to use the Internet. The aim would be to run tele-audiology services in parallel to other currently provided tinnitus interventions.

A key strategy of implementation is involving stakeholders from the inception in the choice of research design to identify elements relevant to decision-making, such as benefits, harms, and costs. Outlining the intended intervention effects are also required. In addition ensuring health professionals are positive about implementing these services is important.

Interventions will also require tailoring according to the specific implementation context. Strategies to ensure continued evaluation and monitoring need to be in place (Andrews and Williams, 2015). These innovations require dedicated practitioners to integrate forms of tele-audiology into healthcare using innovate solutions.

FUTURE RESEARCH DIRECTIONS

There are numerous future research themes still required before Internet-interventions can be integrated into clinical care. One is to identify for whom these Internet interventions are most suitable. To date, there are no established predictors for outcomes of guided iCBT (Andersson and Hedman, 2013).

Although support within Internet interventions both from health professionals and peers with tinnitus is important, the optimal way to provide support requires further attention. The degree and form of guidance required still needs to be established. Factors aiding implementation of Internet-based interventions will also strengthen implementation of new interventions. One challenge is keeping up with the dynamic nature of the field by continually updating these interventions according to advances in the research. Perhaps the greatest research challenge is identifying factors that can aid acceptability and credibility of these interventions by health professionals and stakeholders. It is also important to ensure that end-users value these services and are satisfied with what they offer.

CONCLUSION

Much potential exists for tele-audiology. One form of tele-audiology, namely an Internet-based intervention for tinnitus has been discussed. The process from development to implementation is outlined and a framework is provided that can be used by those interested in further developing tele-audiology, an area filled with potential.

ACKNOWLEDGMENT

We are grateful to the British Society of Audiology for funding the effectiveness trial in the UK. We would like to thank Linköping University, Anglia Ruskin University, Lamar University and the University of Nottingham for supporting work related developing Internet-Interventions for Tinnitus. We thank George Vlaescu for his expertise in web design and technical support.

DISCLAIMER

The involvement of the authors was supported by their institutions, Anglia Ruskin University, Lamar University, Linköping University, National Institute of Health Research, but the views expressed are made by the authors and do not represent those of these institutions nor the UK Department of Health. These organisations had no role in the approval or preparation of this chapter.

REFERENCES

Abbott, J. M., Kaldo, V., Klein, B., Austin, D., Hamilton, C., Piterman, L., ... Andersson, G. (2009). A cluster randomised trial of an internet-based intervention program for tinnitus distress in an industrial setting. *Cognitive Behaviour Therapy, 38*(3), 162–173. doi:10.1080/16506070902763174 PMID:19675959

Altman, D. G., & Bland, J. M. (1999). How to randomise. *BMJ (Clinical Research Ed.), 319*(7211), 703–704. doi:10.1136/bmj.319.7211.703 PMID:10480833

Andersson, G. (2002). Psychological aspects of tinnitus and the application of cognitive–behavioral therapy. *Clinical Psychology Review, 22*(7), 977–990. doi:10.1016/S0272-7358(01)00124-6 PMID:12238249

Andersson, G., Carlbring, P., Berger, T., Almlöv, J., & Cuijpers, P. (2009). What makes internet therapy work? *Cognitive Behaviour Therapy, 38*(sup1S1), 55–60. doi:10.1080/16506070902916400 PMID:19675956

Andersson, G., Carlbring, P., Ljótsson, B., & Hedman, E. (2013). Guided internet-based CBT for common mental disorders. *Journal of Contemporary Psychotherapy, 43*(4), 223–233. doi:10.100710879-013-9237-9

Andersson, G., Estling, F., Jakobsson, E., Cuijpers, P., & Carlbring, P. (2011). Can the patient decide which modules to endorse? an open trial of tailored internet treatment of anxiety disorders. *Cognitive Behaviour Therapy, 40*(1), 57–64. doi:10.1080/16506073.2010.529457 PMID:21337215

Andersson, G., & Hedman, E. (2013). Effectiveness of guided internet-based cognitive behavior therapy in regular clinical settings. *Verhaltenstherapie, 23*(3), 140–148. doi:10.1159/000354779

Andersson, G., & Kaldo, V. (2004). Internet-based cognitive behavioral therapy for tinnitus. *Journal of Clinical Psychology, 60*(2), 171–178. doi:10.1002/jclp.10243 PMID:14724924

Andersson, G., Paxling, B., Wiwe, M., Vernmark, K., Felix, C. B., Lundborg, L., ... Carlbring, P. (2012). Therapeutic alliance in guided internet-delivered cognitive behavioural treatment of depression, generalized anxiety disorder and social anxiety disorder. *Behaviour Research and Therapy, 50*(9), 544–550. doi:10.1016/j.brat.2012.05.003 PMID:22728647

Andersson, G., Strömgren, T., Ström, L., & Lyttkens, L. (2002). Randomized controlled trial of internet-based cognitive behavior therapy for distress associated with tinnitus. *Psychosomatic Medicine, 64*(5), 810–816. PMID:12271112

Andersson, G., & Titov, N. (2014). Advantages and limitations of internet-based interventions for common mental disorders. *World Psychiatry; Official Journal of the World Psychiatric Association (WPA)*, *13*(1), 4–11. doi:10.1002/wps.20083 PMID:24497236

Andrews, G., & Williams, A. D. (2015). Up-scaling clinician assisted internet cognitive behavioural therapy (iCBT) for depression: A model for dissemination into primary care. *Clinical Psychology Review*, *41*, 40–48. doi:10.1016/j.cpr.2014.05.006 PMID:25043445

Arnberg, F. K., Linton, S. J., Hultcrantz, M., Heintz, E., & Jonsson, U. (2014). Internet-delivered psychological treatments for mood and anxiety disorders: A systematic review of their efficacy, safety, and cost-effectiveness. *PLoS One*, *9*(5), e98118. doi:10.1371/journal.pone.0098118 PMID:24844847

Baguley, D., Andersson, G., McFerran, D., & McKenna, L. (2013). A multidisciplinary synthesis. Tinnitus: A Multidisciplinary Approach, 221-224.

Barak, A., Klein, B., & Proudfoot, J. G. (2009). Defining internet-supported therapeutic interventions. *Annals of Behavioral Medicine*, *38*(1), 4–17. doi:10.100712160-009-9130-7 PMID:19787305

Baranowski, T., & Stables, G. (2000). Process evaluations of the 5-a-day projects. *Health Education & Behavior: The Official Publication of the Society for Public Health Education*, *27*(2), 157–166. doi:10.1177/109019810002700202 PMID:10768797

Baumeister, H., Reichler, L., Munzinger, M., & Lin, J. (2014). The impact of guidance on internet-based mental health interventions—A systematic review. *Internet Interventions*, *1*(4), 205–215. doi:10.1016/j.invent.2014.08.003

Bendelin, N., Hesser, H., Dahl, J., Carlbring, P., Nelson, K. Z., & Andersson, G. (2011). Experiences of guided internet-based cognitive-behavioural treatment for depression: A qualitative study. *BMC Psychiatry*, *11*(1), 107. doi:10.1186/1471-244X-11-107 PMID:21718523

Bennett, K., Bennett, A. J., & Griffiths, K. M. (2010). Security considerations for e-mental health interventions. *Journal of Medical Internet Research*, *12*(5), e61. doi:10.2196/jmir.1468 PMID:21169173

Beukes, E. W., Allen, P. A., Baguley, D. M., Manchaiah, V., & Andersson, G. (2018a). Long-term efficacy of audiologist-guided internet-based cognitive behaviour therapy for tinnitus. *American Journal of Audiology*, *27*(3S). doi:10.1044/2018_AJA-IMIA3-18-0004

Beukes, E. W., Allen, P. M., Manchaiah, V., Baguley, D. M., & Andersson, G. (2017b). Internet-based intervention for tinnitus: Outcome of a single-group open trial. *Journal of the American Academy of Audiology*, *28*(4), 340–351. doi:10.3766/jaaa.16055 PMID:28418328

Beukes, E. W., Andersson, G., Allen, P., Manchaiah, V., & Baguley, D. M. (2018). Effectiveness of Guided Internet-Based Cognitive Behavioral Therapy vs Face-to-Face Clinical Care for Treatment of TinnitusA Randomized Clinical Trial. *JAMA Otolaryngology-Head & Neck Surgery*. Published online October 04, 2018. doi:10.1001/jamaoto.2018.2238

Beukes, E. W., Baguley, D. M., Allen, P. M., Manchaiah, V., & Andersson, G. (2017c). Audiologist-guided internet-based cognitive behaviour therapy for adults with tinnitus in the United Kingdom: A randomized controlled trial. *Ear and Hearing*, *39*, 423–433. doi:10.1097/AUD.0000000000000505 PMID:29095725

Beukes, E. W., Manchaiah, V., Andersson, G., Allen, P. M., Terlizzi, P. M., & Baguley, D. M. (2017a). Situationally influenced tinnitus coping strategies: A mixed methods approach. *Disability and Rehabilitation*, 1–11. doi:10.1080/09638288.2017.1362708 PMID:28793790

Beukes, E. W., Manchaiah, V., Baguley, D. M., Allen, P. M., & Andersson, G. (2017). Process evaluation of internet-based cognitive behavioural therapy for adults with tinnitus in the context of a randomised control trial. *International Journal of Audiology*, *57*(2), 98–109. doi:10.1080/14992027.2017.1384858 PMID:28990807

Beukes, E. W., Vlaescu, G., Manchaiah, V., Baguley, D. M., Allen, P. M., Kaldo, V., & Andersson, G. (2016). Development and technical functionality of an internet-based intervention for tinnitus in the UK. *Internet Interventions*, *6*, 6–15. doi:10.1016/j.invent.2016.08.002 PMID:30135809

Bhatt, J. M., Lin, H. W., & Bhattacharyya, N. (2016). Prevalence, severity, exposures, and treatment patterns of tinnitus in the United States. *JAMA Otolaryngology-Head & Neck Surgery*, *142*(10), 959–965. doi:10.1001/jamaoto.2016.1700 PMID:27441392

Campbell, M., Fitzpatrick, R., Haines, A., & Kinmonth, A. L. (2000). Framework for design and evaluation of complex interventions to improve health. *British Medical Journal*, *321*(7262), 694–696. doi:10.1136/bmj.321.7262.694 PMID:10987780

Chiang, L., Chen, W., Dai, Y., & Ho, Y. (2012). The effectiveness of telehealth care on caregiver burden, mastery of stress, and family function among family caregivers of heart failure patients: A quasi-experimental study. *International Journal of Nursing Studies*, *49*(10), 1230–1242. doi:10.1016/j.ijnurstu.2012.04.013 PMID:22633448

Chiauzzi, E., Rodarte, C., & DasMahapatra, P. (2015). Patient-centered activity monitoring in the self-management of chronic health conditions. *BMC Medicine, 13*(1), 77. doi:10.118612916-015-0319-2 PMID:25889598

Cima, R., Joore, M., Maes, I., Scheyen, D., Refaie, A. E., Baguley, D. M., Vlaeyen, J.W., & Anteunis, L. (2009). Cost-effectiveness of multidisciplinary management of tinnitus at a specialized tinnitus centre. *BMC Health Services Research, 9*, 29-6963-9-29.

Cima, R. F., Vlaeyen, J. W., Maes, I. H., Joore, M. A., & Anteunis, L. J. (2011). Tinnitus interferes with daily life activities: A psychometric examination of the tinnitus disability index. *Ear and Hearing, 32*(5), 623–633. doi:10.1097/AUD.0b013e31820dd411 PMID:21336139

Cochrane, A. (1972). *Effectiveness and efficiency: Random reflections on health services*. London: Academic Press.

Craig, P., Dieppe, P., Macintyre, S., Michie, S., Nazareth, I., Petticrew, M., & Medical Research Council Guidance. (2008). Developing and evaluating complex interventions: The new medical research council guidance. BMJ (Clinical Research Ed.), 337.

Cuijpers, P., van Straten, A., & Andersson, G. (2008). Internet-administered cognitive behavior therapy for health problems: A systematic review. *Journal of Behavioral Medicine, 31*(2), 169–177. doi:10.100710865-007-9144-1 PMID:18165893

Davis, A., & Rafaie, E. A. (2000). Epidemiology of tinnitus. *Tinnitus Handbook,*, 1-23.

Day, S. X., & Schneider, P. L. (2002). Psychotherapy using distance technology: A comparison of face-to-face, video, and audio treatment. *Journal of Counseling Psychology, 49*(4), 499–503. doi:10.1037/0022-0167.49.4.499

Donkin, L., & Glozier, N. (2012). Motivators and motivations to persist with online psychological interventions: A qualitative study of treatment completers. *Journal of Medical Internet Research, 14*(3), e91. doi:10.2196/jmir.2100 PMID:22743581

Eikelboom, R. H., & Swanepoel, D. W. (2016). International survey of audiologists' attitudes toward telehealth. *American Journal of Audiology, 25*(3S), 295–298. doi:10.1044/2016_AJA-16-0004 PMID:27768191

Eldridge, S. M., Lancaster, G. A., Campbell, M. J., Thabane, L., Hopewell, S., Coleman, C. L., & Bond, C. M. (2016). Defining feasibility and pilot studies in preparation for randomised controlled trials: Development of a conceptual framework. *PLoS One*, *11*(3), e0150205. doi:10.1371/journal.pone.0150205 PMID:26978655

Elgoyhen, A. B., Langguth, B., De Ridder, D., & Vanneste, S. (2015). Tinnitus: Perspectives from human neuroimaging. *Nature Reviews. Neuroscience*.

Ferguson, M., & Henshaw, H. (2015). Computer and internet interventions to optimize listening and learning for people with hearing loss: Accessibility, use, and adherence. [PubMed]. *American Journal of Audiology*, *24*(3), 338–343. doi:10.1044/2015_AJA-14-0090

Gander, P. E., Hoare, D. J., Collins, L., Smith, S., & Hall, D. A. (2011). Tinnitus referral pathways within the national health service in England: A survey of their perceived effectiveness among audiology staff. *BMC Health Services Research*, *11*(1), 1. doi:10.1186/1472-6963-11-162 PMID:21733188

Glasgow, R. E., Lichtenstein, E., & Marcus, A. C. (2003). Why don't we see more translation of health promotion research to practice? rethinking the efficacy-to-effectiveness transition. *American Journal of Public Health*, *93*(8), 1261–1267. doi:10.2105/AJPH.93.8.1261 PMID:12893608

Glasgow, R. E., Vogt, T. M., & Boles, S. M. (1999). Evaluating the public health impact of health promotion interventions: The RE-AIM framework. *American Journal of Public Health*, *89*(9), 1322–1327. doi:10.2105/AJPH.89.9.1322 PMID:10474547

Greenwell, K., Featherstone, D., & Hoare, D. J. (2015). The application of intervention coding methodology to describe the tinnitus e-programme, an internet-delivered self-help intervention for tinnitus. *American Journal of Audiology*, *24*(3), 311–315. PMID:26649537

Grewal, R., Spielmann, P., Jones, S., & Hussain, S. (2014). Clinical efficacy of tinnitus retraining therapy and cognitive behavioural therapy in the treatment of subjective tinnitus: A systematic review. *The Journal of Laryngology and Otology*, *128*(12), 1028–1033. doi:10.1017/S0022215114002849 PMID:25417546

Griffiths, F., Lindenmeyer, A., Powell, J., Lowe, P., & Thorogood, M. (2006). Why are health care interventions delivered over the internet? A systematic review of the published literature. *Journal of Medical Internet Research*, *8*(2), e10. doi:10.2196/jmir.8.2.e10 PMID:16867965

Griffiths, K. M., & Christensen, H. (2007). Internet-based mental health programs: A powerful tool in the rural medical kit. *The Australian Journal of Rural Health*, *15*(2), 81–87. doi:10.1111/j.1440-1584.2007.00859.x PMID:17441815

Grimshaw, J. M., Eccles, M. P., Lavis, J. N., Hill, S. J., & Squires, J. E. (2012). Knowledge translation of research findings. *Implementation Science; IS*, *7*(1), 1. doi:10.1186/1748-5908-7-50 PMID:22651257

Grol, R. (2001). Successes and failures in the implementation of evidence-based guidelines for clinical practice. *Medical Care*, *39*(8), II-46–II-54. PMID:11583121

Hadjistavropoulos, H. D., Thompson, M. J., Klein, B., & Austin, D. W. (2012). Dissemination of therapist-assisted internet cognitive behaviour therapy: Development and open pilot study of a workshop. *Cognitive Behaviour Therapy*, *41*(3), 230–240. doi:10.1080/16506073.2011.645550 PMID:22428582

Hall, D. A., Fackrell, K., Li, A. B., Thavayogan, R., Smith, S., Kennedy, V., ... Haider, H. F. (2018). A narrative synthesis of research evidence for tinnitus-related complaints as reported by patients and their significant others. *Health and Quality of Life Outcomes*, *16*(1), 61. doi:10.118612955-018-0888-9 PMID:29642913

Hall, D. A., Láinez, M. J., Newman, C. W., Sanchez, T. G., Egler, M., Tennigkeit, F., ... Langguth, B. (2011). Treatment options for subjective tinnitus: Self reports from a sample of general practitioners and ENT physicians within Europe and the USA. *BMC Health Services Research*, *11*(1), 302. doi:10.1186/1472-6963-11-302 PMID:22053947

Hallam, R., Rachman, S., & Hinchcliffe, R. (1984). Psychological aspects of tinnitus. *Contributions to Medical Psychology*, *3*, 31–53.

Harvey, G., & Kitson, A. (2015). Translating evidence into healthcare policy and practice: Single versus multi-faceted implementation strategies–is there a simple answer to a complex question? *International Journal of Health Policy and Management*, *4*(3), 123–126. doi:10.15171/ijhpm.2015.54 PMID:25774368

Hayes, S. C., Wilson, K. G., Gifford, E. V., Follette, V. M., & Strosahl, K. (1996). Experiential avoidance and behavioural disorders: A functional dimensional approach to diagnosis and treatment. *Journal of Consulting and Clinical Psychology*, *64*(6), 1152–1168. doi:10.1037/0022-006X.64.6.1152 PMID:8991302

Hedman, E., El Alaoui, S., Lindefors, N., Andersson, E., Rück, C., Ghaderi, A., ... Ljótsson, B. (2014). Clinical effectiveness and cost-effectiveness of internet-vs. group-based cognitive behavior therapy for social anxiety disorder: 4-year follow-up of a randomized trial. *Behaviour Research and Therapy*, *59*, 20–29. doi:10.1016/j.brat.2014.05.010 PMID:24949908

Heinrich, S., Rozental, A., Carlbring, P., Andersson, G., Cotter, K., & Weise, C. (2016). Treating tinnitus distress via the internet: A mixed methods approach of what makes patients seek help and stay motivated during internet-based cognitive behavior therapy. *Internet Interventions*, *4*, 120–130. doi:10.1016/j.invent.2016.04.001 PMID:30135798

Henry, J. L., & Wilson, P. H. (2001). *The psychological management of chronic tinnitus: A cognitive-behavioral approach*. Allyn & Bacon.

Hesser, H., Weise, C., Westin, V. Z., & Andersson, G. (2011). A systematic review and meta-analysis of randomized controlled trials of cognitive–behavioral therapy for tinnitus distress. *Clinical Psychology Review*, *31*(4), 545–553. doi:10.1016/j.cpr.2010.12.006 PMID:21237544

Hill, J. W., & Powell, P. (2009). The national healthcare crisis: Is eHealth a key solution? *Business Horizons*, *52*(3), 265–277. doi:10.1016/j.bushor.2009.01.006

Hoare, D. J., Kowalkowski, V. L., Kang, S., & Hall, D. A. (2011). Systematic review and meta-analyses of randomized controlled trials examining tinnitus management. *The Laryngoscope*, *121*(7), 1555–1564. doi:10.1002/lary.21825 PMID:21671234

James, J. A. (2013). *Patient engagement: People actively involved in their health and health care tend to have better outcomes--and, some evidence suggests, lower costs*. Project HOPE.

Jasper, K., Weise, C., Conrad, I., Andersson, G., Hiller, W., & Kleinstaeuber, M. (2014). Internet- based guided self-help versus group cognitive behavioral therapy for chronic tinnitus: A randomized controlled trial. *Psychotherapy and Psychosomatics*, *83*(4), 234–246. doi:10.1159/000360705 PMID:24970708

Jastreboff, M. M. (2007). Sound therapies for tinnitus management. *Progress in Brain Research*, *166*, 435–440. doi:10.1016/S0079-6123(07)66042-7 PMID:17956808

Johansson, R., & Andersson, G. (2012). Internet-based psychological treatments for depression. *Expert Review of Neurotherapeutics*, *12*(7), 861–870. doi:10.1586/ern.12.63 PMID:22853793

Kaldo, V., Cars, S., Rahnert, M., Larsen, H. C., & Andersson, G. (2007). Use of a self-help book with weekly therapist contact to reduce tinnitus distress: A randomized controlled trial. *Journal of Psychosomatic Research*, *63*(2), 195–202. doi:10.1016/j.jpsychores.2007.04.007 PMID:17662757

Kaldo, V., Haak, T., Buhrman, M., Alfonsson, S., Larsen, H., & Andersson, G. (2013). Internet-based cognitive behaviour therapy for tinnitus patients delivered in a regular clinical setting: Outcome and analysis of treatment dropout. *Cognitive Behaviour Therapy*, *42*(2), 146–158. doi:10.1080/16506073.2013.769622 PMID:23432207

Kaldo, V., Levin, S., Widarsson, J., Buhrman, M., Larsen, H. C., & Andersson, G. (2008). Internet versus group cognitive-behavioral treatment of distress associated with tinnitus: A randomized controlled trial. *Behavior Therapy*, *39*(4), 348–359. doi:10.1016/j.beth.2007.10.003 PMID:19027431

Kaldo-Sandström, V., Larsen, H. C., & Andersson, G. (2004). Internet- based cognitive-behavioral self-help treatment of tinnitus: Clinical effectiveness and predictors of outcome. *American Journal of Audiology*, *13*(2), 185–192. doi:10.1044/1059-0889(2004/023) PMID:15903144

Kaltenthaler, E., Sutcliffe, P., Parry, G., Beverley, C., Rees, A., & Ferriter, M. (2008). The acceptability to patients of computerized cognitive behaviour therapy for depression: A systematic review. *Psychological Medicine*, *38*(11), 1521–1530. doi:10.1017/S0033291707002607 PMID:18205964

Kaplan, K., Salzer, M. S., Solomon, P., Brusilovskiy, E., & Cousounis, P. (2011). Internet peer support for individuals with psychiatric disabilities: A randomized controlled trial. *Social Science & Medicine*, *72*(1), 54–62. doi:10.1016/j.socscimed.2010.09.037 PMID:21112682

Khedr, E. M., Ahmed, M. A., Shawky, O. A., Mohamed, E. S., El Attar, G. S., & Mohammad, K. A. (2010). Epidemiological study of chronic tinnitus in Assiut, Egypt. *Neuroepidemiology*, *35*(1), 45–52. doi:10.1159/000306630 PMID:20389124

Kreuter, M. W., Strecher, V. J., & Glassman, B. (1999). One size does not fit all: The case for tailoring print materials. *Annals of Behavioral Medicine*, *21*(4), 276–283. doi:10.1007/BF02895958 PMID:10721433

Landgrebe, M., Azevedo, A., Baguley, D., Bauer, C., Cacace, A., Coelho, C., ... Langguth, B. (2012). Methodological aspects of clinical trials in tinnitus: A proposal for an international standard. *Journal of Psychosomatic Research*, *73*(2), 112–121. doi:10.1016/j.jpsychores.2012.05.002 PMID:22789414

Langguth, B. (2011). A review of tinnitus symptoms beyond 'ringing in the ears': A call to action. *Current Medical Research and Opinion*, *27*(8), 1635–1643. doi:10.1185/03007995.2011.595781 PMID:21699365

Laplante-Lévesque, A., Brännström, K. J., Andersson, G., & Lunner, T. (2012). Quality and readability of English-language internet information for adults with hearing impairment and their significant others. *International Journal of Audiology*, *51*(8), 618–626. doi:10.3109/14992027.2012.684406 PMID:22731921

Lustria, M. L. A., Noar, S. M., Cortese, J., Van Stee, S. K., Glueckauf, R. L., & Lee, J. (2013). A meta-analysis of web-delivered tailored health behavior change interventions. *Journal of Health Communication*, *18*(9), 1039–1069. doi:10.1080/10810730.2013.768727 PMID:23750972

Lutz, W. (2003). Efficacy, effectiveness, and expected treatment response in psychotherapy. *Journal of Clinical Psychology*, *59*(7), 745–750. doi:10.1002/jclp.10169 PMID:12808581

Manchaiah, V., Danermark, B., Ronnberg, J., & Lunner, T. (2014). Importance of "process evaluation" in audiological rehabilitation: Examples from studies on hearing impairment. *International Journal of Otolaryngology*, *2014*, 168684. doi:10.1155/2014/168684 PMID:25276135

Martinez, C., Wallenhorst, C., McFerran, D., & Hall, D. A. (2015). Incidence rates of clinically significant tinnitus: 10-year trend from a cohort study in England. *Ear and Hearing*, *36*(3), e69–e75. doi:10.1097/AUD.0000000000000121 PMID:25470370

McFerran, D., Hoare, D. J., Carr, S., Ray, J., & Stockdale, D. (2018). Tinnitus services in the united kingdom: A survey of patient experiences. *BMC Health Services Research*, *18*(1), 110. doi:10.118612913-018-2914-3 PMID:29433479

Michikawa, T., Nishiwaki, Y., Kikuchi, Y., Saito, H., Mizutari, K., Okamoto, M., & Takebayashi, T. (2010). Prevalence and factors associated with tinnitus: A community-based study of japanese elders. *Journal of Epidemiology*, *20*(4), 271–276. doi:10.2188/jea.JE20090121 PMID:20501961

Moore, G., Audrey, S., Barker, M., Bond, L., Bonell, C., Hardeman, W., … & Baird, J. (2015). Process evaluation of complex interventions. *Complex Interventions in Health: An Overview of Research Methods,* 222 - 231.

Morrison, L. G., Yardley, L., Powell, J., & Michie, S. (2012). What design features are used in effective e-health interventions? A review using techniques from critical interpretive synthesis. *Telemedicine Journal and e-Health*, *18*(2), 137–144. doi:10.1089/tmj.2011.0062 PMID:22381060

Muñoz, R. F. (2010). Using evidence-based internet interventions to reduce health disparities worldwide. *Journal of Medical Internet Research*, *12*(5), e60. doi:10.2196/jmir.1463 PMID:21169162

Musiat, P., Goldstone, P., & Tarrier, N. (2014). Understanding the acceptability of e-mental health-attitudes and expectations towards computerised self-help treatments for mental health problems. *BMC Psychiatry*, *14*(1), 109. doi:10.1186/1471-244X-14-109 PMID:24725765

Nyenhuis, N., Golm, D., & Kröner-Herwig, B. (2013). A systematic review and meta-analysis on the efficacy of self-help interventions in tinnitus. *Cognitive Behaviour Therapy*, *42*(2), 159–169. doi:10.1080/16506073.2013.803496 PMID:23777192

Nyenhuis, N., Zastrutzki, S., Weise, C., Jäger, B., & Kröner-Herwig, B. (2013). The efficacy of minimal contact interventions for acute tinnitus: A randomised controlled study. *Cognitive Behaviour Therapy*, *42*(2), 127–138. doi:10.1080/16506073.2012.655305 PMID:22413736

Palmqvist, B., Carlbring, P., & Andersson, G. (2007). *Internet-delivered treatments with or without therapist input: Does the therapist factor have implications for efficacy and cost?* Academic Press.

Păsărelu, C. R., Andersson, G., Bergman Nordgren, L., & Dobrean, A. (2017). Internet-delivered transdiagnostic and tailored cognitive behavioral therapy for anxiety and depression: A systematic review and meta-analysis of randomized controlled trials. [PubMed]. *Cognitive Behaviour Therapy*, *46*(1), 1–28.

Paxling, B., Lundgren, S., Norman, A., Almlöv, J., Carlbring, P., Cuijpers, P., & Andersson, G. (2013). Therapist behaviours in internet-delivered cognitive behaviour therapy: Analyses of e-mail correspondence in the treatment of generalized anxiety disorder. *Behavioural and Cognitive Psychotherapy*, *41*(03), 280–289. doi:10.1017/S1352465812000240 PMID:22717145

Perle, J. G., Langsam, L. C., Randel, A., Lutchman, S., Levine, A. B., Odland, A. P., ... Marker, C. D. (2013). Attitudes toward psychological telehealth: Current and future clinical psychologists' opinions of Internet-Based interventions. *Journal of Clinical Psychology*, *69*(1), 100–113. doi:10.1002/jclp.21912 PMID:22975897

Pflug, J. (2011). Contextuality and computer-mediated communication: A cross cultural comparison. *Computers in Human Behavior*, *27*(1), 131–137. doi:10.1016/j.chb.2009.10.008

Piaggio, G., Elbourne, D. R., Pocock, S. J., Evans, S. J., Altman, D. G., & CONSORT Group. (2012). Reporting of noninferiority and equivalence randomized trials: Extension of the CONSORT 2010 statement. *Journal of the American Medical Association, 308*(24), 2594–2604. doi:10.1001/jama.2012.87802 PMID:23268518

Pizer, S. D., & Prentice, J. C. (2011). What are the consequences of waiting for health care in the veteran population? *Journal of General Internal Medicine, 26*(2), 676–682. doi:10.100711606-011-1819-1 PMID:21989621

Polisena, J., Coyle, D., Coyle, K., & McGill, S. (2009). Home telehealth for chronic disease management: A systematic review and an analysis of economic evaluations. *International Journal of Technology Assessment in Health Care, 25*(3), 339–349. doi:10.1017/S0266462309990201 PMID:19619353

Reavley, N. J., & Jorm, A. F. (2011). The quality of mental disorder information websites: A review. *Patient Education and Counseling, 85*(2), e16–e25. doi:10.1016/j.pec.2010.10.015 PMID:21087837

Riach, E. (2003). The privacy and electronic communications directive. *The New Law Journal, 1*(7071), 379–380.

Ritter, P., Lorig, K., Laurent, D., & Matthews, K. (2004). Internet versus mailed questionnaires: A randomized comparison. *Journal of Medical Internet Research, 6*(3).

Saunders, R. P., Evans, M. H., & Joshi, P. (2005). Developing a process-evaluation plan for assessing health promotion program implementation: A how-to guide. *Health Promotion Practice, 6*(2), 134-147.

Schulz, K. F., Altman, D. G., & Moher, D. (2010). CONSORT 2010 statement: Updated guidelines for reporting parallel group randomised trials. *BMC Medicine, 8*(1), 18. doi:10.1186/1741-7015-8-18 PMID:20334633

Scott, K. M., Lim, C., Al-Hamzawi, A., Alonso, J., Bruffaerts, R., Caldas-de-Almeida, J. M., ... Kessler, R. C. (2016). Association of mental disorders with subsequent chronic physical conditions: World mental health surveys from 17 countries. *JAMA Psychiatry, 73*(2), 150–158. doi:10.1001/jamapsychiatry.2015.2688 PMID:26719969

Shargorodsky, J., Curhan, G. C., & Farwell, W. R. (2010). Prevalence and characteristics of tinnitus among US adults. *The American Journal of Medicine, 123*(8), 711–718. doi:10.1016/j.amjmed.2010.02.015 PMID:20670725

Shore, J. H., Mishkind, M. C., Bernard, J., Doarn, C. R., Bell, I. Jr, Bhatla, R., ... Vo, A. (2014). A lexicon of assessment and outcome measures for telemental health. *Telemedicine Journal and e-Health*, *20*(3), 282–292. doi:10.1089/tmj.2013.0357 PMID:24476192

Smith, P., McKeon, A., Blunt, I., & Edwards, N. (2014). *NHS hospitals under pressure: Trends in acute activity up to 2022*. London, UK: Nuffield Trust.

Stockdale, D., McFerran, D., Brazier, P., Pritchard, C., Kay, T., Dowrick, C., & Hoare, D. J. (2017). An economic evaluation of the healthcare cost of tinnitus management in the UK. *BMC Health Services Research*, *17*(1), 577. doi:10.118612913-017-2527-2 PMID:28830503

Thabane, L., Ma, J., Chu, R., Cheng, J., Ismaila, A., Rios, L. P., ... Goldsmith, C. H. (2010a). A tutorial on pilot studies: The what, why and how. *BMC Medical Research Methodology*, *10*(1), 1. doi:10.1186/1471-2288-10-1 PMID:20053272

Thompson, P., Pryce, H., & Refaie, E. (2011). Group or individual tinnitus therapy: What matters to participants? *Audiological Medicine*, *9*(3), 110–116. doi:10.3109/1651386X.2011.604470

Thoren, E. S., Andersson, G., & Lunner, T. (2012). The use of research questionnaires with hearing impaired adults: Online vs. paper-and-pencil administration. *BMC Ear, Nose, and Throat Disorders, 12*.

Thorén, E. S., Öberg, M., Wänström, G., Andersson, G., & Lunner, T. (2014). A randomized controlled trial evaluating the effects of online rehabilitative intervention for adult hearing-aid users. *International Journal of Audiology*, *53*(7), 452–461. doi:10.3109/14992027.2014.892643 PMID:24749664

Titov, N., Andrews, G., Davies, M., McIntyre, K., Robinson, E., & Solley, K. (2010). Internet treatment for depression: A randomized controlled trial comparing clinician vs. technician assistance. *PLoS One*, *5*(6), e10939. doi:10.1371/journal.pone.0010939 PMID:20544030

Titov, N., Andrews, G., Schwencke, G., Solley, K., Johnston, L., & Robinson, E. (2009). An RCT comparing effect of two types of support on severity of symptoms for people completing internet-based cognitive behaviour therapy for social phobia. *The Australian and New Zealand Journal of Psychiatry*, *43*(10), 920–926. doi:10.1080/00048670903179228

Tomlinson, M., Rotheram-Borus, M. J., Swartz, L., & Tsai, A. C. (2013). Scaling up mHealth: Where is the evidence? *PLoS Medicine*, *10*(2), e1001382. doi:10.1371/journal.pmed.1001382 PMID:23424286

Totten, A. M., Womack, D. M., Eden, K. B., McDonagh, M. S., Griffin, J. C., Grusing, S., & Hersh, W. R. (2016). *Telehealth: mapping the evidence for patient outcomes from systematic reviews*. Rockville, MD: Agency for Healthcare Research and Quality (US). Technical Briefs, No. 26. Available from: https://www.ncbi.nlm.nih.gov/books/NBK379320/

Tulbure, B. T. (2011). The efficacy of internet-supported intervention for social anxiety disorder: A brief meta-analytic review. *Procedia: Social and Behavioral Sciences*, *30*, 552–557. doi:10.1016/j.sbspro.2011.10.108

UK Parliament. (1998). *Data Protection*. Retrieved 15 February 2016, from: http://www.legislation.gov.uk/ukpga/1998/29/contents

van Beugen, S., Ferwerda, M., Hoeve, D., Rovers, M. M., Spillekom-van Koulil, S., van Middendorp, H., & Evers, A. W. (2014). Internet-based cognitive behavioral therapy for patients with chronic somatic conditions: A meta-analytic review. *Journal of Medical Internet Research*, *16*(3), e88. doi:10.2196/jmir.2777 PMID:24675372

Vlaescu, G., Alasjö, A., Miloff, A., Carlbring, P., & Andersson, G. (2016). Features and functionality of the iterapi platform for internet-based psychological treatment. *Internet Interventions*, *6*, 107–114. doi:10.1016/j.invent.2016.09.006 PMID:30135819

Vlaescu, G., Carlbring, P., Lunner, T., & Andersson, G. (2015). An e-platform for rehabilitation of persons with hearing problems. *American Journal of Audiology*, *24*(3), 271–275. doi:10.1044/2015_AJA-14-0083 PMID:26649528

Weise, C., Kleinstauber, M., & Andersson, G. (2016). Internet-delivered cognitive-behavior therapy for tinnitus: A randomized controlled trial. *Psychosomatic Medicine*, *78*(4), 501–510. doi:10.1097/PSY.0000000000000310 PMID:26867083

West, D. (2012). How mobile devices are transforming healthcare. *Issues in Technology Innovation*, *18*(1), 1–11.

Williams, C., & Whitfield, G. (2001). Written and computer-based self-help treatments for depression. *British Medical Bulletin*, *57*(1), 133–144. doi:10.1093/bmb/57.1.133 PMID:11719913

Wise, K., Rief, W., & Goebel, G. (1998). Meeting the expectations of chronic tinnitus patients: Comparison of a structured group therapy program for tinnitus management with a problem-solving group. *Journal of Psychosomatic Research*, *44*(6), 681–685. doi:10.1016/S0022-3999(97)00310-3 PMID:9678749

KEY TERMS AND DEFINITIONS

Cognitive Behavioral Therapy (CBT): A form of psychological therapy that is directed at modifying unhelpful thought patterns and behaviors to help manage specific problems.

Digital Healthcare: Providing healthcare in formats other than face-to-face contact, such as internet and computer-based interventions.

E-Health: Utilization of information and communication technologies to deliver healthcare.

Guided Intervention: Real-time or asynchronous professional support while undertaking an intervention.

Habituation: Becoming accustomed to perceiving tinnitus to the point that it does not affect day-to-day functioning and has no associated negative emotional response.

Internet-Based Cognitive Behavioral Therapy (iCBT): Cognitive behavioral therapy provided via the internet.

Internet Intervention: Using the internet as means of delivering healthcare.

Tailored Intervention: Interventions that include aspects such as personalized messages or content that can be adapted for an individual.

Tinnitus: The perception of a sound in the absence of an identifiable external sound source.

Usual Face-to-Face (F2F) Tinnitus Care: Receiving individual or group-based care in a clinic from a hearing-care practitioner.

Chapter 7
Apps for Hearing Healthcare: Trends, Challenges, and Potential Opportunities

Alessia Paglialonga
Consiglio Nazionale delle Ricerche (CNR-IEIIT), Italy

Francesco Pinciroli
Politecnico di Milano, Italy

Gabriella Tognola
Consiglio Nazionale delle Ricerche (CNR-IEIIT), Italy

ABSTRACT

This chapter provides a picture of the evolution of mobile applications (apps) for hearing health care (HHC) in terms of availability, variety, penetration, offered services, and target users. Special emphasis is given to newly developed methods that might assist audiologists and hearing professionals to get meaningful information and guidance for informed adoption of apps for themselves as well as for patients and their families. The chapter also shows how these novel methods can be used to characterize and compare a variety of apps across a wide range of services and target user groups. A representative sample of apps, assessed by using such a standardized framework, is analyzed to derive a multifaceted picture of apps for HHC. The chapter outlines and discusses emerging trends and needs in the area and highlights the open challenges as well as potential opportunities for professionals, researchers, developers, and stakeholders at large.

DOI: 10.4018/978-1-5225-8191-8.ch007

INTRODUCTION

In the growing area of digitally enabled audiology, the emerging mHealth (mobile Health) branch is extremely promising and opens novel opportunities for professionals and hearing health care (HHC) providers. In the past years we have witnessed a rapid growth of the number and variety of mHealth solutions in HHC. Especially, mobile applications (apps) are rising growing interest. The debate about the potential benefits of these novel solutions, the existing gaps and challenges, as well as the emerging opportunities is open and lively (Bright and Pallawela, 2016; Paglialonga, Pinciroli, and Tognola, 2017a; Paglialonga, Tognola, and Pinciroli, 2015a; Paglialonga, Tognola, and Pinciroli, 2015b; Tognola, Paglialonga, Chiaramello, and Pinciroli, 2015; Wong and Fung, 2015).

This Chapter describes the recent evolution of apps for HHC and assesses the current scenario in terms of availability, variety, penetration, offered services, and target user groups. The Chapter also shows how newly developed methods for app characterization and assessment can support audiologists and hearing professionals. These methods can enable them to get meaningful knowledge about apps, understand their peculiar features, and, in turn, help their patients to get increased benefit from informed, effective use of these solutions. Specifically, the Chapter describes a recently developed method that is able to characterize apps for HHC, regardless the operating system and hardware platform, by using a core set of features: the *ALFA4Hearing* model (Paglialonga et al., 2017a; Paglialonga et al., 2015a). Then, the Chapter describes the multifaceted picture obtained by using the *ALFA4Hearing* model on a representative sample of apps. Finally, the Chapter discusses the main emerging trends and needs in this area and highlight the open challenges as well as some potential opportunities for professionals, researchers, developers, and stakeholders at large.

BACKGROUND

mHealth is a broad term that encompasses any use of mobile and wearable technology to address key health care challenges (e.g., access, quality, affordability, matching of resources, and behavioral norms) through the exchange of information (Qiang, Yamamichi, Hausman, Miller and Altman, 2012). It becomes thus clear that mHealth can be an entirely novel facilitator to try to address health care challenges. Within the broad area of mHealth, mobile applications (apps) are rising growing interest. Apps are software applications designed for use on mobile devices, such as smartphones and tablets, rather than desktop or laptop computers. As such, they have core characteristics that are specific to the mobile environment. Specifically: (i) penetration into populations, due to communication access to population and subgroups; (ii) large availability due to increasing smartphone capabilities, functionality, and sensors integration and due to an increasing number of health-related devices; (iii) wireless broadband access to the Internet thanks to increasing communication speed and device connectivity; and (iv) ability to be tethered to individuals due to increasing capability of locating, measuring data, monitoring function, and communicating with others (Davis, diClemente and Prietula, 2016). Moreover, use of apps presents specific potential benefits in terms of, for example: increased patient motivation towards behavior change, promotion of preventive behaviors and health monitoring in the general population, enhanced patient-doctor engagement, tailored patient-reported measures and Ecological Momentary Assessment, improved service delivery in resource limited settings, patient empowerment, and patient centered care (Mosa, Yoo, and Sheets, 2012; van Kerkhof, van der Laar, de Jong, Weda, and Hegger, 2016; Zhao, Freeman, and Li, 2016; Liao, Chien, Chen, Hsiung, Chen, Hsieh, and Wu, 2017; Kim and Lee, 2017; Rehman, Kamal, Morris, Sayani, Merchant, and Virani, 2017; Scherer, Ben-Zeev, Li, and Kne, 2017; Burke, et al., 2017; Groshek, Oldenburg, Sarasohn-Kahn and Sitler, 2015; Bastawrous, and Armstrong, 2013; Ozdalga, Ozdalga, and Ahuja, 2012; Paglialonga, Mastropietro, Scalco, Rizzo, in press). On the other hand, important challenges exist that are specific to the field, including: concerns about security, data protection and data reuse (Mantovani and Quinn, 2014; Privacy Rights Clearinghouse, 2016); risks about safety or misuse (Misra, Lewis, and Aungst, 2013), quality and effectiveness (Lewis, 2013; Murfin, 2013), responsibility (Charani, Castro-Sánchez, Moore, and Holmes, 2014), regulation of informed use and trust (Albrecht, Von Jan, and Pramann, 2013; Albrecht, 2013; Barton, 2012), as well as integration and interoperability among different platforms and services (Federal Communications Commission, 2012).

Mobile apps are now making the leap from early adopters to mainstream (IMS Institute for Healthcare Informatics, 2013) and they can become more than just a novel way of service delivery: a cost- and clinically-effective means for addressing challenges in health care (Steinhubl, Muse, and Topol, 2015; Federal Communications Commission, 2012; Qiang et al., 2012; World Health Organization, 2011). Smartphone applications are growing rapidly, with increasing penetration into clinical practice, and they can potentially become leading edge technology in today's mobile environment. Over 325,000 health-related apps are available on major app stores, according to 2017 estimates (Research2guidance, 2017).

Apps are used frequently and with proven success in several medical specialties. A number of examples can be found in the literature, for example in asthma risk management (e.g., Kenner, 2016), cardiology (e.g., Martínez-Pérez, de la Torre-Díez, López-Coronado, and Herreros-González, 2013), diabetes management (e.g., Huckvale, Adomaviciute, Prieto, Leow, and Car, 2015), emergency medicine (e.g.,

Wallis, Fleming, Hasselberg, Laflamme, and Lundin, 2016), nutrition (e.g., Bardus, van Beurden, Smith, and Abraham, 2016), as well as psychology and mental health (e.g., Helf and Hlavacs, 2016).

On the other hand, in HHC the clinical use of medical apps is at its early stages (Martínez-Pérez, de la Torre-Díez, and López-Coronado, 2013). A larger and larger number of apps for hearing are made available on the market, covering a very wide range of functions and services for the different target user groups, from professional and patient education to hearing screening, from remote counseling to auditory training, from personal sound amplification to support tools for parents and significant others (Paglialonga et al., 2017a; Paglialonga et al., 2015a, 2015b; Tognola et al., 2015), as described in detail in the following section. Nowadays, the several apps available can support the patients throughout the whole journey: in hearing loss prevention and education, in assessment and diagnosis, as well as in intervention and rehabilitation. Interest is growing among audiologists, scientists, patients, and citizens around these novel solutions– and getting these solutions can be as simple as getting into an app store and typing some search words.

So, on the one hand it is clear that the scenario of apps for HHC is complex, very dynamic, and promising but, on the other hand, it is also clear that the risk for the users (patients, audiologists, physicians, significant others, as well as citizens with no diagnosed hearing loss seeking for advice) is to be left with no clear guidance or reliable app information. A large amount of research has addressed this need and the debate is open. Some of the most significant results in this area are presented throughout the Chapter.

APPS FOR HEARING HEALTH CARE

A Variety of Solutions and Services

The growing interest in the area of mHealth for HHC and, in particular, in the area mobile apps, is demonstrated by an increasing number of apps and mobile-based services available and documented by a significant number of studies published in the recent years. Recent reviews have shown the large variety of services and functionalities of apps (Paglialonga et al., 2017a; Paglialonga et al., 2015a). Overall, the distribution of apps for HHC was described across four main service application areas, i.e., (i) *education & information*, (ii) *screening & assessment*, (iii) *intervention & rehabilitation*, and (iv) *assistive tools* (Paglialonga et al., 2017a).

(i) *education & information*. Apps in the area of *education and information* included services such as, e.g., continuing education programs, anatomy pictures and atlases, reference guides (for professionals, for students, or for patients), question banks, interactive tools for hearing loss awareness promotion (including, e.g., simulations of hearing loss and hearing amplification), or tools for hearing loss prevention and noise monitoring (Paglialonga et al., 2017a; Paglialonga et al., 2015a). In principle, these services are not only app based and can be ideally delivered through the internet – but the use of apps for information & education opens new opportunities for ubiquitous use, customization, and ultimately user engagement,

In this area, Wong and Fung (2015) provided important evidence by reviewing educational apps relating to otolaryngology–head and neck surgery specialty. They searched for apps related to the specialty on the App Store, Google Play, BlackBerry World, and Windows Store in January 2014 and found 75 apps overall. They organized apps into four main categories corresponding to the main function. The 'education' category comprised apps aimed at educating medical students, residents, physicians, and other health care professionals. This category included question banks, reference texts, and anatomy pictures and atlases. In the 'journal/conference' category they classified apps containing abstracts and articles for journals and apps designed for conferences and meetings. In the 'clinical' category they included apps designed for use in clinical settings by physicians and other health care professionals to support clinical activities and patient-doctor interactions. Apps in this category included, e.g., clinical reference guides, cancer staging tools, and apps intended to aid in procedures. Apps designed for use by patients were placed into a fourth category, labeled 'patients', which included, e.g., specific patient-oriented clinic and hospital information, and apps designed for educating patients. The review concluded that several high-quality apps were available at that time for education and clinical use that could potentially be integrated into everyday clinical use. However, the authors underlined the need for appropriate guidance from the specialty to ensure app quality and accuracy of content. A study aimed at ensuring quality of apps for *education and information* addressed the problem of developing an app to deliver health information to deaf people, trying to overcome the disparity that deaf people face when accessing health information because of social and language barriers (Chininthorn, Glaser, Tucker, and Diehl, 2016). The study investigated the current modalities of health information delivery to deaf people, addressed the sources they preferred and their reasons, and searched for effective techniques for delivering understandable information to identify specifications for developing a health app for this target user group. As a result, the study identified three techniques to deliver understandable health information to deaf people and that should be used in a Health Knowledge Transfer System for this population, specifically: signed language (including dialects), health drama techniques, and use of pictures and simple text descriptions to enhance their understanding.

(ii) *screening & assessment.* Among the several services available in the area of *screening & assessment*, the app market currently provides pure-tone tests, speech-

and speech-in-noise tests, video otoscopy, measures of tinnitus pitch and loudness, self-reported measures of tinnitus or hearing handicap and disability (ranging from standardized structured questionnaires to simpler lists of questions, or single-question measures) and, also, some apps to manage or complement clinical equipment and instrumentation (Bright and Pallawela, 2016; Paglialonga et al., 2017a; Paglialonga et al., 2015a).

Several studies have been published in this service application area, providing several examples of app-based screening and assessment in hearing (see, e.g., Abu-Ghanem, Handzel, Ness, Ben-Artzi-Blima, Fait-Ghelbendorf, and Himmelfarb, 2016; Derin, Cam, Beydilli, Acar, Elicora, and Sahan, 2016; Larrosa, et al., 2015; Livshitz, et al., 2017; Mahomed-Asmail, Swanepoel, Eikelboom, Myburgh, and Hall, 2016; Thompson, Sladen, Borst, and Still, 2015). A recent review (Bright and Pallawela, 2016) assessed the evidence about validated apps for ear and hearing assessment. The study identified 30 apps through a commercial review of the two leading app stores (Google Play and Apple App Store) and searched six databases (EMBASE, MEDLINE, Global Health, Web of Science, CINAHL, and mHealth Evidence) to look for evidence about their validation against gold standard measures. Overall, the study identified 11 eligible peer-reviewed studies that examined 6 different apps. By the analysis of this studies in terms of methods, participants, outcomes, results, and study quality (as measured using the Quality Assessment for Diagnostic Accuracy Studies tool, QUADAS-2), the review concluded that, for the very few validated apps, further research is still required to assess accuracy for use in ear and hearing assessment (including self- or tester-administered pure-tone audiometry as well as screening audiometry).

The area of validation and calibration of apps for HHC is an important subject of research. Significant efforts have been done recently to try to address - and improve - the reliability and accuracy of mobile solutions for hearing assessment in non-clinical settings such as, for example, noisy environments or underserved contexts. For example, to try to limit the effects of environmental noise on hearing screening, Na, Joo, Yang, Kang, Hong, and Woo (2014) have developed a system combining a smartphone, an *ad hoc* app, consumer earphones, and an automated correction algorithm that compensates the hearing threshold values based on the noise measured by the built-in microphone. The study showed that the system was able to compensate for the effects of environmental noise and provided reliable estimates of hearing levels in the twenty-one adult subjects tested. Sandström, Swanepoel, Carel Myburgh, and Laurent (2016) used a repeated-measure within-subject study to validate smartphone-based audiometry (using calibrated low-cost headphones) compared to conventional audiometry in a sound booth and a primary health-care clinic environment. They found accurate results for smartphone-based audiometry in the two tested settings and concluded that smartphone-based threshold audiometry could be useful in underserved primary health-care contexts, provided that calibrated headphones are used. Encouraging findings were also shown by a recent study (Louw, Swanepoel, Eikelboom, and Myburgh, 2017) that demonstrated the accuracy and time efficiency of a smartphone hearing screening app in primary health care clinics on 1,236 participants screened. Similarly, other studies have demonstrated the accuracy of apps for hearing screening and testing in different settings (soundproof and waiting room settings) to explore the possible application in developing countries and underserved contexts (e.g., Khoza-Shangase and Kassner, 2013; Peer and Fagan, 2015). Smartphone apps are typically used with consumer earphones. Some studies investigated the reliability of using consumer technology and suggested potential improvements. For example, a preliminary evaluation of test–retest reliability and accuracy of an audiometer app for iPad by using commercial earphones as a low-cost alternative to a clinical audiometer was conducted recently in a restricted sample of normal hearing participants (Corry, Sanders, and Searchfield, 2017). The study showed good test–retest reliability but the app using Apple earbud earphones provided different hearing thresholds compared to the clinical audiometer with insert earphones. Research to address the issue of calibration of consumer headphones is ongoing. For example, Masalski, Kipiński, Grysiński, and Kręcicki (2016) have proposed procedures for biological calibration of reference sound levels for Android-based mobile devices, i.e., in relation to the normal-hearing threshold of the subjects. The study was able to characterize the differences and variability of reference sound levels for different models of mobile devices, suggesting the possibility of using biological calibration for determining predefined reference sound level, thus encouraging further research in this area.

In addition to the many studies about apps-based audiometry and screening mentioned above, in the area of *screening & assessment* the literature also shows some examples of apps addressing different services, for example otoscopy (Richards, Gaylor, and Pilgrim, 2015) and tinnitus assessment (Probst, Pryss, Langguth, and Schlee, 2016; Schlee, et al., 2016). An otoscope app was compared to traditional otoscopy by Richards et al. (2015) in a prospective cross-sectional study involving patients younger than 18 years. The study showed substantial intra-rater agreement between the two methods. A survey among physicians, parents, and patients revealed that all of them tended to prefer the otoscopy app due to ease of use, precision, improved view of tympanic membrane, and usefulness as an educational tool. As for tinnitus assessment, although several apps are available on the market, a small number of studies have been published so far. Specifically, two studies monitored patients in daily life by using an app that tracks users' perceptions of tinnitus, thus allowing for Ecological Momentary Assessment (EMA) (Probst et al., 2016; Schlee et al., 2016). Specifically, the app measured tinnitus along several dimensions, including subjective perception and loudness, distress, emotional valence and arousal, stress and concentration levels, and general degree of symptoms compared to the user 'worst' experience. The first study (Probst et al., 2016) investigated emotion dynamics in 306 users of the app and provided evidence that emotion dynamics are associated with tinnitus-related distress and with the time course of tinnitus loudness. The second study (Schlee et al., 2016) involved 857 patients and showed the viability of a tinnitus tracking app as a safe instrument for longitudinal assessment of tinnitus perception in daily life.

(iii) *intervention & rehabilitation.* Apps in the area of *intervention & rehabilitation* include a large variety of services, e.g., remote consultation, hearing aid fitting and control, auditory training, speech and language rehabilitation, personal sound amplification, as well as tinnitus masking and tinnitus relief tools. The literature available in this area is related mainly to apps for sound amplification and auditory training. Galster (2012) described apps designed for personal sound amplification through the smartphone or tablet, based on amplification and frequency shaping of the acoustic input (the apps used either the measured audiogram or pre-set configurations). In some apps, there are also options to introduce a high- or low-cutoff to the input signal and to adjust for volume and maximum output limiting. Amlani, Taylor, Levy, and Robbins (2013) investigated whether smartphone-based hearing-aid apps could serve as an alternative to hearing aids. Performance was measured via behavioral (as measured by speech recognition in noise) and self-report (as measured by self-assessment responses on benefit, quality of life, and satisfaction) measures. The results showed similar speech-in-noise recognition performance for the two methods. From the subjective measures, the results showed that the clients favoured the apps in terms of benefits, but still preferred the traditional hearing aids when considering satisfaction. The Authors remarked that the intended use of smartphone-based hearing aid applications is to provide temporary assistance to individuals with hearing deficits. Based on this study, the Authors also suggested that it would be important that hearing aid manufacturers provide patients with adjustable controls. In fact, several apps have been put on the market recently by hearing aid manufacturers to provide recipients of hearing aids some control over their devices. In the area of smartphone hearing aid apps, Grebel, Dang, Ma, Payne, and Cooper (2015) developed a smartphone-based hearing aid app on Android, including both gain (volume) increases and frequency compression techniques. The app required user input to tailor its parameters and set an individualized target bandwidth to compress signals to the desired frequency ranges using linear frequency compression. However, the authors concluded that the proposed app needed improvements and further developments because there were distortions in the output audio and latency of output beyond the desired limit – so caution should be taken in considering smartphones as potential substitutes of hearing aids. Evidence and technology developments in this area are likely to grow in the near future.

An interesting development in the field of mobile technologies for sound amplification has been proposed by Panahi, Kehtarnavaz, and Thibodeau (2016). The study proposed a novel noise adaptive speech enhancement solution able to run in real-time on smartphones and able to interface with commercially available hearing aids. Testing with different noise types in participants with normal hearing and hearing impairment showed significant improvements in speech recognition in noise (on average, 30% increase), suggesting the viability of the proposed smartphone-based speech enhancement approach for improving speech understanding in environmental noise. Another interesting technical solution in this area is a mobile based, wireless, stigma-free implementation for personal frequency modulation (FM) for people with mild-to-moderate hearing loss developed by Lin et al. (2018). This smartphone-based hearing assistive system consisted of a smartphone running a mobile application and a Bluetooth handset coupled with the smartphone. The study showed an average 20% improvement of speech intelligibility in four signal-to-noise ratio conditions, and a favorable user experience compared to the conventional FM systems, as measured in five participants with various degrees of hearing loss.

In the area of rehabilitation apps, Olson (2015) reviewed auditory training programs that are readily accessible for adults with hearing loss, hearing aids, or cochlear implants via web-based formats or smartphone technology. The study identified some issues such as, for example: memory for storage on mobile devices, which can limit the range of stimuli available on mobile platforms compared to computer training or web-based programs; unwanted noise within smartphone technology that might create additional distortion; and small visual layout that may not be adequate for adults over 50-years-old, even with large font. Nevertheless, the study concluded that mobile-based auditory training programs can be important in clinical practice, for example to introduce clients to auditory training given the modest cost of apps and the large availability of smartphones.

(iv) *assistive tools*. In the fourth application area, *assistive tools*, several apps are available on the market, overall providing a variety of services to help deaf and hard of hearing people in their daily living. Examples are: captioning and transcription, communication services, sign language dictionaries, sign language learning tools, as well as visual or vibrotactile alerts (Paglialonga et al., 2017a; Paglialonga et al., 2015a). The attitudes and needs of families of children with communication disabilities towards mobile technology, including iPads, as a form of augmentative and alternative communication (AAC) were assessed by Meder and Wegner (2015). The study conducted a survey among 64 parents or caregivers of children with communication-related disabilities, recruited from online family communities and websites. Important needs were identified such as ease of use and affordability, the integration of multiple functions into the mobile device (e.g., access to information, social opportunities, and entertainment), suggesting practical directions for development in the area.

Concerning the accuracy of smartphone-based speech-to-text applications for communication with profoundly deaf patients, Lyall, Clamp, and Hajioff (2016) conducted a preliminary study involving thirty doctors and medical students and showed that smartphone dictation was faster but less accurate, but that slow speech may improve accuracy. Research is recommended to try to improve accuracy and reliability of smartphone-based assistive tools. For example, in the field of smartphone-based alerts for deaf and hard of hearing people, research has been done to try to develop reliable algorithms to develop pattern recognition application for detecting non-speech environmental sounds and identify potential hazards and events outside of the field of view of people with hearing loss, both outdoor and indoor, providing results that encourage further developments (Mielke and Brueck, 2016; Mielke and Brueck, 2015; Mielke, Grunewald, and Brueck, 2013).

To sum up, the reviewed literature as well as the analysis of the app markets revealed that, on the one hand, there is a large amount of apps that are available for a variety of services and needs but also that, on the other hand, a large amount of research is still needed to fully understand the feasibility and benefits of introducing these solutions into clinical practice. A particularly interesting area of research is devoted to the development of methods to characterize and assess apps, as discussed in the followings.

CHARACTERIZATION AND ASSESSMENT OF HEALTH APPS

The rapid growth in the number and variety of health apps has inspired a significant amount of research to try to devise methods to characterize and assess apps (reviewed by Paglialonga, Lugo, and Santoro, 2018). This is a very timely and important field of research as, to date, potential app users (patients, physicians, as well as citizens seeking for health information or services) cannot find comprehensive, reliable resources to guide them in informed adoption of health apps. In the ongoing digital transformation in health care, it would be particularly important to provide physicians and health care professionals with proper means to characterize and assess apps, supporting them in the identification of the most appropriate solutions. For potential app users, the main source of information still remains the web. Relevant sources include not only the app stores but, also, the developers' websites, health-related web-portals, expert communities, and some health app clearinghouses that were developed to inform consumers and health care providers through voluntary review and evaluation systems (see, e.g., Aungst, Clauson, Misra, Lewis, and Husain, 2014; Boudreaux, Waring, Hayes, Sadasivam, Mullen, and Pagoto, 2014). Unfortunately, the attempts made so far, by public or private organizations, to develop general certification frameworks for apps have failed (Boulos, Brewer, Karimkhani, Buller, and Dellavalle, 2014). For example, the HACP, Happtique Health App Certification Program was suspended in 2013 due to security shortcomings. In general, certification and standardization are difficult to achieve due to key market factors such as the number of features, diversity of information, and rapid pace of development (Chan and Misra, 2014). Nevertheless, it would be very important that guidelines for app development, marketing, and use are introduced as these may be highly effective to improve the quality standards of apps on the market (Paglialonga et al., 2018).

In general, online resources can be a first filter to gather knowledge about health apps and, as such, they can be helpful to support users in the identification of apps to answer specific needs. However, online resources may fail to provide users with deep understanding of the relevant features and functions of apps. The recent literature provides several examples of methods for the characterization and assessment of health apps that, overall, introduced a variety of modalities to classify and evaluate health apps. Some of these methods focused on specific medical domains (e.g., diabetes care, cardiology, oncology, pharmacology, and hearing) whereas others are more general in scope and can be used across several specialties (BinDhim, Hawkey, and Trevena, 2015; Hussain, et al., 2015). Some researchers proposed classification schemes based on users' outcomes such as, for example, methods based on health management strategies, user engagement approaches, or the potential to influence behavior change in fitness apps (Sama, Eapen, Weinfurt, Shah, and Schulman, 2014; West, Hall, Hanson, Barnes, Giraud-Carrier, and Barrett, 2012). Some others focused on the enabling drivers for behavior change in apps to prevent and manage disease in older adults (Wang, An, Lu, Chen, Li, and Levkoff, 2014). In some other studies, the apps assessed were coded and characterized not only for the enabling driver mechanisms and services/functions but, also, for their content, e.g., adherence to clinical guidelines (e.g., Abroms, Padmanabhan, Thaweethai, and Phillips, 2011), completeness of information (Muessig, Pike, LeGrand, and Hightow-Weidman, 2013), availability of data analysis features for diabetes self-care (Huckvale et al., 2015), or medical professional involvement and inclusion of evidence-based content (Connor, Brady, Beaux, and Tulloh, 2014; Pandey, Hasan, Dubey, and Sarangi, 2013; O'Neill and Brady, 2012). Another important area of research is the assessment of app safety and trustworthiness. Some studies have tried to develop organized frameworks in this area, but these aspects are difficult to standardize (Albrecht, 2013; Lewis, 2013; Murfin 2013; Wicks and Chiauzzi, 2015). Noticeably, when dealing with user-oriented app attributes, there are some important elements related to app use that are difficult to identify and measure, such as, e.g., operability, usability, depth of understanding, and quality of experience. A large amount of research has been conducted in this direction and some expert-based evaluations have been developed

(Arnhold, Quade, and Kirch, 2014; Demidowich, Lu, Tamler, and Bloomgarden, 2012) as well as easy-to-use tools for the apps' end users (e.g., Martínez-Pérez, de la Torre-Díez, Candelas-Plasencia, and López-Coronado, 2013; Reynoldson,et al., 2014; Stoyanov, Hides, Kavanagh, Zelenko, Tjondronegoro, and Mani, 2015; Stoyanov, Hides, Kavanagh, and Wilson, 2016).

Important efforts have been done recently to develop user-oriented assessment methods that are informative and easy-to-understand. For example, a list of miscellaneous features was introduced by Gosnell, Costello, and Shane (2011) to describe various apps developed for people with communication problems, as relevant to the specific category of apps. Similarly, a 'pictorial' approach was introduced recently to identify apps for cardiology, oncology, pharmacology, and diabetes self-care apps (Bonacina, Marceglia, and Pinciroli, 2014; Basilico, Marceglia, Bonacina, and Pinciroli, 2016). The rationale behind these approaches was to collect meaningful information about a core set of attributes, grouped into main domains, and to use a 'traffic-light' color code to represent the quality and reliability of the attributes. The 'pictorial' approach, with its straightforward color code representation and its easy-to-understand organization of information (attributes grouped into main domains), inspired the development of a novel method to characterize apps for HHC, the *ALFA4Hearing* model (At-a-glance Labelling for Features of Apps for Hearing health care) (Paglialonga et al., 2017a). The *ALFA4Hearing* model organizes information about a core set of app features, as relevant to hearing, that are grouped into main components and uses a color code representation to highlight the relevance of each of the model features. The rationale of this method is to characterize apps by using a core set of features that are related to the medical specialty and meaningful to HHC and that, at the same time, belong to more general components that are related to health apps in general, i.e., the app's promoters, offered services, implementation features, target user groups, and descriptive information. The use of a color code representation has the advantage of being easier to read and able to code features on a scale (e.g., relevant, partially relevant, not relevant in the model) compared to, for example, a checklist of features with binary yes/no information.

The ALFA4 Hearing Model to Characterize Apps for HHC

The *ALFA4Hearing* model (At-a-glance Labelling for Features of Apps for Hearing health care) organizes relevant information about apps for HHC over an easy-to-use graphical representation, so that different apps can be assessed and compared over a common model, regardless the operating system and hardware platform (Paglialonga et al., 2017a). The model (Figure 1) includes a core set of 29 features that are grouped into five main components, i.e., (1) *Promoters*; (2) *Services*; (3) *Implementation*; (4) *Users*; and (5) *Descriptive information*. The five components highlight information about: (1) "who promoted the app?" (Promoters); (2) "which service(s) is/are provided by the app?" (Services); (3) "how is the app implemented?" (Implementation); (4) "whom is the app targeted to?" (Users); and (5) "what are the general user-oriented features?" (*Descriptive information*). Each of the model components includes a variable number of features. Specifically, the component *Promoters* includes seven features: Hardware/Software (HW/SW) company, Drug company, Government services (Public Health), Clinics and HHC providers, Professional, scientific and educational institutions, Publisher, and Independent promoter. The component *Services* includes four features: Education & Information, Screening & Assessment, Intervention & Rehabilitation, and Assistive Tools. *Implementation* includes nine features: Text & readings display, Pictures & video streaming, Audio playback, Pictures and video recording, Audio recording, Interaction with the user, Interaction with external devices, Interaction with other apps, services, or web, and Wireless data transmission. This component allows, for example, to highlight the nature of apps as 'stand-alone' or 'hybrid', the use of transducers, the degree of interaction with the user, the input/output modalities (e.g., audio, pictures, video, text on screen), or the use of Internet. The component *Users* includes four features: Citizens, Patients with hearing problems, Physicians and HHC professionals, and Families and significant others. The last component *Descriptive information* includes five features: App description, User manual, User support, App version, User ratings.

Each feature in the *ALFA4Hearing* model can be coded by using a color representation. Specifically, the color of the features in any of the components *Promoters*, *Services*, *Implementation*, or *Users* will be *green* if the feature is relevant, *yellow* if partially relevant, or *white* if not relevant. For example, the feature audio playback is coded *green* if audio playback is essential, *yellow* if it is optional, and *white* if it is not used. The color of the features in the component *Descriptive information* follows slightly different criteria. For example, the features *App description* will be *green* if the description is provided in detail, *yellow* if it is partially provided, and *white* if it is not provided. The same holds for the feature *User manual*, whereby user manual is intended as any kind of guide or in-app instructions for use (e.g., text, pictures, videos, or tutorial). The feature *User support* will be *green* if the app provides personal support assistance (for example, by using e-mail, phone, or chat), *yellow* if the app provides general support information (for example, by using forums, websites, or FAQs), or *white* if the app does not provide any support. The feature *App version* will be *green* if the app evaluated is a full version, *yellow* if it is a lite version (i.e., providing core functionalities but requiring upgrades for being fully operational), or *white* if it is a demo version. Finally, the feature *User ratings* will be *green* if the average value of ratings, as reported on the app store, is higher than or equal to 4 stars, *yellow* if it is between 2 and 4 stars, *red* if it is equal to or lower than 2 stars, or *white* if no ratings are available on the app store. For this last feature, a slightly different coding scheme (*green*, *yellow*, *red*, and *white*) was introduced to account for the usual color code adopted for users' reviews on the online stores. In addition, for the feature *User ratings* the model also shows details about the number of available ratings and, for those app stores that provide country-specific review data (e.g., the iOS store), the country code of the specific market (e.g., UK, US, IT).

Figure 1 shows, as an example, the *ALFA4Hearing* model in two apps: *Audiogram Mobile* for iOS (panel A) and *Speech Assistant AAC* for Android (panel B). *Audiogram Mobile* is an app for professional hearing testing developed and promoted by an independent developer. The app administers pure-tone audiometry (air- and bone-conduction, manual and automated testing, and noise masking) by using professional, calibrated headphones. *Speech Assistant AAC* is a text-to-speech AAC aid for patients with communication problems developed and promoted by a software development company.

As shown in Figure 1, the *green* (relevant) features in the component *Promoters* were *Independent promoter* and *HW/SW company*, respectively. In the component *Services*, the relevant features were *Screening & Assessment* in the former (audiogram app) and *Assistive Tools* in the latter (communication app). In the component *Implementation*, both apps included *Audio playback* and *Interaction with the user* as *green* as they are essential features. *Interaction with external devices* was *green* in *Audiogram Mobile* (headphones required) and *yellow* in *Speech Assistant AAC* (headphones/earphones optional). In *Speech Assistant AAC*, the feature *Interaction with other apps, services, or web* is *yellow* as the app uses the device built-in service for text-to-speech voices. As for the component *Users*, *Audiogram Mobile* is intended for use by audiologists and hearing professionals (so, the feature *Physicians and HHC professionals* is *green*) whereas *Speech Assistant AAC* was specifically developed for deaf patients (so, the feature *Patients with hearing problems* is *green*). The analysis of the remaining features in the component *Descriptive information*, is straightforward. The *App description* and *App manual* were *green* in *Audiogram Mobile* and *yellow* in *Speech Assistant AAC* because the former provides concise information about the app description and user manual whereas the latter provided detailed information. This is likely due to the fact that the target user groups are different. On the one hand, *Audiogram Mobile* is an app for hearing professionals, who are highly familiar with audiometry and do not need extensive information about the app functions, nor detailed instructions for use. On the other hand, *Speech Assistant AAC* is an app for patients so the developers included a detailed app description and user manual. *User support* is *green* in the two apps as both provide personal support assistance to users (e-mail contact). The feature *App version* was *green* in *Audiogram Mobile* and *yellow* in *Speech Assistant AAC* because the former was tested in full version whereas the latter was tested in lite version. Finally, the feature *User ratings* was

Figure 1. Examples of the ALFA4Hearing model in Audiogram Mobile for iOS (panel A) and Speech Assistant AAC for Android (panel B)

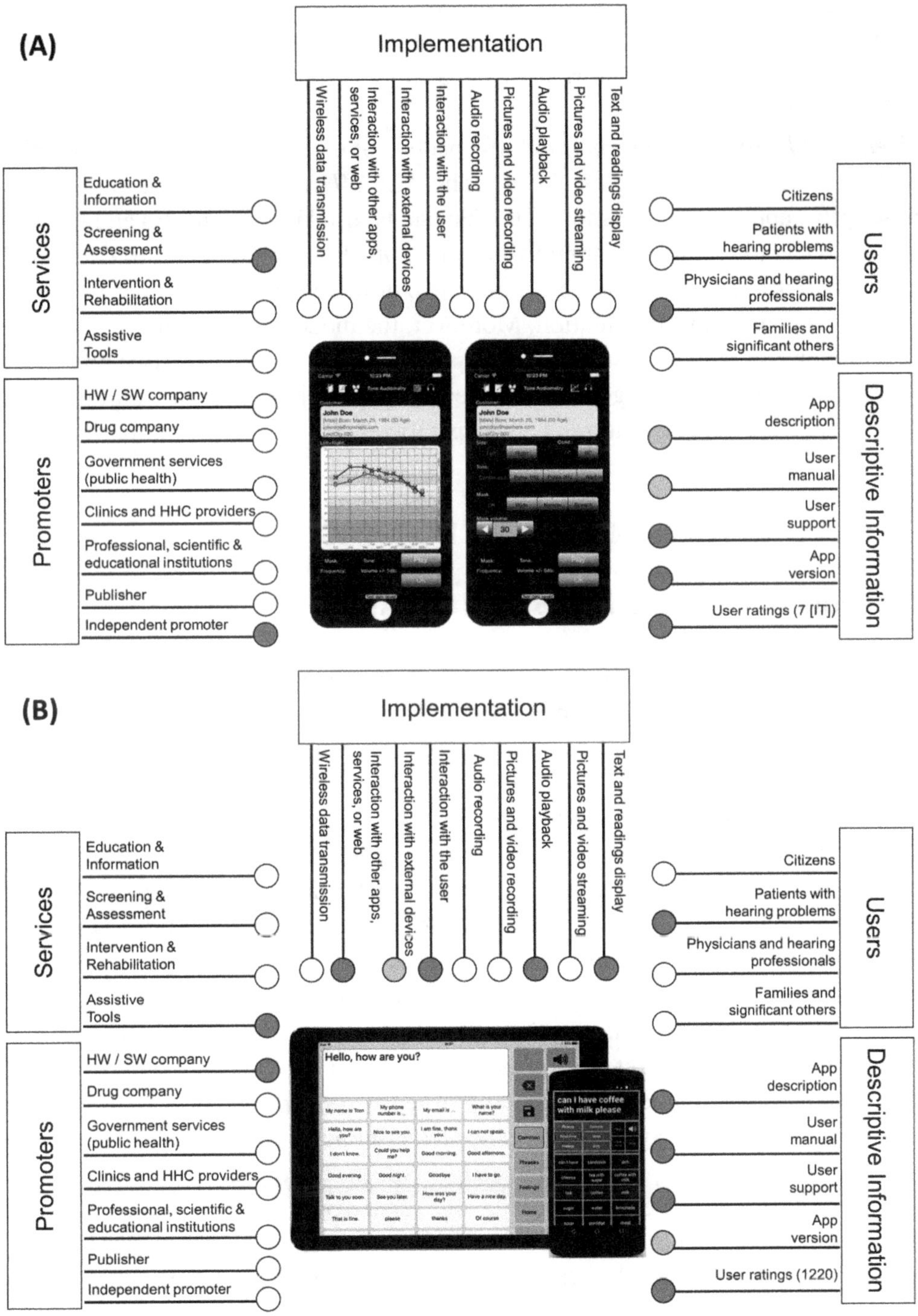

green in the two apps, both rated 4/5 stars on the respective market (*Audiogram Mobile* had 7 ratings on the Italian [IT] Apple App Store, *Speech Assistant AAC* had 1,220 ratings globally on Google Play).

So, overall, as shown in Figure 1 and discussed above, the *ALFA4Hearing* model can provide, at a glance, an informative picture of specific apps by collecting relevant information along the five main components *Promoters*, *Services*, *Implementation*, *Users*, and *Descriptive information*, irrespective of the operating system (e.g., iOS and Android in the examples above). The *ALFA4Hearing* model is basically a descriptive approach of apps for HHC that can be used by researchers and hearing professionals to identify meaningful information about apps. As such, the model can also be used, for example, to compare two or more apps with similar functions by using a common representation. Moreover, the model can be used to assess the distribution of features in samples of apps (e.g., apps for specific user groups or for specific conditions, or generic samples of apps for HHC, as shown in the next section) and extract relevant trends in a specific area or in the general market.

CHARACTERIZATION OF APPS FOR HHC

Analysis of Features in a Sample of Apps

This section outlines some quantitative results obtained from the analysis of the *ALFA4Hearing* features in a large, representative sample of apps for HHC. Based on the distribution of features in the tested sample, the trends, challenges, and potential opportunities are discussed.

The tested sample included 120 apps (60 from the iOS store, 60 from the Android store) distributed across a wide range of services and functions. Apps were found on Google Play and Apple App Store by using the following search keywords: assistive technology, assistive tool, assistive device, audiology, audio, auditory, auditory training, cochlear implant, implantable device, hearing, hearing aid, hearing consultation, hearing loss, hearing rehabilitation, hearing screening, hearing system, language, noise, speech, tinnitus. Apps that had not been updated in the past two years were excluded. In fact, an analysis of all apps in the 'Medical' and 'Health & Fitness' categories on the US iTunes app store (80,490 apps overall, as of May 31 2017) revealed that the average time since the last update was 1 year and 4 months and that about 25% of apps had no updates in the past two years.

Apps were tested in their original language version by downloading and reviewing the app content to identify all the relevant features, as listed in the *ALFA4Hearing* model. An iPad 2 (model A1396, 64 Gb) on iOS 9.2 and a Samsung Galaxy Tab 10.1 3G (model GT-P7500, 32Gb) on Android 5.1.1 were used. In the sample of

120 apps, the number of apps that were coded *green* and *yellow* (and, for the only feature *User ratings*, the number of apps that were *red*) was computed (Paglialonga et al., 2017a). The distribution of features is reported in Table 1.

Table 1 shows that in the component *Promoters*, most of the apps were promoted by HW/SW companies or independent promoters. A smaller set of apps were promoted by professional, scientific & educational institutions, clinics and hearing providers, publishers, government services (public health), and no app in the tested sample was promoted by drug companies. The *Services* delivered by the tested apps covered the four application areas of Education & Information, Screening & Assessment, Intervention & Rehabilitation, and Assistive Tools. In the component *Implementation*, the Table shows that several apps used text & readings as well as pictures & videos as major (37 and 23 *green*, respectively) or minor element (18 and 17 *yellow*, respectively). Audio playback was used in most of the apps as it is typically essential, e.g., in hearing testing, in hearing rehabilitation, as well as in communication tools. Audio recording was found to be relevant in apps that record the user's voice e.g., for hearing rehabilitation and auditory training or for communication, or in apps that record incoming speech or sounds for sound enhancement through the smartphone. Interaction with the user was an important element in apps for hearing testing, rehabilitation, or auditory training. Interaction with external devices was found in apps that need external transducers (headphones or earplugs), and apps that communicate with hearing aids. A non-negligible number of apps included interactions with other apps, services, or web such as, for example, apps that used GPS or maps applications to find services, apps that used web browsers to provide additional resources, apps connected to social network apps, or with the smartphone music library and music player. Finally, wireless data transmission was used in a small number of apps, specifically in apps that communicate with hearing aids or with communication devices or other tools. As for the app *Users*, the Table shows that most of the apps were intended for use by patients and citizens (113 *green* combined), and a smaller number for professionals and for families and significant others. The last five features in the component *Descriptive information* showed that: a high number of apps included a description of the app in a user manual, either detailed (48 and 49 *green*, respectively) or partial (15 and 23 *yellow*, respectively); apps frequently provided user support, either direct (49 *green*) or general (24 *yellow*); most of the apps (i.e., 98) were in full version, 14 lite, and 8 demo (i.e., *white*); and many apps were rated above 4 stars (46 *green*) or between 2 and 4 stars (45 *yellow*), only two apps were rated below 2 stars (2 *red*), whereas the remaining apps had no ratings (27 *white*). Overall, the information reported in Table 1 can be seen as a general descriptive picture of the tested sample and suggests important trends as well as emerging challenges in this area that might translate in potential opportunities for research and clinical practice or for technology developments, as outlined below.

Table 1. Number of apps that were coded green and yellow in each the 29 features of the ALFA4Hearing model (N=120)

Components	Features	*Green*	*Yellow*	*Red*
Promoters	HW/SW company	44	1	
	Drug company	0	0	
	Government services (public health)	2	0	
	Clinics and HHC providers	11	1	
	Professional, scientific & educational institutions	16	5	
	Publisher	8	1	
	Independent promoter	41	1	
Services	Education & information	32	14	
	Screening & assessment	28	4	
	Intervention & rehabilitation	38	7	
	Assistive tools	22	0	
Implementation	Text & readings display	37	18	
	Pictures & video streaming	23	17	
	Audio playback	71	5	
	Pictures and video recording	0	1	
	Audio recording	23	12	
	Interaction with the user	50	45	
	Interaction with external devices	44	37	
	Interaction with other apps, services, web	15	30	
	Wireless data transmission	6	2	
Users	Citizens	42	15	
	Patients with hearing problems	71	34	
	Physicians & HHC professionals	22	19	
	Families and significant others	12	18	
Descriptive information	App description	48	15	
	User manual	49	23	
	User support	49	24	
	App version	98	14	
	User ratings	46	45	2

Trends, Challenges, and Potential Opportunities

The analysis of apps' features in the tested sample, as shown in Table 1, suggests several important trends as well as potential gaps in the area of apps for HHC, in each of the five model components.

Specifically, as shown by the analysis of the component *Promoters*, the number of apps promoted by HW/SW companies was much higher than the number of apps promoted by professional/scientific institutions, clinics and HHC providers, or government services. It is thus clear that companies (including, e.g., manufacturers of hearing aids, cochlear implants, implantable devices, as well as manufacturers and providers of audiological equipment), along with independent developers, are the most active promoters in the current market of apps for HHC and that scientific and professional institutions are relatively absent – in terms of number of available apps. In fact, publication of apps can be a means for companies to provide improved and more tailored services to patients, to enable client empowerment and loyalty management and, ultimately, to leverage their market (for example, by engaging clients, selling more products, providing additional services to healthcare professionals). On the other hand, stakeholders from the public, non-for-profit, as well as from private healthcare sectors (including professional and scientific institutions, hospitals, clinics, and government services) still seem to have limited impact on the app market. As suggested by the large amount of literature in the field as reviewed above, the interest by the several stakeholders in this area is growing. So, probably, the number of apps promoted by the scientific and clinical communities and by governmental bodies is likely to increase in the near future. Other potential opportunities can be foreseen for drug companies (0 apps promoted in the tested sample) and publishers (8 apps promoted in the tested sample). There is room for greater involvement of these categories of promoters and a large potential market that will grow in the future due to the increasing population of people with hearing problems, especially in the older age groups. On the one hand, drug companies might enter this promising market by providing apps for drug management and adherence. On the other hand, publishers (including conventional as well as web-publishers) can act as key players, for example, by delivering apps with reliable, evidence-based educational content for the different target users groups (patients, citizens, or professionals).

In the area of app *Services*, the apps tested were distributed throughout the four service application areas, with a slightly higher proportion in the areas of Education & information and Intervention & rehabilitation (32 and 38 apps coded *green*, respectively) and a slightly lower number of apps in the areas of Screening & assessment and Assistive tools (28 and 22 apps coded *green*, respectively). The range of services and functions offered in each of these areas is large as shown by the market and literature reviews discussed above. So there are apps for the several potential needs of the different target user groups. At the same time, in the current market of apps for HHC, the large majority of apps deliver only one specific function (e.g., hearing testing, or hearing aid maintenance, or auditory training, and so on) and, only in a small number of cases, they combine more than one function (e.g., hearing screening combined with hearing loss information, or sound amplification combined with hearing testing). This might again suggest another potential opportunity for app promoters, i.e., the development of apps that include several functions across more than one service application area, as relevant to the different user groups such as, for example, deaf and hard of hearing patients, with their several needs. This can also suggest an important opportunity for researchers and clinicians, i.e., addressing whether multiple-service apps can be more effective to support patients with hearing loss throughout their journey. In fact, the combination of services is not necessarily an advantage in and of itself. Rather, it would be important to identify which services are more effective and how to deliver them in a truly integrated way for improved patients' benefit and satisfaction.

In the component *Implementation* an evident trend was that apps for HHC, as expected, make ample use of audio playback (e.g., for hearing testing, auditory training, or rehabilitation) but that, at the same time, they do not necessarily require the use of transducers. Only a very small number of apps in the tested sample included requirements for standardized transducers, suggesting that calibration of output levels in apps for HHC is still an open challenge, and research in this field is needed. Moreover, it is worth noting that only a small number of the tested apps included audio recordings, typically for speech rehabilitation and, only in a few apps, for environmental noise recording. This points to another open challenge, i.e., how to use apps in controlled ambient noise. This might translate in a potential opportunity for app promoters, i.e., developing reliable apps for hearing testing and hearing rehabilitation that check for environmental noise levels to be within the acceptable limits and, if needed, are able to compensate for the effects of noise. Another trend emerging from the analysis of the component *Implementation* is that apps for HHC frequently tend to include some degree of interaction with the users (50 *green*, 45 *yellow*). This is a timely opportunity as interaction with patients can promote the individual's active role and ultimately increase engagement and awareness. At the same time, this can point to some open challenges, specifically in terms of usability and ease-of-use - especially for the growing population of older patients. Similarly, text & readings are used frequently in apps for HHC (37 *green*, 18 *yellow*), for example to deliver information, provide detailed app description and instructions, or administer texts in speech and language rehabilitation apps. Again, this can be helpful to help users to gain improved knowledge but, at the same time, this can be an issue as readability of content and user literacy might be limitations, especially for the elderly. These challenges, overall, point to the importance of some principles for app developers. For example, to implement usable, easy-to-understand procedures and to optimize the app screens and interfaces for the specific target group, especially for the older ones. Use of available guidelines, such as the WCAG (Web Content Accessibility Guidelines) or ARIA (Accessible Rich Internet Applications), can be of help to warrant accessibility to people with disabilities.

In the component *Users*, an important trend observed was that, in addition to the high number of apps developed for patients with hearing loss (71 *green*, 34 *yellow*), many apps are developed for citizens, i.e., individuals with no diagnosed hearing loss (42 *green*, 15 *yellow* in the tested sample). This suggests that there is growing interest to provide apps for hearing loss awareness promotion, hearing loss prevention, hearing screening, and, in general, education for the general population. On the other hand, the number of apps that were specifically intended for use by audiologists and hearing professionals was relatively small (22 *green* out of 120) and the number of apps for families, relatives, and significant others was even smaller (12 *green*, 18 *yellow*). Therefore, a significant opportunity for app promoters might be to develop more apps that deliver a wider range of services to be used by professionals, either in clinical as well as in non-clinical settings or underserved contexts, so to take full advantage of the potential of mobile solutions in the field. Moreover, another opportunity can be to give more attention to the potential role of patients' families and significant others, and develop more apps that can enable them to support patients for improved outcomes, for example apps to educate and enable parents of children with hearing aids or cochlear implants, apps to involve parents in auditory training and speech and language rehabilitation in children, or apps to empower families and significant others to help patients with hearing loss, especially the older ones.

In the component *Descriptive Information*, it is worth noting that many apps tend to include a detailed description, complete user manual, and direct support for users. In this area it would be thus important that future research addresses the usability, reliability, and readability of the supporting information, so to define whether minimum requirements can be set for the quality and readability of supporting information.

From the analysis of the distribution of features in the tested sample of apps, a number of challenges and gaps can be highlighted, and several directions for developments can be outlined, for the ultimate aim to develop more reliable, effective, powerful mobile-based solutions able to improve patients' outcomes, engagement, and overall satisfaction.

FUTURE RESEARCH DIRECTIONS

Several research directions have been highlighted throughout this Chapter from a literature review and a market review of apps for HHC. The analysis of the app market suggests that there are still some gaps and challenges that need to be tackled. Future research as well as efforts in clinical practice and technology developments shall try to fill in these gaps and address the most relevant challenges in the field.

Deeper involvement of stakeholders from the public, non-for-profit, as well as from private sectors (including professional and scientific institutions, hospitals, clinics, and government services) is recommended throughout the process of app concept, design and development, and promotion. This can be a potential, significant opportunity for delivering novel apps that, through the involvement of researchers, clinicians, hearing professionals, as well as policy makers, can be built upon pillars of evidence base, reliability, and overall quality.

The concept of quality of health apps is complex in nature and a matter of debate in and of itself. Future research shall try to identify the core domains of app quality and develop methods to assess them. As discussed above, the literature about the assessment of health apps is large and there is still a need for a clear definition of approaches, measures, or methods to guarantee app quality. For example, in the area of apps for HHC, elements such as calibration of output levels, monitoring of environmental noise levels, and compliance with audiometric standards are extremely important, and still far from being fully addressed, so important efforts should be put in this direction. Closely related to the concept of quality, other general elements (with implications well beyond the area of hearing) such as usability, readability of information, ease-of-use, as well as evidence base, are very important and future research shall try to identify guiding principles to try to set minimum requirements for health apps and the information/services delivered.

The *ALFA4Hearing* model here shown is a useful method to characterize and compare apps for HHC and to analyze specific sets of apps. There are several potential research directions in this area. For example, from the point of view of app characterization, the model can be used to try to answer specific questions, for example to analyze what are the recurrent features and feature patterns of apps used for specific purposes (e.g., apps for hearing testing, for rehabilitation, for auditory training, or for professional education) or for specific target groups (e.g., apps for patients with hearing loss, apps for patients with tinnitus, or for children with hearing and communication problems, apps for older adults). This would be of value to get more insight into the peculiar needs in specific application areas, to understand the underlying trends in more detail, so to get further guidance for further developments. Another promising direction for research might be to combine the *ALFA4Hearing* model with some methods for app quality assessment to try to gain deeper knowledge about the drivers and facilitators to effective use of apps in this area. This is very important and, at the same time, this is challenging as quality is complex, largely subjective in nature, and can hardly be standardized. Nevertheless, it is possible that some methods, as available from the literature, could combined with the descriptive approach provided by the *ALFA4Hearing* model. Future studies shall try to understand which quality assessment methods may complement the *ALFA4Hearing* model into a combined evaluation framework and, also, how they should be adapted or further developed for this purpose.

Last, but not least, other research directions that might enhance the potential of the *ALFA4Hearing* model to extract app information concern the application of advanced methods for data visualization and cognitive computing (Paglialonga, Pinciroli, Barbieri, Caiani, Riboldi, and Tognola, 2017b). Specifically, graph analysis theory show great promise in this sense as it is able to represent a large amount of information from multiple perspectives and can be used to take a closer look at the several, complex relationships among the many app features (Paglialonga, Barbieri, Malgara, Rosati, Pinciroli, and Tognola G., 2017c). Cognitive computing (Noor, 2015) is a promising area for app characterization as it might be used to extract meaningful information from unstructured text on the web (e.g., from the apps' webpages on the app stores, from the developers' websites, from app clearinghouses, and so on) and might be used to extract the apps' features and fill out the model in an automated way (Paglialonga, Riboldi, Tognola, and Caiani, 2017d; Paglialonga, Schiavo, and Caiani, in press).

CONCLUSION

This Chapter has outlined the recent evolution of apps for HHC and the current availability of services and functions for the different target user groups. Evidence from the literature combined with the analysis of the current market suggest a dynamic, rapidly evolving scenario where the number of app-based solutions is growing along with the amount of clinical evidence. The area of apps for HHC shows great promise but there are challenges that should not be overlooked. Significant efforts in research and clinical practice are needed to try to fully address the benefits of apps and to define optimal modalities for service delivery. To take full advantage of the potential benefits of apps, the involvement of audiologists and professionals is essential. The path towards effective adoption and use of apps needs that all the relevant stakeholders join forces towards the common goal of providing apps that guarantee evidence base, reliability, and quality for the benefit of patients.

REFERENCES

Abroms, L. C., Padmanabhan, N., Thaweethai, L., & Phillips, T. (2011). iPhone apps for smoking cessation: A content analysis. *American Journal of Preventive Medicine*, *40*(3), 279–285. doi:10.1016/j.amepre.2010.10.032 PMID:21335258

Abu-Ghanem, S., Handzel, O., Ness, L., Ben-Artzi-Blima, M., Fait-Ghelbendorf, K., & Himmelfarb, M. (2016). Smartphone-based audiometric test for screening hearing loss in the elderly. *European Archives of Oto-Rhino-Laryngology*, *273*(2), 333–339. doi:10.100700405-015-3533-9 PMID:25655259

Albrecht, U. V. (2013). Transparency of health-apps for trust and decision making. *Journal of Medical Internet Research*, *15*(12), e277. doi:10.2196/jmir.2981 PMID:24449711

Albrecht, U. V., Von Jan, U., & Pramann, O. (2013). Standard reporting for medical apps. *Studies in Health Technology and Informatics*, *190*, 201–203. PMID:23823422

Amlani, A., Taylor, B., Levy, C., & Robbins, L. (2013). Utility of smartphone-based hearing aid applications as a substitute to traditional hearing aids. *Hearing Review*, *20*, 16–18.

Arnhold, M., Quade, M., & Kirch, W. (2014). Mobile applications for diabetics: A systematic review and expert-based usability evaluation considering the special requirements of diabetes patients age 50 years or older. *Journal of Medical Internet Research*, *16*(4), e104. doi:10.2196/jmir.2968 PMID:24718852

Aungst, T. D., Clauson, K. A., Misra, S., Lewis, T. L., & Husain, I. (2014). How to identify, assess and utilise mobile medical applications in clinical practice. *International Journal of Clinical Practice*, *68*(2), 155–162. doi:10.1111/ijcp.12375 PMID:24460614

Bardus, M., van Beurden, S. B., Smith, J. R., & Abraham, C. (2016). A review and content analysis of engagement, functionality, aesthetics, information quality, and change techniques in the most popular commercial apps for weight management. *The International Journal of Behavioral Nutrition and Physical Activity*, *13*(1), 35. doi:10.118612966-016-0359-9 PMID:26964880

Barton, A. J. (2012). The regulation of mobile health applications. *BMC Medicine*, *10*(1), 46. doi:10.1186/1741-7015-10-46 PMID:22569114

Basilico, A., Marceglia, S., Bonacina, S., & Pinciroli, F. (2016). Advising patients on selecting trustful apps for diabetes self-care. *Computers in Biology and Medicine, 71*, 86–96. doi:10.1016/j.compbiomed.2016.02.005 PMID:26897071

Bastawrous, A., & Armstrong, M. J. (2013). Mobile health use in low- and high-income countries: An overview of the peer-reviewed literature. *Journal of the Royal Society of Medicine, 106*(4), 130–142. doi:10.1177/0141076812472620 PMID:23564897

BinDhim, N. F., Hawkey, A., & Trevena, L. (2015). A systematic review of quality assessment methods for smartphone health apps. *Telemedicine Journal and e-Health, 21*(2), 97–104. doi:10.1089/tmj.2014.0088 PMID:25469795

Bonacina, S., Marceglia, S., & Pinciroli, F. (2014). A pictorial schema for a comprehensive user-oriented identification of medical apps. *Methods of Information in Medicine, 53*(03), 208–224. doi:10.3414/ME13-01-0093 PMID:24727980

Boudreaux, E. D., Waring, M. E., Hayes, R. B., Sadasivam, R. S., Mullen, S., & Pagoto, S. (2014). Evaluating and selecting mobile health apps: Strategies for healthcare providers and healthcare organizations. *Translational Behavioral Medicine, 4*(4), 363–371. doi:10.100713142-014-0293-9 PMID:25584085

Boulos, M. N., Brewer, A. C., Karimkhani, C., Buller, D. B., & Dellavalle, R. P. (2014). Mobile medical and health apps: State of the art, concerns, regulatory control and certification. *Online Journal of Public Health Informatics, 5*(3), 229. PMID:24683442

Bright, T., & Pallawela, D. (2016). Validated smartphone-based apps for ear and hearing assessments: A Review. *JMIR Rehabilitation and Assistive Technology, 3*(2), e13. doi:10.2196/rehab.6074 PMID:28582261

Burke, L. E., Shiffman, S., Music, E., Styn, M. A., Kriska, A., Smailagic, A., ... Rathbun, S. L. (2017). Ecological Momentary Assessment in Behavioral Research: Addressing Technological and Human Participant Challenges. *Journal of Medical Internet Research, 19*(3), e77. doi:10.2196/jmir.7138 PMID:28298264

Chan, S. R., & Misra, S. (2014). Certification of mobile apps for health care. *Journal of the American Medical Association, 312*(11), 1155–1156. doi:10.1001/jama.2014.9002 PMID:25226486

Charani, E., Castro-Sánchez, E., Moore, L. S. P., & Holmes, A. (2014). Do smartphone applications in healthcare require a governance and legal framework? It depends on the application! *BMC Medicine, 12*(1), 29. doi:10.1186/1741-7015-12-29 PMID:24524344

Chininthorn, P., Glaser, M., Tucker, W. D., & Diehl, J. C. (2016). Exploration of deaf people's health information sources and techniques for information delivery in Cape Town: A qualitative study for the design and development of a mobile health app. *JMIR Human Factors*, *3*(2), e28. doi:10.2196/humanfactors.6653 PMID:27836819

Connor, K., Brady, R. R. W., Beaux, A., & Tulloh, B. (2014). Contemporary hernia smartphone applications (apps). *Hernia*, *18*, 557–561. PMID:23801277

Corry, M., Sanders, M., & Searchfield, G. D. (2017). The accuracy and reliability of an app-based audiometer using consumer headphones: Pure tone audiometry in a normal hearing group. *International Journal of Audiology*, *56*(9), 706–710. doi:10.1080/14992027.2017.1321791 PMID:28485673

Davis, T. L., DiClemente, R., & Prietula, M. (2016). Taking mHealth Forward: Examining the Core Characteristics. *JMIR mHealth and uHealth*, *4*(3), e97. doi:10.2196/mhealth.5659 PMID:27511612

Demidowich, A. P., Lu, K., Tamler, R., & Bloomgarden, Z. (2012). An evaluation of diabetes self-management applications for Android smartphones. *Journal of Telemedicine and Telecare*, *18*(4), 235–238. doi:10.1258/jtt.2012.111002 PMID:22604278

Derin, S., Cam, O. H., Beydilli, H., Acar, E., Elicora, S. S., & Sahan, M. (2016). Initial assessment of hearing loss using a mobile application for audiological evaluation. *The Journal of Laryngology and Otology*, *130*(3), 248–251. doi:10.1017/S0022215116000062 PMID:26781699

Federal Communications Commission (FCC). (2012). *mHealth Task Force findings and recommendations*. Retrieved June 12, 2018, from http://www2.itif.org/2012-mhealth-taskforce-recommendations.pdf

Galster, J. A. (2012). Apps for audiology. *Audiology Practices*, *4*, 16–19.

Gosnell, J., Costello, J., & Shane, H. (2011). Using a clinical approach to answer "What communication apps should we use?" *ASHA SIG 12. Perspectives on Augmentative and Alternative Communication*, *20*(3), 87–96. doi:10.1044/aac20.3.87

Grebel, K., Dang, D., Ma, L., Payne, D., & Cooper, B. (2015). iSound: A smartphone based intelligent sound fusion system for the hearing impaired. *Lecture Notes in Computer Science*, *9204*, 155–164. doi:10.1007/978-3-319-21837-3_16

Groshek, M. R., Oldenburg, J., Sarasohn-Kahn, J., & Sitler, B. (2015). *mHealth app essentials: patient engagement, considerations, and implementation*. Healthcare Information and Management Systems Society (HIMSS) News. Retrieved June 12, 2018 from http://www.himss.org/ResourceLibrary/genResourceFAQ.aspx?ItemNumber=39175

Helf, C., & Hlavacs, H. (2016). Apps for life change: Critical review and solution directions. *Entertainment Computing*, *14*, 17–22. doi:10.1016/j.entcom.2015.07.001

Huckvale, K., Adomaviciute, S., Prieto, J. T., Leow, M. K., & Car, J. (2015). Smartphone apps for calculating insulin dose: A systematic assessment. *BMC Medicine*, *13*(1), 106. doi:10.118612916-015-0314-7 PMID:25943590

Hussain, M., Al-Haiqi, A., Zaidan, A. A., Zaidan, B. B., Kiah, M. L., Anuar, N. B., & Abdulnabi, M. (2015). The landscape of research on smartphone medical apps: Coherent taxonomy, motivations, open challenges and recommendations. *Computer Methods and Programs in Biomedicine*, *122*(3), 393–408. doi:10.1016/j.cmpb.2015.08.015 PMID:26412009

IMS Institute for Healthcare Informatics. (2013). *Patient Apps for Improved Healthcare: From Novelty to Mainstream*. Retrieved June 12, 2018 from http://moodle.univ-lille2.fr/pluginfile.php/128248/mod_resource/content/0/patients%20apps%20for%20improved%20healthcare%20IMS.pdf

Kenner, A. (2016). Asthma on the move: How mobile apps remediate risk for disease management. *Health Risk & Society*, *17*(7-8), 510–529. doi:10.1080/13698575.2015.1136408

Khoza-Shangase, K., & Kassner, L. (2013). Automated screening audiometry in the digital age: Exploring uHear™ and its use in a resource-stricken developing country. *International Journal of Technology Assessment in Health Care*, *29*(1), 42–47. doi:10.1017/S0266462312000761 PMID:23298579

Kim, B. Y., & Lee, J. (2017). Smart Devices for Older Adults Managing Chronic Disease: A Scoping Review. *JMIR mHealth and uHealth*, *5*(5), e69. doi:10.2196/mhealth.7141 PMID:28536089

Larrosa, F., Rama-Lopez, J., Benitez, J., Morales, J. M., Martinez, A., Alañon, M. A., ... Rey-Martinez, J. (2015). Development and evaluation of an audiology app for iPhone/iPad mobile devices. *Acta Oto-Laryngologica*, *135*(11), 1119–1127. doi:10.3109/00016489.2015.1063786 PMID:26144548

Lewis, T. L. (2013). A systematic self-certification model for mobile medical apps. *Journal of Medical Internet Research, 15*(4), e89. doi:10.2196/jmir.2446 PMID:23615332

Liao, G. Y., Chien, Y. T., Chen, Y. J., Hsiung, H. F., Chen, H. J., Hsieh, M. H., & Wu, W. J. (2017). What to Build for Middle-Agers to Come? Attractive and Necessary Functions of Exercise-Promotion Mobile Phone Apps: A Cross-Sectional Study. *JMIR mHealth and uHealth, 5*(5), e65. doi:10.2196/mhealth.6233 PMID:28546140

Lin, Y., Lai, Y., Chang, H., Tsao, Y., Chang, Y., & Chang, R. Y. (2018). SmartHear: A smartphone-based remote microphone hearing assistive system using wireless technologies. *IEEE Systems Journal, 12*(1), 20–29. doi:10.1109/JSYST.2015.2490104

Livshitz, L., Ghanayim, R., Kraus, C., Farah, R., Even-Tov, E., Avraham, Y., ... Gilbey, P. (2017). Application-based hearing screening in the elderly population. *The Annals of Otology, Rhinology, and Laryngology, 126*(1), 36–41. doi:10.1177/0003489416672873 PMID:27913721

Louw, C., Swanepoel, D. W., Eikelboom, R. H., & Myburgh, H. C. (2017). Smartphone-based hearing screening at primary health care clinics. *Ear and Hearing, 38*(2), e93–e100. doi:10.1097/AUD.0000000000000378 PMID:27764002

Lyall, F. C., Clamp, P. J., & Hajioff, D. (2016). Smartphone speech-to-text applications for communication with profoundly deaf patients. *The Journal of Laryngology and Otology, 130*(1), 104–106. doi:10.1017/S0022215115003151 PMID:26611260

Mahomed-Asmail, F., Swanepoel, D. W., Eikelboom, R. H., Myburgh, H. C., & Hall, J. III. (2016). Clinical validity of hearScreen™ smartphone hearing screening for school children. *Ear and Hearing, 37*(1), e11–e17. doi:10.1097/AUD.0000000000000223 PMID:26372265

Mantovani, E., & Quinn, P. (2014), mHealth and data protection – the letter and the spirit of consent legal requirements. *International Review of Law, Computers and Technology, 20*(2), 222-236.

Martínez-Pérez, B., de la Torre-Díez, I., Candelas-Plasencia, S., & López-Coronado, M. (2013). Development and evaluation of tools for measuring the quality of experience (QoE) in mHealth applications. *Journal of Medical Systems, 37*(5), 9976. doi:10.100710916-013-9976-x PMID:24014255

Martínez-Pérez, B., de la Torre-Díez, I., & López-Coronado, M. (2013). Mobile health applications for the most prevalent conditions by the World Health Organization: Review and analysis. *Journal of Medical Internet Research, 15*(6), e120. doi:10.2196/jmir.2600 PMID:23770578

Martínez-Pérez, B., de la Torre-Díez, I., López-Coronado, M., & Herreros-González, J. (2013). Mobile Apps in Cardiology [Review]. *JMIR mHealth and uHealth, 1*(2), e15. doi:10.2196/mhealth.2737 PMID:25098320

Masalski, M., Kipiński, L., Grysiński, T., & Kręcicki, T. (2016). Hearing tests on mobile devices: Evaluation of the reference sound level by means of biological calibration. *Journal of Medical Internet Research, 18*(5), e130. doi:10.2196/jmir.4987 PMID:27241793

Meder, A. M., & Wegner, J. R. (2015). iPads, mobile technologies, and communication applications: A survey of family wants, needs, and preferences. *Augmentative and Alternative Communication, 31*(1), 27–36. doi:10.3109/07434618.2014.995223 PMID:25685882

Mielke, M., & Brueck, R. (2015). Design and evaluation of a smartphone application for non-speech sound awareness for people with hearing loss. In *Proceedings of the 2015 Annual International Conference of the IEEE Engineering in Medicine and Biology Society (IEEE EMBC 2015).* IEEE Press.

Mielke, M., & Brueck, R. (2016). A home automation based environmental sound alert for people experiencing hearing loss. In *Proceedings of the 2016 Annual International Conference of the IEEE Engineering in Medicine and Biology Society (IEEE EMBC 2016).* IEEE Press.

Mielke, M., Grunewald, A., & Brueck, R. (2013). An assistive technology for hearing-impaired persons: analysis, requirements and architecture. In *Proceedings of the 2013 Annual International Conference of the IEEE Engineering in Medicine and Biology Society (IEEE EMBC 2013).* IEEE Press.

Misra, S., Lewis, T. L., & Aungst, T. D. (2013). Medical application use and the need for further research and assessment for clinical practice: Creation and integration of standards for best practice to alleviate poor application design. *JAMA Dermatology, 149*(6), 661–662. doi:10.1001/jamadermatol.2013.606 PMID:23783150

Mosa, A. S. M., Yoo, I., & Sheets, L. (2012). A systematic review of healthcare applications for smartphones. *BMC Medical Informatics and Decision Making, 12*(1), 67. doi:10.1186/1472-6947-12-67 PMID:22781312

Muessig, K. E., Pike, E. C., LeGrand, S., & Hightow-Weidman, L. B. (2013). Mobile phone applications for the care and prevention of HIV and other sexually transmitted diseases: A review. *Journal of Medical Internet Research, 15*(1), e1. doi:10.2196/jmir.2301 PMID:23291245

Murfin, M. (2013). Know your apps: An evidence-based approach to evaluation of mobile clinical applications. *The Journal of Physician Assistant Education: the Official Journal of the Physician Assistant Education Association, 24*(3), 38–40. doi:10.1097/01367895-201324030-00008 PMID:24261171

Na, Y., Joo, H. S., Yang, H., Kang, S., Hong, S. H., & Woo, J. (2014). Smartphone-based hearing screening in noisy environments. *Sensors (Basel), 14*(6), 10346–10360. doi:10.3390140610346 PMID:24926692

Noor, A. K. (2015). Potential of cognitive computing and cognitive systems. *Ocean Engineering, 5*(1), 75–88.

O'Neill, S., & Brady, R. R. W. (2012). Colorectal smartphone apps: Opportunities and risks. *Colorectal Disease, 14*(9), e530–e534. doi:10.1111/j.1463-1318.2012.03088.x PMID:22646729

Olson, A. D. (2015). Options for auditory training for adults with hearing loss. *Seminars in Hearing, 36*(4), 284–295. doi:10.1055-0035-1564461 PMID:27587915

Ozdalga, E., Ozdalga, A., & Ahuja, N. (2012). The smartphone in medicine: A review of current and potential use among physicians and students. *Journal of Medical Internet Research, 14*(5), e128. doi:10.2196/jmir.1994 PMID:23017375

Paglialonga, A., Barbieri, R., Malgara, F., Rosati, R., Pinciroli, F., & Tognola, G. (2017c). Multidimensional characterization of mobile apps for hearing health care by using the ALFA4Hearing (At-a-glance Labelling for Features of Apps for Hearing health care) model combined with data visualization methods. In *Proceedings of the 2017 Medical Informatics Europe (EFMI MIE 2017)*. IOS Press.

Paglialonga, A., Lugo, A., & Santoro, E. (2018). An overview on the emerging area of identification, characterization, and assessment of health apps. *Journal of Biomedical Informatics, 83*, 97–102. doi:10.1016/j.jbi.2018.05.017 PMID:29852318

Paglialonga, A., Mastropietro, A., Scalco, E., & Rizzo, G. (in press). The mHealth. In G. Andreoni & G. Perego (Eds.), *Present, present continuous and future of mHealth: a reference grammar for next healthcare*. London: Springer.

Paglialonga, A., Pinciroli, F., Barbieri, R., Caiani, E. G., Riboldi, M., & Tognola, G. (2017b). E-Health solutions for better care: Characterization of health apps to extract meaningful information and support users' choices. In *Proceedings of the 3rd IEEE International Forum on Research and Technologies for Society and Industry* (*IEEE RTSI 2017*). IEEE Press.

Paglialonga, A., Pinciroli, F., & Tognola, G. (2017a). The *ALFA4Hearing* model (At-a-glance Labelling for Features of Apps for Hearing healthcare) to characterize mobile apps for hearing healthcare. *American Journal of Audiology*, *26*(3S), 408–425. doi:10.1044/2017_AJA-16-0132 PMID:29049624

Paglialonga, A., Riboldi, M., Tognola, G., & Caiani, E. G. (2017d). Automated Identification of Health Apps' Medical Specialties and Promoters from the Store Webpages. In *Proceedings of the 6th IEEE International Conference on E-Health and Bioengineering* (*IEEE EHB 2017*). IEEE Press.

Paglialonga, A., Schiavo, M., & Caiani, E. G. (in press). Automated Characterization of Mobile Health Apps' Features by Extracting Information from the Web: An Exploratory Study. *American Journal of Audiology*.

Paglialonga, A., Tognola, G., & Pinciroli, F. (2015a). Apps for hearing sciences and care. *American Journal of Audiology*, *24*, 293-298.

Paglialonga, A., Tognola, G., & Pinciroli, F. (2015b). Apps for hearing healthcare. *Studies in Health Technology and Informatics*, *210*, 666–668. PMID:25991233

Panahi, I., Kehtarnavaz, N., & Thibodeau, L. (2016). Smartphone-based noise adaptive speech enhancement for hearing aid applications. In *Proceedings of the 2016 Annual International Conference of the IEEE Engineering in Medicine and Biology Society (IEEE EMBC 2016)*. IEEE Press.

Pandey, A., Hasan, S., Dubey, D., & Sarangi, S. (2013). Smartphone apps as a source of cancer information: Changing trends in health information-seeking behavior. *Journal of Cancer Education*, *28*(1), 138–142. doi:10.100713187-012-0446-9 PMID:23275239

Peer, S., & Fagan, J. J. (2015). Hearing loss in the developing world: Evaluating the iPhone mobile device as a screening tool. *South African Medical Journal*, *105*(1), 35–39. doi:10.7196/SAMJ.8338 PMID:26046161

Privacy Rights Clearinghouse. (2016). *Mobile Health and Fitness Apps: What Are the Privacy Risks?* Retrieved June 12, 2018 from https://www.privacyrights.org/consumer-guides/mobile-health-and-fitness-apps-what-are-privacy-risks

Probst, T., Pryss, R., Langguth, B., & Schlee, W. (2016). Emotion dynamics and tinnitus: Daily life data from the "TrackYourTinnitus" application. *Scientific Reports*, *6*(1), 31166. doi:10.1038rep31166 PMID:27488227

Qiang, C. Z., Yamamichi, M., Hausman, V., Miller, R., & Altman, D. (2012). *Mobile applications for the health sector*. Washington, DC: World Bank. Retrieved June 12, 2018 from http://documents.worldbank.org/curated/en/2012/04/16742613/mobile-applications-health-sector

Rehman, H., Kamal, A. K., Morris, P. B., Sayani, S., Merchant, A. T., & Virani, S. S. (2017). Mobile Health (mHealth) Technology for the Management of Hypertension and Hyperlipidemia: Slow Start but Loads of Potential. *Current Atherosclerosis Reports*, *19*(3), 12. doi:10.100711883-017-0649-y PMID:28210974

Research2guidance. (2017). *mHealth app developer economics 2017 -The state of the art of mHealth app publishing*. Retrieved June 12, 2018 from https://research2guidance.com/product/mhealth-economics-2017-current-status-and-future-trends-in-mobile-health

Reynoldson, C., Stones, C., Allsop, M., Gardner, P., Bennett, M. I., Closs, S. J., ... Knapp, P. (2014). Assessing the quality and usability of smartphone apps for pain self-management. *Pain Medicine*, *15*(6), 898–909. doi:10.1111/pme.12327 PMID:24422990

Richards, J. R., Gaylor, K. A., & Pilgrim, A. J. (2015). Comparison of traditional otoscope to iPhone otoscope in the pediatric ED. *The American Journal of Emergency Medicine*, *33*(8), 1089–1092. doi:10.1016/j.ajem.2015.04.063 PMID:25979304

Sama, P. R., Eapen, Z. J., Weinfurt, K. P., Shah, B. R., & Schulman, K. A. (2014). An evaluation of mobile health application tools. *JMIR mHealth and uHealth*, *2*(2), e19. doi:10.2196/mhealth.3088 PMID:25099179

Sandström, J., Swanepoel, D. W., Carel Myburgh, H., & Laurent, C. (2016). Smartphone threshold audiometry in underserved primary health-care contexts. *International Journal of Audiology*, *55*(4), 232–238. doi:10.3109/14992027.2015.1124294 PMID:26795898

Scherer, E. A., Ben-Zeev, D., Li, Z., & Kne, J. M. (2017). Analyzing mHealth Engagement: Joint Models for Intensively Collected User Engagement Data. *JMIR mHealth and uHealth*, *5*(1), e1. doi:10.2196/mhealth.6474 PMID:28082257

Schlee, W., Pryss, R. C., Probst, T., Schobel, J., Bachmeier, A., Reichert, M., & Langguth, B. (2016). Measuring the moment-to-moment variability of tinnitus: The TrackYourTinnitus smart phone app. *Frontiers in Aging Neuroscience*, *8*, 294. doi:10.3389/fnagi.2016.00294 PMID:28018210

Steinhubl, S. R., Muse, E. D., & Topol, E. J. (2015). The emerging field of mobile health. *Science Translational Medicine*, *7*(283), 283rv3. doi:10.1126citranslmed.aaa3487 PMID:25877894

Stoyanov, S. R., Hides, L., Kavanagh, D. J., & Wilson, H. (2016). Development and validation of the user version of the Mobile Application Rating Scale (uMARS). *JMIR mHealth and uHealth*, *4*(2), e72. doi:10.2196/mhealth.5849 PMID:27287964

Stoyanov, S. R., Hides, L., Kavanagh, D. J., Zelenko, O., Tjondronegoro, D., & Mani, M. (2015). Mobile App Rating Scale: A new tool for assessing the quality of health mobile apps. *JMIR mHealth and uHealth*, *3*(1), e27. doi:10.2196/mhealth.3422 PMID:25760773

Thompson, G. P., Sladen, D. P., Borst, B. J., & Still, O. L. (2015). Accuracy of a tablet audiometer for measuring behavioral hearing thresholds in a clinical population. *Otolaryngology - Head and Neck Surgery*, *153*(5), 838–842. doi:10.1177/0194599815593737 PMID:26183518

Tognola, G., Paglialonga, A., Chiaramello, E., & Pinciroli, F. (2015). eHealth for Hearing – new views and apps practicalities. *European Journal of Biomedical Informatics*, *11*(3), en43–en49.

van Kerkhof, L. W. M., van der Laar, C. W. E., de Jong, C., Weda, M., & Hegger, I. (2016). Characterization of apps and other e-tools for medication use: Insights into possible benefits and risks. *JMIR mHealth and uHealth*, *4*(2), e34. doi:10.2196/mhealth.4149 PMID:27052946

Wallis, L. A., Fleming, J., Hasselberg, M., Laflamme, L., & Lundin, J. (2016). A smartphone app and cloud-based consultation system for burn injury emergency care. *PLoS One*, *11*(2), e0147253. doi:10.1371/journal.pone.0147253 PMID:26918631

Wang, A., An, N., Lu, X., Chen, H., Li, C., & Levkoff, S. (2014). A classification scheme for analyzing mobile apps used to prevent and manage disease in late life. *JMIR mHealth and uHealth, 2*(1), e6. doi:10.2196/mhealth.2877 PMID:25098687

West, J. H., Hall, P. C., Hanson, C. L., Barnes, M. D., Giraud-Carrier, C., & Barrett, J. (2012). There's an app for that: Content analysis of paid health and fitness apps. *Journal of Medical Internet Research, 14*(3), e72. doi:10.2196/jmir.1977 PMID:22584372

Wicks, P., & Chiauzzi, E. (2015). 'Trust but verify'--five approaches to ensure safe medical apps. *BMC Medicine, 13*(1), 205. doi:10.118612916-015-0451-z PMID:26404791

Wong, M. C., & Fung, K. (2015). Mobile applications in otolaryngology-head and neck surgery. *Otolaryngology - Head and Neck Surgery, 152*(4), 638–643. doi:10.1177/0194599815568946 PMID:25628367

World Health Organization. (2011). *mHealth: New horizons for health through mobile technologies*. Retrieved June 12, 2018 from www.who.int/goe/publications/ehealth_series_vol3/en/

Zhao, J., Freeman, B., & Li, M. (2016). Can Mobile Phone Apps Influence People's Health Behavior Change? An Evidence Review. *Journal of Medical Internet Research, 18*(11), e287. doi:10.2196/jmir.5692 PMID:27806926

KEY TERMS AND DEFINITIONS

ALFA4 Hearing Model: A descriptive method to characterize apps for hearing healthcare.

App: An application software designed to run on mobile devices such as smartphones and tablets.

Assessment: The evaluation of quality components.

Characterization: The identification of relevant characteristic features.

eHealth: The use of information and communication technologies (ICT) for health.

mHealth: The branch of eHealth that makes use of mobile devices.

Service Area: Each of the four categories in which the app functions can be classified (education and information, screening and assessment, intervention and rehabilitation, and assistive tools).

Chapter 8
Tele-Audiology and Security Management:
Is Anyone Hearing the Threats?

Rick Harvey
Layer Security, Australia

Ingo Mueller
Hochschule für Telekommunikation Leipzig, Germany

ABSTRACT

Security is a huge topic and not at all fun. It's hard to understand. It can be scary. It is always lurking. And poor security can bring down any system, regardless of how useful or important it is. Understanding the risks and vulnerabilities in systems and the motivations and methods of attackers is important in designing and operating secure and robust systems. This chapter aims to give a perspective on how to think about information technology (IT) security, how it applies to telehealth and audiology, and finally gives some recommendations about important considerations for tele-audiology systems that include devices, data housing, smartphone applications, and patient records.

DOI: 10.4018/978-1-5225-8191-8.ch008

INTRODUCTION

Security matters. It's the flip-side of all the significant advances in technology, communications, business and social interactions. For every new way that society finds to make use of technology for better efficiencies and outcomes, the bad guys find a way to abuse it. This is the reason why there seems to be an endless series of new cyber-attacks, privacy breaches and organizations being compromised.

Any system can fail. This may be because of poor design, accident, human error, misconfiguration or improper use. But assuming all this is correct, then an attacker will put the system under pressure looking for just one weak point. If the attacker finds one, then there has been a security failure. With Information Technology (IT) systems, the attacker has many advantages. Attackers can attack any of the components of a system: computers, devices, networks, applications and the people and processes around them. Each of those components may have multiple vulnerabilities. Attacks can be automated and launched from anywhere in the world via the Internet. Consequently, the Internet today experiences a continuous and never-ending flood of attacks (Kaspersky, 2017). The defenders must defend everything, but the attackers just need to find the tiniest vulnerability.

Tele-audiology is a microcosm of the world of attackers and defenders. At the device level, the hearing aid and associated configuration software may have weaknesses. At the business level, the audiology practice may have weaknesses or may be connected to external IT systems that have weaknesses.

Any attack has its consequences. Attacking a medical device may be life-threatening (e.g. pace-makers, dialysis machines etc.). Attacking a business may be also be detrimental due to economic losses, loss of reputation, litigation or stress on patients with a breach of their privacy.

This chapter aims to give an overview of security and areas that need to be considered when running a tele-audiology system. Section 2 gives a background and overview to security, why it is such a difficult area and most importantly, why it matters to tele-audiology. Section 3 provides a security analysis of tele-audiology systems. Section 4 outlines a framework for security management to ensure a reasonable level of security for a tele-audiology practice and highlights important aspects that need to be considered when implementing it.

Finally, this chapter closes with some conclusions with an emphasis on the following points:

- Security is not only a technical issue, it is a business concern.
- Every system is breakable, but it is the weak and least defended systems that get hacked first.
- Attackers go after the assets of most value. In tele-audiology, this is probably the patient data.
- All aspects of all IT related systems need to be defended. This includes people and processes.
- Make use of security professionals and industry best practices.

BACKGROUND

Security is a vast subject. Areas include computer security, information security, physical security, national security, economic security, just to name a few. The reasons why security can fail are numerous and varied. They cut across many fields including psychology, sociology, economics, biology, neuroscience, game theory, political science, law, philosophy, theology, cognitive science, and, many others (Schneier, 2012).

This chapter limits itself to computer and information security. Even this area is huge, covering every aspect of technology, people and processes including all the computers, devices, networks, applications, operations, and all the different types of interactions between people, systems, networks and information. Clearly all of this is not going to be explained. But this section does try to give a perspective on why an understanding of security is so important.

What Is Information Security?

Information security has many names. Two common ones are computer security and cybersecurity. At its core, the aim of information security is to protect computer systems and the information they process against unauthorized access, manipulation, theft, loss or other types of failures such as denial of service.

The scope of information security covers nearly every aspect of an IT system. For example, computers, smartphones, laptops, wireless networks, Internet communications, the software that runs on computers, the people that use these computers and the processes that are performed by these systems.

There are three key properties of information security often referred to as the CIA triad – confidentiality, integrity, availability.

Confidentiality is concerned with the protection of information against unauthorized access, e.g. only the audiologist should be able to access contact details or health records of a patient but not another patient or an outsider. This also relates to a patient's privacy. If confidentiality cannot be guaranteed, neither can privacy.

Integrity is concerned with the protection of information against unauthorized manipulation, e.g. only the audiologist should be able to change a patient record, add or delete contact details, or change a diagnosis.

Availability is concerned with ensuring ongoing authorized access to information, e.g. the audiologist should be able to access patient records or payment information whenever and wherever they need to be able to react to patient's requests or to adjust treatment in a timely manner.

How Big Is the Security Problem?

The security problem has grown as fast as the computing industry has grown.

Back in the 1960s, there were mainframes. These were expensive, hard to use computers that were operated by expert users within large organizations. This made mainframes relatively easy to secure, and ensure confidentiality, integrity and availability of information. In the 1970s mini computers started to be used in business, but again the businesses had them well controlled as they too were still operated mainly in isolation. In the 1980s personal computers and simple networking using telephone lines and modems started to become widespread and the first computer viruses started to appear. In the 1990s, the Internet brought computing to much of the world and so began new types of scams and computer crime.

The trend of rapid advancements in both computing and security problems has continued as depicted in Figure 1.

Figure 1. Advances in information technology verses the rise of security problems

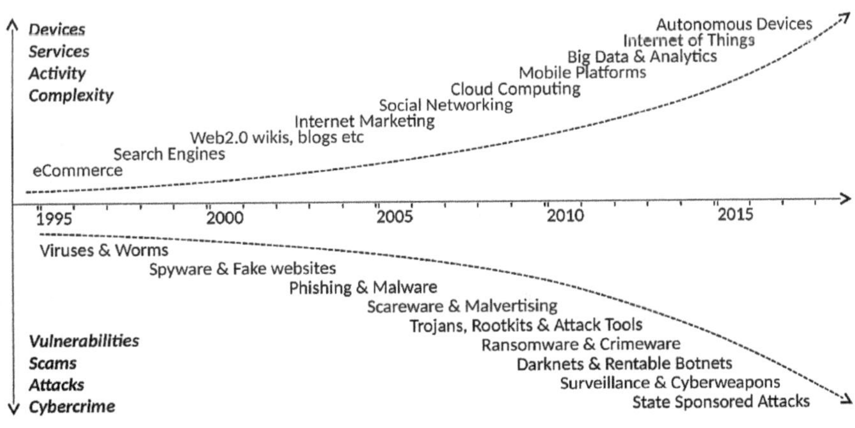

Why Is Security So Hard?

In many ways, breaking security is like the art of cheating. It is probably the only endeavour that has no rules. Think of securing a house. The owner will start by locking the house when they go out. If there is a break in, then the owner might strengthen the doors and windows. If burglars pick or break the locks, then the owner might put in bigger or more locks. If thieves come through the roof or the floor, then the house may be further fortified with bars and other reinforcements. But just trying to defend the perimeter is not enough. Clever adversaries will find other devious ways of getting into the house. Criminals could trick the owner and simply knock on the front door dressed as a policeman. Or they could hide in the driveway and threaten the owner with a knife or gun when they arrive home. They could even hack into any Internet connected camera or smart TV inside the house and observe the owner's every move or eavesdrop on their every conversation.

As can be seen, this is a game of escalation. The defenders apply more defences. The attackers find new ways of attacking. The more complexity in a system, the harder it is to defend, and the easier it is to attack. The defender must be ready for every possible scenario. But the attacker simply needs to find just one single weakness. As technology advances, the odds are increasingly stacked against the defenders. This is because technology and the Internet give attackers leverage and scale.

In essence, the attackers have a lot in their favour. Nearly every aspect of society relies on computing so the attacker has a myriad of systems to attack. Any given system has vulnerabilities so there is a vast array of ways to attack it. If that system is broken, then the attacker can attack any similar system at the same time. Attackers can cloak their identity and hide where they operate from by making use of compromised machines in a different part of the world. The attacker does not even need to be skilled. They can simply make use of malicious software written by someone else and run it as many times as they like.

All the above together makes it very easy for an attacker to attack millions of computers around the globe with little knowledge and skill from the comfort of their hideout. Given that law enforcement in the digital world of the Internet is extremely difficult due to a lack of mandate and competing jurisdictions, the risk to be caught is low which further increases the incentive for criminals to commit computer crime. Too many systems. Too many ways to attack them. Too easy to do the attack from anywhere, by anyone, as often as required. And no market incentive or laws to make companies do the right thing about security. Sadly, the defenders aren't keeping pace with the attackers. In fact, it could be argued that, in the age of ongoing advances in nearly every profession, that security is the only profession that is going backwards.

Will the Security Problem Ever Be Solved?

Unfortunately, no. But the security problem does not need to be completely solved, because security is a *trade-off.*

Nearly everything about security is a trade-off. What is gained verses what is lost. For example, a tele-audiology business may not employ a security guard at their premise. Not because guards do not stop crime, but because the business owner has made a trade-off. The cost of employing the guard is not worth the risk of someone stealing things from their office.

In this way, security is like insurance. Some people do not have any and simply take the risk. Some people have lots because they fear the worst. Security is a subjective feeling which may or may not match reality. People who feel safe take unnecessary risks. People who do not feel safe may make costly decisions.

There is a whole industry that is dedicated to the theory of this security trade-off. It is called *risk analysis*. The essence is to try to prioritize how to best spend the time and money on a mitigation. For example, a power failure may be tolerable in a business. But in a hospital, it cannot be tolerated and so back-up generators need to be put in place. In a risk assessment, the critical assets will be identified, the likelihood of failure determined and the impact on the system or business of any failure will be assessed.

The trade-offs also apply to the attacker. A burglar walking down a street will choose the "easy" targets first. There is a cost-benefit to him. This means that to be safe, a business does not need to have perfect security, it just needs to be better than similar businesses. However, a business may be more of a target if it has high value assets. Just like in a block of shops, the thief will spend extra time and effort to go after the jewellery store in preference to the pizza shop because the prize is so much greater. This means that it is unwise to concentrate high value information in a single place, for example all medical data in a single database.

How Harmful Can a Break in Security Be?

Computing is controlling more and more of society. The more it controls, the greater the scope for things to go badly wrong.

Until recently, attacks have mainly been financially motivated. Information may get stolen, money may be scammed, Web sites may be taken down, but this typically is not a catastrophic loss. The victims may lose some privacy, or money or be embarrassed by leaks, but the consequences are not directly life threatening.

As computing progressively connects the virtual and the physical world, the security landscape changes because of the "consequences of failure". In particular, safety critical industries including power, transport and medical. In these industries, the consequences of failure are much grimmer. Losing a credit card is nowhere near as bad as a hack on a self-driving car which could cause accidents or even fatalities.

Devices with computing capabilities continue to get smaller, faster, cheaper and more powerful. It is estimated that around 20 billion IoT (Internet of Things) devices could be online by 2020 (Gartner, 2017). Flipping the view, the world is getting more computers that do more things. A microwave is really a computer that cooks food. Smart phones are really computers that can make phone calls. A car is really a collection of computers that transport people. And a hearing aid is really a very small computer that amplifies sound.

This brings medical devices to the forefront of concern (Newman, 2017). They are becoming increasingly computerized and networked in order to improve patient care, treatment or monitoring. But medical devices also have vulnerabilities. Researchers have found vulnerabilities in nearly every device they examine, ranging from CT scanners, MRI machines to insulin pumps, pacemakers and defibrillators (Sametinger, Rozenblit, Lysecky & Ott, 2015; Li, Raghunathan & Jha, 2011; Halperin, Heydt-Benjamin, Ransford, Clark, Defend, Morgan, Fu, Kohno, & Maisel, 2008; Rios, 2017). If exploited by attackers, the consequences of failure may be death.

Another important factor is "consequences for the industry". That is, even if a given business does the right thing, if another industry related business is broken, the net result could affect all the businesses in that industry. For example, in February 2015, Anthem health insurance provider in the US was hacked and nearly 80 million people's detailed health history was stolen (Abelson & Goldstein, 2015). The after effects were many including wide-scale fraud using stolen identities and a new black market of prescription drugs being obtained by impersonation.

Why Does Security Matter to Tele-Audiology Practices?

There are different types of attackers and their motivations to attack a tele-audiology system differ. As a tele-audiology practice is unlikely to be a target for state-sponsored hackers, industrial espionage and cyber warfare activities, it is most likely financial gain that attracts attackers to tele-audiology systems. In this context, a tele-audiology practice offers various assets and properties that may be used by an attacker to generate a profit.

There are three key assets related to patients:

1. Health records and other patient-related data. Here the privacy of patients is at stake. Other concerns include identity theft, blackmail (e.g. medical history), fraud (e.g. order medication using a patients account) or the interference with treatment of patient.
2. Payment details. For example, attackers may sell credit card information on the black market (also known as the Dark Web) or may attempt to empty a patient's account.
3. Patient access credentials and contact details. When patients register with a medical practice they typically leave an email address, a phone number and other contact details. They may also have access to a practice Web portal for which they require a username and password. Phone numbers may be used by an attacker to call patients and to trick them into revealing other personal information, transfer money, e.g. by pretending to collect tax debts or government fines. Since passwords are frequently reused, an attacker may be able to use the email address and password of a patient to take control of their mailbox, online banking accounts, etc.

There are other assets in a tele-audiology practice's IT system that are of value to attackers. For example:

- Access credentials to practice IT systems and applications. If an attacker can get hold of them they may gain unauthorized access, manipulate, erase or steal patient-related data.
- Information essential for running the business including accounting, pay roll and tax information as well as payment provider information and access credentials. This information may be used by an attacker to steal money from the practice, alter or erase records or block access to this information and claim a ransom.
- Tele-audiology practices are small businesses that often integrate their IT system with larger businesses, such as banks or hearing aid manufacturers and vendors. Since small businesses have less money and resources to spend on security they are the ideal backdoor for attacks on larger businesses.
- Point-of-sale devices such as credit card readers or contactless payment systems may be compromised by an attacker to record and steal credit card information including pin codes with the aim to sell this information on the Dark Web or to empty outpatient accounts.
- The IT system itself is an asset. It can be abused to run attacks on other businesses and organizations or computer systems in general, e.g. spam campaigns or denial of service attacks.

There are many other assets of lesser importance that still require protection, but they are out of scope here. To make sure all assets in a tele-audiology practice are properly identified and protected, a detailed risk analysis needs to be performed. For more information see Landoll (2011).

SECURITY ANALYSIS OF TELE-AUDIOLOGY SYSTEMS

This section outlines the main components of a typical tele-audiology system and discusses security concerns relevant to tele-audiology practitioners. Note, this analysis is not exhaustive. To assess the security of a concrete tele-audiology system in depth, a detailed analysis of all system components as well as relevant policies and procedures is required.

The key components of a tele-audiology system are the hearing aids, the connector devices, the hearing aid management software and the backend IT systems, as depicted in Figure 2.

Hearing Aids

The key component of any tele-audiology system is the hearing aid device that typically comprise an internal microphone, a digital processor also called digital amplifier, a set of digital filters and a receiver component. It further contains a built-in battery, an on/off switch and a volume control.

A hearing aid usually operates as follows. The microphone picks up ambient sounds from the patient's environment and passes them on to the amplifier. The digital amplifier: (1) converts analogue input signals into a digital audio stream; (2) applies various filters to reduce background noise and to emphasize spoken words or other sounds of interested, and; (3) amplifies the volume to accommodate the

Figure 2. Components in a tele-audiology system for security analysis

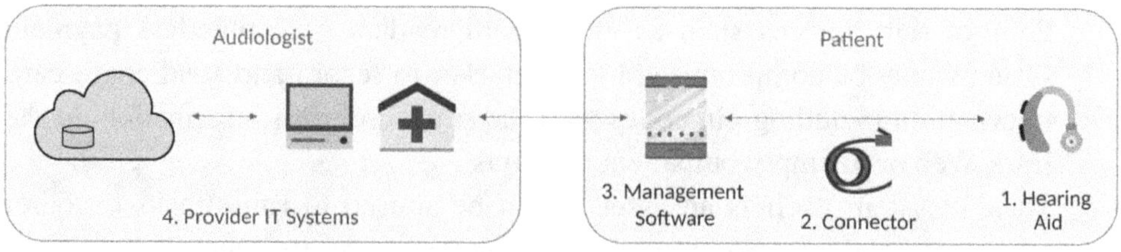

patient's hearing loss. The manipulated audio stream is then transferred to the receiver that converts it back into an analogue signal and outputs it to the patient's inner ear.

Security Considerations

The digital components of a hearing aid are purpose-built and have been optimized for size, weight and battery longevity. This means that they: (1) have limited computing power; (2) cannot be easily reprogrammed, and; (3) do not offer recording/storage facilities for large quantities of data (audio or otherwise). Moreover, hearing aids operate in isolation and are not connected to a computer network such as the Internet. If a conventional hearing aid is connected to another computing device, it is usually only for short periods of time (e.g. the duration of a patient consultation) and via a cable connection.

These properties of a hearing aid lead to a very small attack surface. This means that attackers find it difficult to connect to a hearing aid to use it for malicious activities such as manipulating the device, stealing information or using the device to attack other computer systems.

From an economic perspective, a hearing aid also provides only a low-value target. All an attacker may achieve is to prevent the hearing aid from operating normally. Since conventional hearing aids operate in isolation, such an attack does not scale (i.e. the costs to perform the attack on many devices is higher than the expected gain) which makes it very unlikely.

The most serious theoretical attack on a hearing aid is to overhear conversations of a patient. Even though the latter would constitute a serious security and privacy breach, it is very unlikely. Firstly, the attacker would need to add further components to the hearing aid which the patient would likely notice. Secondly, there are many easier ways to overhear and record conversations.

The potential impact of a compromised hearing aid on the patient's well-being is low if we assume that vendors adhere to strict health regulations and standards that ensure that hearing aids can never emit electromagnetic or other radiation levels that harm a patient or the people around them. Distorted sounds and white noise that is unpleasant to the ear, draining the battery or destroying the hearing aid altogether are the most likely outcomes of an attack.

Various Web sites detail the experiences of hobby inventors that extended their hearing aids, e.g. to connect them to, and to reconfigure them via, smartphones (Hack & Hear, 2016; Ward, 2012). This shows that some patients may tamper with their own hearing aids but given the limited capabilities of a hearing aid it is unlikely that they pose, inadvertently or intentionally, security risks on other components of a tele-audiology system.

There are no obvious attacks in which an attacker uses a hearing aid to attack another computer system. It has been reported that hearing aids can be reprogrammed to replay wireless network signals as sounds (Stinson, 2014). However, even if such a wireless network is unsecured and transfers data unprotected, a hearing aid alone cannot be used to recover the actual data.

In summary, hearing aids are unlikely to be attacked by attackers and the expected impact of such attacks is low. Only a very determined, skilled and well-funded attacker with a high value target will explore attacks on hearing aids in their current form. At the time of writing, no known attacks or vulnerabilities of hearing aids have been reported in academic literature or industry forums.

Next Generation Hearing Aids

The ongoing miniaturization of integrated computer chips have paved the way for the development of next generation hearing aids that integrate additional components that offer a range of additional features such as Bluetooth connectivity to smartphones, smartwatches or TV sets, spatially directed hearing and the ability to zoom into important sounds or conversations. The patient can control these new features via an application on their smartphone.

Security Considerations

From a security point of view the most significant of these features is the support for continuous wireless connectivity to a smartphone. Various versions of the Bluetooth standard are known to have security flaws that may enable an attacker to recover the data that is transmitted between a hearing aid and a connected smartphone (Lekowski, 2016). However, the hearing aid mainly transmits control data which is of low value for an attacker. Moreover, attacks on Bluetooth are local attacks that do not scale well and are, therefore, of little interest to attackers.

Connected hearing aids open one interesting avenue of attack. By attacking patients' smartphones, an attacker may be able to perform a so-called denial of service (DOS) attack which switches off or damages the hearing aids of a particular vendor with the aim to extort money from them. If hearing aids from this vendor can only be controlled via smartphones this attack can be extended to claim a ransom from patients as well.

Other attacks on a hearing aid may be possible, including tracking a patient's movements, remotely profiling their encounters and record conversations (Grantcharov, 2016). However, these attacks can be realized more easily and more effectively by simply compromising a patient's smartphone.

Current next-generation hearing aids are not directly connected to the Internet and thus remain an unlikely element in attacks on other computer systems.

Overall, next generation hearing aids provide an increased attack surface but remain a low-value target given the data they transmit to a connected smartphone. The pairing with smartphones does not add significant new security concerns to a tele-audiology system as long as smartphones are not used to transfer data between a hearing aid and other components of a tele-audiology system.

Connector Devices

Hearing aids offer a range of parameters that need to be adjusted to the concrete needs of a patient. To adjust these parameters, a connector device is required. A typical connector is a purpose-built cable that is plugged into the hearing aid and connected to a computer in a tele-audiology practice, usually a desktop PC or laptop, that runs a specific hearing aid management software. The connection to the computer may be wired as well or realized with a wireless Bluetooth connection.

Security Considerations

Potential security concerns involving the connector are very limited in number and impact. A typical connector does not have many processing capabilities and in the simplest case constitutes only a cable. If the connector provides wired connectivity, an attacker may replace the original connector or manipulate the desktop PC or laptop that is connected to it. If the connector provides wireless connectivity, an attacker has the additional option to remotely interfere or eavesdrop on the data transmission through the connector. As mentioned earlier, various versions of the Bluetooth standard have known security issues.

However, the data exchanged through the connector poses a low value target as it comprises only hearing aid configuration data. Furthermore, the connector is not continuously plugged in to the hearing aid which significantly reduces the scalability of attacks. In summary, the connector provides a very limited attack surface and is unlikely to be targeted by attackers.

Hearing Aid Management Software

A hearing aid is programmed by an audiologist with the help of a specific hearing aid management software. This software typically runs on a desktop PC or laptop in an audiology practice and correlates information about the configuration of a hearing aid and possibly other patient data. In this way, a long-term history of the patient's configuration changes is recorded that may be used for diagnostic purposes.

Security Considerations

The management software may contain software bugs or inadequate access controls that allow an attacker to obtain unauthorized access to hearing aid configuration data. However, this data is of low value for attackers.

The most likely attack on the management software is a substitution attack. This is where a user is tricked into installing what they think is hearing aid software, but is, in fact, malicious software obtained from another apparently innocent site. On installation, the malicious software may install a copy of the legitimate hearing aid software in the foreground, while quietly installing in the background some nasty backdoor that compromises the device.

If in the future hearing aids are configured remotely, via an Internet connection and not a connector device/cable, software bugs or inadequate access controls in the management software may be exploited by an attacker to gain access to other components of a tele-audiology system such as health records, payment details, contact details, etc. Bugs or inadequate access controls may also be exploited by attackers to execute programs that are aimed at attacking other computer systems, e.g. for sending spam emails, run denial of service attacks on Web sites and online portals or to distribute viruses and other computer malware.

In summary, current management software provides a limited attack surface and a low value target. This situation may change if hearing aid management software is extended to enable the remote configuration of hearing aids via the Internet.

Audiology Practice IT System

The remainder and largest part of a tele-audiology system is taken up by the IT system in an audiology practice. It includes all devices such as desktop computers, laptops, tablets, wireless Internet routers, printers, backup system, payment systems and the software they run as well as Cloud-based services they consume or access. It also includes all users, staff and patients, and processes and procedures that are supported by the IT system.

Security Considerations

Given the complexity of an audiology practice IT system, attackers have many avenues of attack at their disposal. In a first step, attackers attempt to gain unauthorized access to the practice IT system. This can be achieved for example by finding software bugs and vulnerabilities in Internet-facing components such as a Web site, a wireless router or an incorrectly configured database. Alternatively, an attacker may trick practice staff to open infected email attachments or to reveal login credentials via phishing emails and Web sites.

Once an attacker gained unauthorized access to a practice IT system, typically they quietly explore its many components to identify further vulnerabilities and items of value. The most valuable target is the patient database. Every audiology practice maintains a patient database that collects health records, including assessment notes, examination results, addresses, contact details, payment details, etc. Other highly valuable targets include the employee payroll system, financial and billing information and records of the practice, payment systems and access credentials such as usernames and passwords.

An attacker may continue to access a computer system for long periods of time undetected and wait for a good opportunity to perform an attack. In the context of an audiology practice, attacks are likely focused on exfiltrating information of value but may also include the wilful destruction of equipment, deletion of data or disruption of normal operations.

Furthermore, an audiology practice IT system may be used to attack other computer systems. For example, so-called botnets may infect desktop PCs, laptops, printers and other networked devices and use them to send out spam and phishing emails or to perform denial of service attacks and Web sites and online portals.

A typical audiology practice is a small business with less expertise and resources for security management than large businesses. This makes them the perfect stepping stone for attackers to infiltrate the computer systems of larger businesses such as partners, banks or hearing aid manufacturers.

If a practice outsources its IT operations or makes use of Cloud-based applications and services, additional security and privacy concerns need to be considered such as who else has access to their and their patients' data, where this data is stored, how this data is backed up, how this data is permanently deleted and what happens if a Cloud solution becomes unavailable.

In summary, an audiology practice IT system offers a large attack surface and provides multiple high value targets. Potential attacks are too numerous to discuss in a single chapter. For further information, refer to Schneier (2004) and Anderson (2008).

SECURITY MANAGEMENT

After a security analysis, such as that discussed in the previous section, a security management plan needs to be defined and implemented. When managing the overall security of an IT system it is important to consider coverage and effectiveness.

Coverage is important to ensure a minimum level of security across all components of an IT system. This can be likened to a roadworthy test for a car. It would not make sense to only concentrate on all the safety features like air bags, anti-lock braking, auto-emergency braking, etc. but ignore the simple things like the tyres being pumped up and the brake lights working. The reason for this is the *weakest link* property of security that states that an attacker only needs to identify and exploit a single weakness to breach an entire system.

Effectiveness is concerned with the extent to which a security risk is being mitigated. The best value in a security trade-off is when the most attention is given to the most critical areas. As described in the Background section, these critical areas in a tele-audiology system are the key assets such as patient data, accounting and payroll systems as well as access credentials and point-of-sale devices. The challenge is to achieve effectiveness in the face of limited resources, expertise, time and budget.

Security management is performed by formulating, implementing and continuously monitoring and updating a *security policy*. A Security Policy represents an organization's plan for managing security. While this is a huge subject covering many information security standards and control frameworks, this section gives an overview of the main areas that a typical security policy covers to protect an organization, such as a tele-audiology business.

Security management generally cover the areas of assets, patching, network, users, monitoring and compliance as depicted in Figure 3. This section also provides examples of essential security measures that every audiology practice should put in place.

Assets and Provisioning

The essence here is:

know what you have.

This means maintaining an inventory including software, hardware and environments of all operational systems.

Figure 3. Security Management Framework

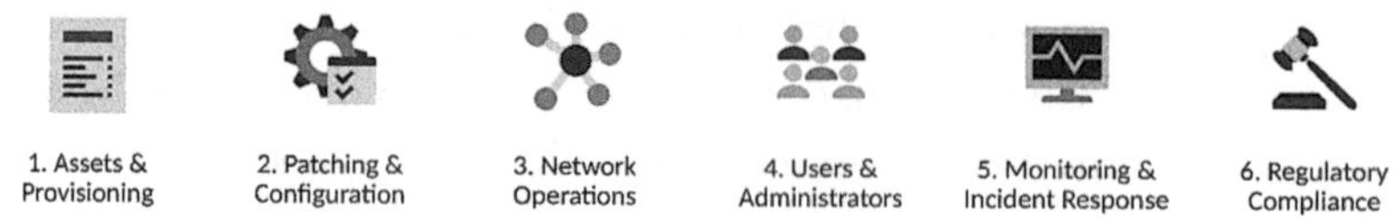

Systems administrators should generally be tracking what computers are connected and what applications are running on a production network. More mature IT departments may use asset management tools that track computers and devices connected to a network.

In a fully controlled environment, only known hardware and known applications should be run. Provisioning is the process of adding new hardware or applications to the IT infrastructure and this process should have approvals and keep records.

Define and Implement a BYOD Policy

A very difficult area is bring-your-own-device (BYOD).

BYOD refers to the recent trend of allowing staff to access applications and network resources from their own portable devices such as tablets and smartphone. Every additional device increases the attack surface and thus provides additional opportunities for attackers to compromise an IT system. Devices that are not owned by a business are particularly dangerous as they are not (fully) covered by the security policy and also often out of the control of system administrators. It may be unknown who has access to the device, what applications the device owner installs and what Web sites the device owner visits. App stores may contain malicious programs or programs with backdoors that leak information to attackers. Web sites may also covertly install malicious code on these devices with all the implications mentioned in earlier sections. Furthermore, portable devices are easily lost or stolen.

To limit potential risks to a tele-audiology practice, it is advisable to restrict access from portable devices to data and resources and to define a plan that outlines what portable devices are allowed, how access to the devices must be controlled by their users and how loss, theft or compromise need to be communicated and acted upon. For example, the window of compromise can be reduced by putting procedures in place that enable the rapid revocation of access rights to critical applications such as a patient database.

Whitelist Applications

Application whitelisting is a technique that enables a system administrator to define which applications can be installed and executed on computers and devices. In this way, the execution of unknown and potentially harmful applications can be restricted. Application whitelisting is a recommendation by the Australian Signals Directorate (ASD) known as the ASD Top 4 and contributes to the mitigation of about 85% of known attacks (Australian Signals Directorate, 2013).

Patching and Configuration

The essence here is:

keep up-to-date what you have.

The most common way that attackers gain access to systems is to exploit a vulnerability in a system that is not up-to-date or misconfigured. IT systems need to be continuously patched and carefully manage configuration settings. Systems should have strong change management processes to prevent misconfigurations and mistakes. For example, there is no point having a protection device, like a firewall, if it is not enabled or not configured properly.

There are many automated tools that can help IT administrators with vulnerability management and configuration management. These tools detect when systems are not fully patched and also when systems deviate from approved configurations.

Regularly Install Updates and Security Patches

Operating systems and application software typically offer many features; each of which adds complexity and potentially contains many software bugs that may be exploited by an attacker. The software industry has slowly reacted to address this issue and recent years have seen a shift in the software development methodology that has resulted in the frequent, sometimes monthly, shipment of software updates and security patches.

To minimize the risk of compromise through software bugs, it is essential to install updates and security patches as soon as they become available. In particular, critical software such as operating systems and Internet browsers need to be updated regularly. It is advisable to turn on auto-update whenever possible. Regularly installing software updates and security patches is another best practice recommended with the ASD Top 4 (Australian Signals Directorate, 2013).

Install Firmware Updates

Computing devices do not only run software in the form of operating and applications that interface with the user and are therefore easily recognized. So-called firmware, small software programs, that provide fundamental services to other software are embedded in every computing device including personal computers, wireless routers and even printers.

Updates for firmware become available from time to time as well, typically to fix security-related bugs in the code. These updates too should be installed in a timely manner to reduce the risk of security breaches through outdated or faulty software.

Network Operations

The essence here is to:

lock-down what you have.

A locked down network is necessary to ensure it is secure and recoverable. Example areas include:

- Security tools such as anti-virus, anti-spam, network firewalls, web application firewalls, intrusion detection systems (IDS).
- Limiting the number of applications, devices and computers.
- Restricting privileges, accounts and administrative entitlements.
- Subdividing networks into segments or data across different databases and systems.
- Subscribing to external threat management systems that can monitor activity on networks.

Recovery means that if a system fails, it needs to be fixed and brought back to an operational state or restarted at an older stable state. For that reason, systems, and in particular all data, should be properly backed up. Backups should be stored offsite and they should be periodically tested to make sure all-important information is being backed up. A typical approach to testing a backup is to use them to bring up a secondary site which may be used as a standby or fail-over site.

Properly Configure Wi-Fi Routers

Most businesses rely on wireless routers to provide network services and to connect computers to the Internet. This means that wireless routers are typically directly connected to the Internet and can be discovered and contacted by external parties. Thus, wireless routers should be considered the first line of defence against attackers.

There are a few basic things that can be done to minimize exposure to such threats. Firstly, the wireless router's default password must be changed to a strong and ideally randomized password that is kept secret. Secondly, the wireless router should be configured to provide only secured connections and allow changes to the router's configuration solely via a local cable connection. Thirdly, the built-in firewall and address filters need to be turned on. It is also recommended to use the latest authentication protocols such as WPA2-Enterprise and strong passwords on each computer that is connected to a wireless router. Access for unknown and unauthorized devices should be denied.

Protect PoS Devices

Point-of-sale (PoS) devices are used to process electronic payments. A PoS device may be a custom-built payment terminal or a mobile application that enables contactless electronic payments. Custom-built terminals are typically connected to a computer that handles the Internet connection for the PoS device and integrates payment transactions into a billing system. This computer needs to be well-protected to minimize the risk that an attacker gains access to the PoS device to skim off credit card details and PIN codes. If a mobile payment app is in use the same applies to the tablet that runs the app. Moreover, this tablet should not be used for any other activities, business or leisure. No other software from unknown or untrustworthy vendors should be installed.

Note, attackers may also attempt to physically tamper with PoS devices. Hence it is essential to ensure that extension slots and ports for connecting external devices are locked down.

Restrict Physical Access

Only authorized personnel should have access to the premises of an audiology practice. This may be enforced, for example with a key card door and gate entry solution. Moreover, all computers need to be turned off, user sessions locked or users logged off whenever computers are not in use. Account passwords and other sensitive information should not be left lying around the office or attached with sticky notes to computer screens. All sensitive information must be locked up in secure drawers and cabinets.

Encrypt All Sensitive Data

All sensitive data on any device should be stored in encrypted form. For example, by turning on disk encryption built into most operating systems, or by turning on data encryption built into most databases. This is particularly important in case devices get lost or stolen. If data is encrypted and the key to unlock this data is provided separately than a thief can only delete data but cannot easily steal and sell it.

It is essential to never share sensitive information including payment details, health records, contact details, etc. via email. Email is a very unsecured communication channel. Emails are transferred in plaintext and copies of emails are kept in plaintext on various services in between the sender and recipient for extended periods of time.

Protecting email attachments with security codes that are derived from personal information of the recipient such as birthdate, initials and so on is also bad practice because an attacker can easily guess such codes and can potentially do so offline – which gives the attacker time to run cracking software.

Ensure the Use of Secure Internet Connections

Many small businesses outsource their IT systems, in particular a number of software applications and services such as the patient database, email, accounting and billing to Cloud-based services. Practice staff as well as patients may have access to these services. It is essential to protect the transfer of data to and from Cloud services with encrypted connections to reduce the risk of breaches. For example, the 'green lock' should appear in the browser's address bar when a user interacts with a Cloud service.

Users and Administrators

The essence here is to:

restrict access to what you have.

This involves authenticating, authorizing and educating staff, especially system administrators. Areas which need to be addressed include ensuring there are no default accounts, strong passwords, logging of all administrative accesses, reviewing accounts and entitlements, and fostering awareness of social engineering (the tricks attackers use to make people fall for scams).

There are many IT tools to manage privileges and audit those privileges. These include anti-virus, anti-spam, content inspection, administrator tracking, etc.

Raise Awareness of Spam and Phishing Emails

Even with recent advances in spam filter and malware scanner technology, spam and phishing emails still pose a significant threat. Spam emails typically try to create traffic to certain Web sites to perform click fraud to rake up advertising money. Phishing emails are aimed at tricking users in revealing sensitive information, such as usernames and passwords or credit card information. This is often done via links that direct the user to a Web site that impersonates a legitimate Web site. Unsuspecting users enter their username and password which are then recorded by the attacker and used to log in on behalf of legitimate users. If Cloud-based software is in use, e.g. for hosting a patient database, this is something to be particularly vigilant about.

Both, spam and phishing emails, may also be used to distribute small malicious programs called malware in the form of attachments or via links to Web sites. Note, popular attachments that carry malware are typically office documents, spreadsheets or PDF files.

There are other forms of social engineering that may coerce or trick audiologists as well as patients into divulging sensitive information such as login credentials or patient-related information. One common trick attackers use is to call up a business and to pretend they provide IT support or tax/accounting advice for which they require access to a computer system or other personal information.

It is very difficult to defend against social engineering attacks. It is advisable to stay abreast of recent developments, e.g. by visiting advisory Web sites and subscribing to newsletters (Stay Smart Online Program, 2017) and to regularly train staff. Using up-to-date spam filters and malware scanners for emails is also essential.

Limit Privileged Access

It is quite common in small businesses that users share accounts or that many user accounts have administrative privileges because it makes it easier to install or remove applications. Privileged access on a computer however means that a user has unrestricted access to all files and folders, can install software, change the configuration of the computer and execute any software program. The problem with this is that it makes it easier for an attacker to compromise a computer system. For example, if an attacker tricks a user into opening an email attachment containing a malicious program, this program is executed without restrictions. In this way, not only one computer is infected, but it is easily possible for the malware to spread laterally through an entire network.

To limit the impact of unauthorized access and execution of software, nominate a system administrator who will have unrestricted access on all computers in your system. However, limit access for all other users by creating restricted user accounts and make sure that each user has their own individual account or accounts.

Limiting access privileges is the last recommendation of the ASD Top 4 (Australian Signals Directorate, 2013).

Ensure the Use of Strong Passwords

Access to computers and applications is typically controlled based on the input of login credentials usually in the form of a username and a password. Passwords have many usability issues. Users forget them easily, share them, reuse them, choose short passwords that are easily remembered but likewise easily guessed. Users need to manage passwords for many different applications, accounts and devices.

All access to critical computers and applications needs to be protected. Define a simple access control policy that outlines the types of valid passwords, their minimum length and how frequently they need to be changed. At the time of writing passwords should have a minimum length of 12 characters to make it harder for attackers to crack them.

If users need to manage multiple passwords, consider the use of password managers or federated identity solutions. A password manager is software that securely stores all passwords of a single user. Instead of having to remember many passwords, now the user only needs to remember one master password. Whenever the user needs to use a password, they login to their password manager and retrieve the required password. Advantages of password managers are: (1) the user can choose one long master password to access the manager and; (2) can use strong randomized passwords for each account password. Federated identity solutions work to the same effect with the added advantage that a user only needs to enter their 'master' password. There is no need to manually copy and paste specific passwords as would be required with a password manager.

However, beware that the master password must be strong because if it is easily guessed or cracked, then an attacker gains access to all accounts and systems that are protected by the passwords inside a password manager or that are integrated in the federated identity solution.

Consider 2-Factor Authentication

Access to particularly critical application or information should be protected with a second factor. For example, the patient database. This means another login credential other than a password is required. A second factor makes it more difficult for an attacker to gain unauthorized access to computers, applications or data. Second factors come in different forms, e.g. as a key fob or portable USB token as well as small mobile applications that generate short 6 to 8-digit access codes every 30-60 seconds.

Monitoring and Incident Response

The essence here is:

watch what you have.

Think of this like the alarm system. The idea is to monitor and look for anomalies and intrusions. If there is a problem, it should be dealt with as soon as possible. This means there needs to be a strong process and tracking of detection, investigation and remediation for all security incidents. In the industry, there are concepts of "time to detect" and "time to remediate" as measures of how effective monitoring and incident response is.

There are many logging and intrusion detection tools. Another important tool here is the help desk, so that issues can be recorded, tracked and reported.

Define and Implement a Ransomware Response Plan

Ransomware attacks are currently widespread and expected to become even more prevalent in coming years. The objective of a ransomware attack is financial gain. An attacker disrupts the victim's business processes by encrypting (scrambling) files on the victim's computers and offers to reinstate them for a payment.

Ransomware is typically distributed with infected emails. Once a victim opens an infected attachment, a small malicious program, called ransomware, is installed on the victim's computer. The ransomware may remain dormant for some time or move laterally in the victim's computer network to infect more computers. Eventually, the ransomware encrypts important files on infected computers and sends the keys that are required to decrypt the files to the command and control centre of an attacker. Afterwards the victim is presented with a ransom note on their computer screen that threatens to throw away these keys permanently if payment is not made by a given deadline.

Victims are advised not to pay because there is no guarantee that the attacker will return the keys or that the attacker does not repeat the attack. To alleviate the impact of ransomware attacks, be prepared. Firstly, run regular backups to be able to recover recent version of files to reduce data loss. Secondly, develop a response plan that clearly defines: (1) who makes the decision whether to pay and how much; (2) how to identify and clean infected computers, and; (3) how to recover from a ransomware attack including where backups are kept and how they are recovered.

Regulatory Compliance

Regulatory compliance is designed to achieve a minimum standard in security management for companies and the way they deal with information. This is a complicated area which will only be touched on here.

The complications are many. There are jurisdictional problems across governments (federal, state, local). There are different laws depending on organization size and type (government, big business, small business and individuals). Some laws may override other laws. Some laws are not necessarily as strong as they sound because of exclusions, escape clauses, and conditions such as consent. The laws move slowly and may not adequately address new problems with technology. New laws may have unintended consequences or may be open to interpretation.

This means that an audiology practice should get legal advice, especially with privacy laws and medical records which have particular attention in these laws (Office of the Australian Information Commissioner, 2017).

Ensure Compliance With Privacy Laws and Regulations

The privacy of patient data is essential. Ensure familiarity with all existing privacy regulations in the local jurisdiction and make sure that relevant controls are implemented. In the context of Cloud-based services, make sure that the Cloud provider also adheres to the privacy laws of the local jurisdiction and determine how they implement necessary controls.

Mandatory Disclosure Regulation

In February 2017, the Australian Senate passed laws that require businesses (and government agencies) to notify the Privacy Commissioner and customers if they have a data breach. The idea of the law is to make public any data breaches. It's designed to address those companies that keep quiet any data breaches to avoid embarrassment and avoid legal action by customers.

Currently, small organizations, with a turnover of less than A$3m per year are exempt. Nevertheless, it is still best practice to take extra steps to avoid data breaches by implementing good security management as described above.

CONCLUSION

Security is a large and complex subject. Given the ever-increasing computerization of all aspects of modern life and the rapid interconnection of computing devices provides a fertile environment for attackers to commit crimes remotely from anywhere in the world in an automated and thus scalable fashion with potentially high gains and a low risk of being caught. The problem will not go away and get worse in the short to medium term.

At the level of audiology-specific devices, including hearing aids and connector devices, there is only a small risk as they offer a very limited attack surface and only contain low value information. Even current trends in the audiology industry towards next generation hearing aids with additional lifestyle features do not significantly change this situation.

However, audiologists must ensure adequate protection of the rest of their IT systems against attackers. Small businesses such as audiology practices need to be vigilant about the security of their IT systems because they have limited expertise in security and budget for addressing security concerns and so are an attractive target to attackers. It is recommended to have a formal security management plan and implement associated controls to protect assets of value such as patient data, payment details, payroll, accounting and billing information, and system credentials.

A tele-audiology business does not need to be an expert in security. There are many security companies that can help a business obtain a good security profile and the practice may choose to outsource much of its operations to reputable IT providers. For advice on suitable outsourcing partners refer to the Australian Signals Directorate Information Security Registered Assessors Program (IRAP) (2017).

Overall, it is important to remember the following:

- Security is not only a technical issue; it is a business concern.
- Every system is breakable, but it is the weak and least defended systems that get hacked first.
- Attackers go after the assets of most value. In tele-audiology, this is likely the patient data, payment details and access credentials.
- All aspects of an IT system need to be defended. This includes people and processes.
- Make use of security professionals and industry best practices.

Security and related threats are moving as fast as technology is being invented. It is in the best interests of professionals to stay informed and ensure the business decision makers properly hear about security risks and get recommendations as to what to do about them. Advice is available from public sources such as government and not-for-profit organizations (Stay Smart Online Program, 2017; Stay Smart Online, 2017; HIMSS Media, 2017; ACCC, 2017).

REFERENCES

Abelson, R., & Goldstein, M. (2015). Anthem Hacking Points to Security Vulnerability of Health Care Industry. *The New York Times*. Retrieved June 1, 2017, from https://www.nytimes.com/2015/02/06/business/experts-suspect-lax-security-left-anthem-vulnerable-to-hackers.html

Anderson, R. (2008). *Security Engineering* (2nd ed.). Indianapolis, IN: Wiley Publishing Inc.

Australian Competition and Consumer Commission (ACCC). (2017). *Scam Watch*. Retrieved June 1, 2017 from https://www.scamwatch.gov.au/

Australian Signals Directorate. (2017). *Information Security Registered Assessors Program*. Retrieved June 1, 2017 from https://www.asd.gov.au/infosec/irap/

Australian Signals Directorate, Australian Cyber Security Centre. (2013). *Top 4 Strategies to Mitigate Targeted Cyber Intrusions: Mandatory Requirement Explained*. Retrieved June 1, 2017 from https://www.asd.gov.au/infosec/top-mitigations/top-4-strategies-explained.htm

Gartner. (2017). *Gartner Says 8.4 Billion Connected "Things" Will Be in Use in 2017, Up 31 Percent From 2016*. Retrieved June 1, 2017 from http://www.gartner.com/newsroom/id/3598917

Grantcharov, C. (2016). *Security of Internet-Connected Hearing Aids*. Retrieved June 1, 2017 from https://www.hearingtracker.com/blog/security-of-internet-connected-hearing-aids/

Hack and Hear. (2016). *Bits around hearing and acoustics*. Retrieved June 1, 2017 from http://www.hackandhear.com/

Halperin, D., Heydt-Benjamin, T. S., Ransford, B., Clark, S. S., Defend, B., Morgan, W., . . . Maisel, W. H. (2008). Pacemakers and Implantable Cardiac Defibrillators: Software Radio Attacks and Zero-Power Defenses. In *Proceedings of the 2008 IEEE Symposium on Security and Privacy* (pp. 129-142). Washington, DC: IEEE Computer Society.

HIMSS Media. (2017). *Healthcare IT News*. Retrieved June 1, 2017 from http://www.healthcareitnews.com/

Kaspersky. (2017). *Cyberthreat Real Time Map*. Retrieved June 1, 2017 from https://cybermap.kaspersky.com/

Landoll, D. (2011). *The Security Risk Assessment Handbook: A Complete Guide for Performing Security Risk Assessments* (2nd ed.). Boca Raton, FL: CRC Press. doi:10.1201/b10937

Lekowski, R. (2016). *Bluetooth: Just How Secure Is It?* Retrieved June 1, 2017 from http://www.lawtechnologytoday.org/2016/05/bluetooth-how-secure-is-it/

Li, C., Raghunathan, A., & Jha, N. K. (2011). Hijacking an Insulin Pump: Security Attacks and Defenses for a Diabetes Therapy System. In *Proceedings of the 2011 IEEE 13th International Conference on e-Health Networking, Applications and Services* (pp. 150-156). Washington, DC: IEEE Computer Society.

Newman, L. H. (2017). *Medical Devices Are the Next Security Nightmare*. Retrieved June 1, 2017, from https://www.wired.com/2017/03/medical-devices-next-security-nightmare/

Office of the Australian Information Commissioner (OAIC). (2017). *Business resource: Handling health information under the Privacy Act: A general overview for health service providers*. Retrieved June 1, 2017 from https://www.oaic.gov.au/engage-with-us/consultations/health-privacy-guidance/business-resource-handling-health-information-under-the-privacy-act-a-general-overview-for-health-service-providers

Rios, B., & Butts, J. (2017). *Security Evaluation of the Implantable Cardiac Device Ecosystem Architecture and Implementation Interdependencies*. Retrieved June 1, 2017 from https://drive.google.com/file/d/0B_GspGER4QQTYkJfaVlBeGVCSW8/view

Sametinger, J., Rozenblit, J., Lysecky, R., & Ott, P. (2015). Security Challenges for Medical Devices. *Communications of the ACM*, *58*(4), 74–82. doi:10.1145/2667218

Schneier, B. (2004). *Secrets and Lies*. Indianapolis, IN: Wiley Publishing Inc.

Schneier, B. (2012). *The Big Idea: Bruce Schneier*. Retrieved June 1, 2017 from https://www.schneier.com/essays/archives/2012/02/the_big_idea_bruce_s.html

Stay Smart Online. (2017). *Small Business Guide*. Retrieved June 1, 2017 from https://www.staysmartonline.gov.au/get-involved/guides/smallbusinessguide

Stay Smart Online Program. (2017). *Stay Smart Online*. Retrieved June 1, 2017 from https://www.staysmartonline.gov.au/

Stinson, E. (2014). *This Guy's Hacked Hearing Aids Let Him Listen to Wi-Fi Networks*. Retrieved June 1, 2017 from https://www.wired.com/2014/12/guys-hacked-hearing-aids-let-listen-wi-fi-networks/

Ward, M. (2012). *Hearing-aid hackers fine-tuning their own devices*. Retrieved June 1, 2017 from http://www.bbc.com/news/technology-18690973

Compilation of References

Abbott, J. M., Kaldo, V., Klein, B., Austin, D., Hamilton, C., Piterman, L., ... Andersson, G. (2009). A cluster randomised trial of an internet-based intervention program for tinnitus distress in an industrial setting. *Cognitive Behaviour Therapy*, *38*(3), 162–173. doi:10.1080/16506070902763174 PMID:19675959

Abelson, R., & Goldstein, M. (2015). Anthem Hacking Points to Security Vulnerability of Health Care Industry. *The New York Times*. Retrieved June 1, 2017, from https://www.nytimes.com/2015/02/06/business/experts-suspect-lax-security-left-anthem-vulnerable-to-hackers.html

Abroms, L. C., Padmanabhan, N., Thaweethai, L., & Phillips, T. (2011). iPhone apps for smoking cessation: A content analysis. *American Journal of Preventive Medicine*, *40*(3), 279–285. doi:10.1016/j.amepre.2010.10.032 PMID:21335258

Abu-Ghanem, S., Handzel, O., Ness, L., Ben-Artzi-Blima, M., Fait-Ghelbendorf, K., & Himmelfarb, M. (2016). Smartphone-based audiometric test for screening hearing loss in the elderly. *European Archives of Oto-Rhino-Laryngology*, *273*(2), 333–339. doi:10.100700405-015-3533-9 PMID:25655259

Access Economics. (2006). *Listen Hear! The economic impact and cost of hearing loss in Australia*. Retrieved from http://www.expression.com.au/files/editor_upload/File/Research%20Reports/listenhearreport.pdf

Agyeman, A. A., & Ofori-Asenso, R. (2015). Perspective: Does personalized medicine hold the future for medicine? *Journal of Pharmacy & Bioallied Sciences*, *7*(3), 239. doi:10.4103/0975-7406.160040 PMID:26229361

Aiello, C. P., & Ferrari, D. V. (2015). Teleaudiology: Efficacy assessment of an online social network as a support tool for parents of children candidates for cochlear implant. *CoDAS*, *27*(5), 411–418. doi:10.1590/2317-1782/20152013061 PMID:26648210

Albrecht, U. V. (2013). Transparency of health-apps for trust and decision making. *Journal of Medical Internet Research*, *15*(12), e277. doi:10.2196/jmir.2981 PMID:24449711

Albrecht, U. V., Von Jan, U., & Pramann, O. (2013). Standard reporting for medical apps. *Studies in Health Technology and Informatics*, *190*, 201–203. PMID:23823422

Altman, D. G., & Bland, J. M. (1999). How to randomise. *BMJ (Clinical Research Ed.)*, *319*(7211), 703–704. doi:10.1136/bmj.319.7211.703 PMID:10480833

AMA encourages telemedicine as part of "med school of the future." (2016). Available at: http://www.hearingreview.com/2016/06/ama-encourages-telemedicine-as-part-of-med-school-of-the-future

American Academy of Child and Adolescent Psychiatry (AACAP) Committee on Telepsychiatry and AACAP Committee on Quality Issues. (2017). Clinical Update: Telepsychiatry With Children and Adolescents. *Journal of the American Academy of Child and Adolescent Psychiatry*, *56*(10), 875–893. doi:10.1016/j.jaac.2017.07.008 PMID:28942810

American National Standards Institute. (1997). *Methods for the calculation of the speech intelligibility index*. New York: Author.

American Speech, Language and Hearing Association. (2014). Teleaudiology Clinical Technicians. Retrieved May 1, 2018, from https://www.asha.org/Practice-Portal/Professional-Issues/Audiology-Assistants/Teleaudiology-Clinical-Assistants/

American Speech-Language-Hearing Association (ASHA). (n.d.) *Teleaudiology Clinical Technicians*. Retrieved September 30, 2018 from https://www.asha.org/Practice-Portal/Professional-Issues/Audiology-Assistants/Teleaudiology-Clinical-Assistants

Amlani, A., Taylor, B., Levy, C., & Robbins, L. (2013). Utility of smartphone-based hearing aid applications as a substitute to traditional hearing aids. *Hearing Review*, *20*, 16–18.

Anderson, R. (2008). *Security Engineering* (2nd ed.). Indianapolis, IN: Wiley Publishing Inc.

Andersson, G. (2002). Psychological aspects of tinnitus and the application of cognitive–behavioral therapy. *Clinical Psychology Review*, *22*(7), 977–990. doi:10.1016/S0272-7358(01)00124-6 PMID:12238249

Andersson, G., Carlbring, P., Berger, T., Almlöv, J., & Cuijpers, P. (2009). What makes internet therapy work? *Cognitive Behaviour Therapy*, *38*(sup1S1), 55–60. doi:10.1080/16506070902916400 PMID:19675956

Andersson, G., Carlbring, P., Ljótsson, B., & Hedman, E. (2013). Guided internet-based CBT for common mental disorders. *Journal of Contemporary Psychotherapy*, *43*(4), 223–233. doi:10.100710879-013-9237-9

Andersson, G., Estling, F., Jakobsson, E., Cuijpers, P., & Carlbring, P. (2011). Can the patient decide which modules to endorse? an open trial of tailored internet treatment of anxiety disorders. *Cognitive Behaviour Therapy*, *40*(1), 57–64. doi:10.1080/16506073.2010.529457 PMID:21337215

Andersson, G., & Hedman, E. (2013). Effectiveness of guided internet-based cognitive behavior therapy in regular clinical settings. *Verhaltenstherapie*, *23*(3), 140–148. doi:10.1159/000354779

Andersson, G., & Kaldo, V. (2004). Internet-based cognitive behavioral therapy for tinnitus. *Journal of Clinical Psychology*, *60*(2), 171–178. doi:10.1002/jclp.10243 PMID:14724924

Andersson, G., Paxling, B., Wiwe, M., Vernmark, K., Felix, C. B., Lundborg, L., ... Carlbring, P. (2012). Therapeutic alliance in guided internet-delivered cognitive behavioural treatment of depression, generalized anxiety disorder and social anxiety disorder. *Behaviour Research and Therapy*, *50*(9), 544–550. doi:10.1016/j.brat.2012.05.003 PMID:22728647

Andersson, G., Strömgren, T., Ström, L., & Lyttkens, L. (2002). Randomized controlled trial of internet-based cognitive behavior therapy for distress associated with tinnitus. *Psychosomatic Medicine*, *64*(5), 810–816. PMID:12271112

Andersson, G., & Titov, N. (2014). Advantages and limitations of internet-based interventions for common mental disorders. *World Psychiatry; Official Journal of the World Psychiatric Association (WPA)*, *13*(1), 4–11. doi:10.1002/wps.20083 PMID:24497236

Andreu-Perez, J., Poon, C. C. Y., Merrifield, R. D., Wong, S. T. C., & Yang, G.-Z. (2015). Big Data for Health. *IEEE Journal of Biomedical and Health Informatics*, *19*(4), 1193–1206. doi:10.1109/JBHI.2015.2450362 PMID:26173222

Andrews, G., & Williams, A. D. (2015). Up-scaling clinician assisted internet cognitive behavioural therapy (iCBT) for depression: A model for dissemination into primary care. *Clinical Psychology Review*, *41*, 40–48. doi:10.1016/j.cpr.2014.05.006 PMID:25043445

Arlinger, S. (2003). Negative consequences of uncorrected hearing loss - a review. *International Journal of Audiology*, *42*(2), S17–S20. doi:10.3109/14992020309074639 PMID:12918624

Arnberg, F. K., Linton, S. J., Hultcrantz, M., Heintz, E., & Jonsson, U. (2014). Internet-delivered psychological treatments for mood and anxiety disorders: A systematic review of their efficacy, safety, and cost-effectiveness. *PLoS One*, *9*(5), e98118. doi:10.1371/journal.pone.0098118 PMID:24844847

Arnhold, M., Quade, M., & Kirch, W. (2014). Mobile applications for diabetics: A systematic review and expert-based usability evaluation considering the special requirements of diabetes patients age 50 years or older. *Journal of Medical Internet Research*, *16*(4), e104. doi:10.2196/jmir.2968 PMID:24718852

Assmann, P., & Summerfield, Q. (2004). The perception of speech under adverse conditions. In *Speech processing in the auditory system* (pp. 231–308). New York, NY: Springer. doi:10.1007/0-387-21575-1_5

Athalye, S., Archbold, S., Mulla, I., Lutman, M., & Nikolopoulous, T. (2015). Exploring views on current and future cochlear implant service delivery: The perspectives of users, parents and professionals at cochlear implant centres and in the community. *Cochlear Implants International*, *16*(5), 241–253. doi:10.1179/1754762815Y.0000000003 PMID:25780991

Aungst, T. D., Clauson, K. A., Misra, S., Lewis, T. L., & Husain, I. (2014). How to identify, assess and utilise mobile medical applications in clinical practice. *International Journal of Clinical Practice*, *68*(2), 155–162. doi:10.1111/ijcp.12375 PMID:24460614

Australia's National Digital Health Strategy. (n.d.). Retrieved from https://conversation.digitalhealth.gov.au/australias-national-digital-health-strategy

Australian Bureau of Statistics. (n.d.). *8146.0 - Household Use of Information Technology, Australia, 2016-17*. Retrieved June 4, 2018, from http://www.abs.gov.au/ausstats/abs@.nsf/mf/8146.0

Australian Competition and Consumer Commission (ACCC). (2017). *Scam Watch.* Retrieved June 1, 2017 from https://www.scamwatch.gov.au/

Australian Competition and Consumer Commission. (2017). *Issues around the sale of hearing aids.* Retrieved 4 September, 2018 from https://www.accc.gov.au/publications/issues-around-the-sale-of-hearing-aids

Australian Digital Health Agency. (2018). *What you told us.* Retrieved August 20, 2018 from https://conversation.digitalhealth.gov.au/what-does-australia-want-digital-health

Australian Parliament: Inquiry into the Hearing Health and Wellbeing of Australia. (2018). Retrieved from http://www.aph.gov.au/Parliamentary_Business/Committees/House/Health_Aged_Care_and_Sport/HearingHealth

Australian Signals Directorate, Australian Cyber Security Centre. (2013). *Top 4 Strategies to Mitigate Targeted Cyber Intrusions: Mandatory Requirement Explained.* Retrieved June 1, 2017 from https://www.asd.gov.au/infosec/top-mitigations/top-4-strategies-explained.htm

Australian Signals Directorate. (2017). *Information Security Registered Assessors Program.* Retrieved June 1, 2017 from https://www.asd.gov.au/infosec/irap/

Baguley, D., Andersson, G., McFerran, D., & McKenna, L. (2013). A multidisciplinary synthesis. Tinnitus: A Multidisciplinary Approach, 221-224.

Bangor, A., Kortum, P. T., & Miller, J. T. (2008). An Empirical Evaluation of the System Usability Scale. *International Journal of Human-Computer Interaction, 24*(6), 574–594. doi:10.1080/10447310802205776

Barak, A., Klein, B., & Proudfoot, J. G. (2009). Defining internet-supported therapeutic interventions. *Annals of Behavioral Medicine, 38*(1), 4–17. doi:10.100712160-009-9130-7 PMID:19787305

Baranowski, T., & Stables, G. (2000). Process evaluations of the 5-a-day projects. *Health Education & Behavior: The Official Publication of the Society for Public Health Education, 27*(2), 157–166. doi:10.1177/109019810002700202 PMID:10768797

Bardus, M., van Beurden, S. B., Smith, J. R., & Abraham, C. (2016). A review and content analysis of engagement, functionality, aesthetics, information quality, and change techniques in the most popular commercial apps for weight management. *The International Journal of Behavioral Nutrition and Physical Activity*, *13*(1), 35. doi:10.118612966-016-0359-9 PMID:26964880

Barton, A. J. (2012). The regulation of mobile health applications. *BMC Medicine*, *10*(1), 46. doi:10.1186/1741-7015-10-46 PMID:22569114

Barton, G. R., Fortnum, H. M., Stacey, P. C., & Summerfield, A. Q. (2006). Hearing-impaired children in the UK IV: Cost-effectiveness of paediatric cochlear implantation. *Ear and Hearing*, *27*(5), 575–588. doi:10.1097/01.aud.0000233967.11072.24 PMID:16957506

Basilico, A., Marceglia, S., Bonacina, S., & Pinciroli, F. (2016). Advising patients on selecting trustful apps for diabetes self-care. *Computers in Biology and Medicine*, *71*, 86–96. doi:10.1016/j.compbiomed.2016.02.005 PMID:26897071

Bastawrous, A., & Armstrong, M. J. (2013). Mobile health use in low- and high-income countries: An overview of the peer-reviewed literature. *Journal of the Royal Society of Medicine*, *106*(4), 130–142. doi:10.1177/0141076812472620 PMID:23564897

Baumeister, H., Reichler, L., Munzinger, M., & Lin, J. (2014). The impact of guidance on internet-based mental health interventions—A systematic review. *Internet Interventions*, *1*(4), 205–215. doi:10.1016/j.invent.2014.08.003

Beckett, R. C., Saunders, E., & Blamey, P. J. (2016). Optimizing Hearing Aid Utilisation using Telemedicine Tools. In I. M. Miranda, R. Martinho, & R. Rijo (Eds.), *Encyclopedia of E-Health and Telemedicine* (pp. 72–85). IGI Global. doi:10.4018/978-1-4666-9978-6.ch007

Beirao, G., Den Ambtman, A., De Pourcq, K., De Regge, M., Simões do Carmo Dias, J., & Kandampully, J. (2016). *The healthcare experience : the supportive role of technology and people in the elderly care sector*. Presented at the Frontiers in Service 2016. Bergen, Norway

Bendelin, N., Hesser, H., Dahl, J., Carlbring, P., Nelson, K. Z., & Andersson, G. (2011). Experiences of guided internet-based cognitive-behavioural treatment for depression: A qualitative study. *BMC Psychiatry*, *11*(1), 107. doi:10.1186/1471-244X-11-107 PMID:21718523

Bennett, K., Bennett, A. J., & Griffiths, K. M. (2010). Security considerations for e-mental health interventions. *Journal of Medical Internet Research*, *12*(5), e61. doi:10.2196/jmir.1468 PMID:21169173

Bentley, T., Johnston, L., & Von Baggo, K. (2002). Putting some emotion into requirements engineering. *Proc. of the 7th Australian Workshop on Requirements Engineering*, 227-244. Melbourne, Australia

Berry, L. L., Davis, S. W., & Wilmet, J. (2015). When the customer is stressed. *Harvard Business Review*, *93*, 86–94.

Beukes, E. W., Allen, P. A., Baguley, D. M., Manchaiah, V., & Andersson, G. (2018a). Long-term efficacy of audiologist-guided internet-based cognitive behaviour therapy for tinnitus. *American Journal of Audiology*, *27*(3S). doi:10.1044/2018_AJA-IMIA3-18-0004

Beukes, E. W., Allen, P. M., Manchaiah, V., Baguley, D. M., & Andersson, G. (2017b). Internet-based intervention for tinnitus: Outcome of a single-group open trial. *Journal of the American Academy of Audiology*, *28*(4), 340–351. doi:10.3766/jaaa.16055 PMID:28418328

Beukes, E. W., Andersson, G., Allen, P., Manchaiah, V., & Baguley, D. M. (2018). Effectiveness of Guided Internet-Based Cognitive Behavioral Therapy vs Face-to-Face Clinical Care for Treatment of TinnitusA Randomized Clinical Trial. *JAMA Otolaryngology-Head & Neck Surgery*. Published online October 04, 2018. doi:10.1001/jamaoto.2018.2238

Beukes, E. W., Baguley, D. M., Allen, P. M., Manchaiah, V., & Andersson, G. (2017c). Audiologist-guided internet-based cognitive behaviour therapy for adults with tinnitus in the United Kingdom: A randomized controlled trial. *Ear and Hearing*, *39*, 423–433. doi:10.1097/AUD.0000000000000505 PMID:29095725

Beukes, E. W., Manchaiah, V., Andersson, G., Allen, P. M., Terlizzi, P. M., & Baguley, D. M. (2017a). Situationally influenced tinnitus coping strategies: A mixed methods approach. *Disability and Rehabilitation*, 1–11. doi:10.1080/09638288.2017.1362708 PMID:28793790

Beukes, E. W., Manchaiah, V., Baguley, D. M., Allen, P. M., & Andersson, G. (2017). Process evaluation of internet-based cognitive behavioural therapy for adults with tinnitus in the context of a randomised control trial. *International Journal of Audiology*, *57*(2), 98–109. doi:10.1080/14992027.2017.1384858 PMID:28990807

Beukes, E. W., Vlaescu, G., Manchaiah, V., Baguley, D. M., Allen, P. M., Kaldo, V., & Andersson, G. (2016). Development and technical functionality of an internet-based intervention for tinnitus in the UK. *Internet Interventions*, *6*, 6–15. doi:10.1016/j.invent.2016.08.002 PMID:30135809

Bexelius, C., Honeth, L., Ekman, A., Eriksson, M., Sandin, S., Bagger-Sjöbäck, D., & Litton, J.-E. (2015). Evaluation of an internet-based hearing test—comparison with established methods for detection of hearing loss. *Journal of Medical Internet Research*, *10*(4), e32. doi:10.2196/jmir.1065 PMID:18940783

Bhatt, J. M., Lin, H. W., & Bhattacharyya, N. (2016). Prevalence, severity, exposures, and treatment patterns of tinnitus in the United States. *JAMA Otolaryngology-Head & Neck Surgery*, *142*(10), 959–965. doi:10.1001/jamaoto.2016.1700 PMID:27441392

BinDhim, N. F., Hawkey, A., & Trevena, L. (2015). A systematic review of quality assessment methods for smartphone health apps. *Telemedicine Journal and e-Health*, *21*(2), 97–104. doi:10.1089/tmj.2014.0088 PMID:25469795

Blamey & Saunders Hearing Pty Ltd. https://www.blameysaunders.com.au/ and http://www.scienceinpublic.com.au/media-releases/backgrounder

Blamey, P. J., & Martin, L. F. A. (2009). Loudness and satisfaction ratings for hearing aid users. *JAAA*, *20*(4), 272–282. PMID:19927699

Blamey, P. J., & Sarant, J. Z. (2003). Development of spoken language by deaf children. Oxford handbook of deaf studies, language, and education, 232-246.

Blamey, P. J., & Saunders, E. (2015). Predicting speech perception from the audiogram and vice versa. *Canadian J Audiology, 2*(2).

Blamey, P. J., Blamey, J. K., & Saunders, E. (2015). Effectiveness of a teleaudiology approach to hearing aid fitting. *J Telemedicine and Telecare, 1*(8), 474-478.

Blamey, P., & Saunders, E. (2015). Predicting Speech Perception from the Audiogram and Vice Versa. *Canadian Audiologist, 2*(1).

Blamey, P., Martin, L. F., & Saunders, E. (2010). *Hearing aid benefit as a function of hearing loss*. Paper presented at the Australasian International Conference on Speech Science and Technology, Melbourne, Australia.

Blamey, P. J. (2005). Adaptive dynamic range optimization (ADRO): A digital amplification strategy for hearing aids and cochlear implants. *Trends in Amplification*, *9*(2), 77–98. doi:10.1177/108471380500900203 PMID:16012705

Blamey, P. J., Blamey, J. K., & Saunders, E. (2015). Effectiveness of a tele-audiology approach to hearing aid fitting. *Journal of Telemedicine and Telecare, 21*(8), 474–478. doi:10.1177/1357633X15611568 PMID:26556060

Blamey, P. J., Sarant, J. Z., Paatsch, L. E., Barry, J. G., Bow, C. P., Wales, R. J., ... Tooher, R. (2001). Relationships among speech perception, production, language, hearing loss, and age in children with impaired hearing. *Journal of Speech, Language, and Hearing Research: JSLHR, 44*(2), 264–285. doi:10.1044/1092-4388(2001/022) PMID:11324650

Blamey, P., Artieres, F., & Başkent, D. (2013). Factors affecting auditory performance of postlinguistically deaf adults using cochlear implants: An update with 2251 patients. *Audiology & Neuro-Otology, 18*, 36–47. doi:10.1159/000343189 PMID:23095305

Blamey, P., & Sarant, J. (2002). Speech perception and language criteria for paediatric cochlear implant candidature. *Audiology & Neuro-Otology, 7*(2), 114–121. doi:10.1159/000057659 PMID:12006739

Blythe, M., Overbeeke, K., Monk, A., & Wright, P. (Eds.). (2004). *Funology: From Usability to Enjoyment*. The Netherlands: Springer.

Boehner, K., DePaula, R., Dourish, P., & Sengers, P. (2007). How emotion is made and measured. *International Journal of Human-Computer Studies, 65*(4), 275–291. doi:10.1016/j.ijhcs.2006.11.016

Bonacina, S., Marceglia, S., & Pinciroli, F. (2014). A pictorial schema for a comprehensive user-oriented identification of medical apps. *Methods of Information in Medicine, 53*(03), 208–224. doi:10.3414/ME13-01-0093 PMID:24727980

Boothroyd, A. (1968). Statistical theory of the speech discrimination score. *The Journal of the Acoustical Society of America, 43*(2), 362–367. doi:10.1121/1.1910787 PMID:5636798

Botasso, M., Sanches, S.G.G., Bento, R.F., & Samelli, A.G. (2015). Teleaudiometry as a screening method in school children. *Clinics SciELO Brasil, 70*(4).

Boudreaux, E. D., Waring, M. E., Hayes, R. B., Sadasivam, R. S., Mullen, S., & Pagoto, S. (2014). Evaluating and selecting mobile health apps: Strategies for healthcare providers and healthcare organizations. *Translational Behavioral Medicine, 4*(4), 363–371. doi:10.100713142-014-0293-9 PMID:25584085

Boulos, M. N., Brewer, A. C., Karimkhani, C., Buller, D. B., & Dellavalle, R. P. (2014). Mobile medical and health apps: State of the art, concerns, regulatory control and certification. *Online Journal of Public Health Informatics*, *5*(3), 229. PMID:24683442

Brennan-Jones, C. G., Eikelboom, R. H., Swanepoel, D. W., Friedland, P. L., & Atlas, M. D. (2016). Clinical validation of automated audiometry with continuous noise-monitoring in a clinically heterogeneous population outside a sound-treated environment. *International Journal of Audiology*, *55*(9), 507–513. doi:10.1080/14992027.2016.1178858 PMID:27206551

Bright, T., & Pallawela, D. (2016). Validated smartphone-based apps for ear and hearing assessments: A Review. *JMIR Rehabilitation and Assistive Technology*, *3*(2), e13. doi:10.2196/rehab.6074 PMID:28582261

Brooke, J. (1996). SUS: "A quick and dirty" usability scale. In P. W. Jordan, B. Thomas, & B. A. Weerdmeester (Eds.), *Usability Evaluation in Industry*. London: Taylor and Francis.

Burke, L. E., Shiffman, S., Music, E., Styn, M. A., Kriska, A., Smailagic, A., ... Rathbun, S. L. (2017). Ecological Momentary Assessment in Behavioral Research: Addressing Technological and Human Participant Challenges. *Journal of Medical Internet Research*, *19*(3), e77. doi:10.2196/jmir.7138 PMID:28298264

Campbell, M., Fitzpatrick, R., Haines, A., & Kinmonth, A. L. (2000). Framework for design and evaluation of complex interventions to improve health. *British Medical Journal*, *321*(7262), 694–696. doi:10.1136/bmj.321.7262.694 PMID:10987780

Campos, P. D., & Ferrari, D. V. (2012). Teleaudiology: Evaluation of teleconsultation efficacy for hearing aid fitting. *Jornal da Sociedade Brasileira de Fonoaudiologia*, *24*(4), 301–308. doi:10.1590/S2179-64912012000400003 PMID:23306678

Carhart, R. (1946). Tests for selection of hearing AIDS. *Laryngoscope*, *56*(12), 780–794. doi:10.1288/00005537-194612000-00004 PMID:20282107

Carhart, R. (1951). Basic principles of speech audiometry. *Acta Oto-Laryngologica*, *40*(1-2), 62–71. doi:10.3109/00016485109138908 PMID:14914512

Chan, S. R., & Misra, S. (2014). Certification of mobile apps for health care. *Journal of the American Medical Association*, *312*(11), 1155–1156. doi:10.1001/jama.2014.9002 PMID:25226486

Charani, E., Castro-Sánchez, E., Moore, L. S. P., & Holmes, A. (2014). Do smartphone applications in healthcare require a governance and legal framework? It depends on the application! *BMC Medicine*, *12*(1), 29. doi:10.1186/1741-7015-12-29 PMID:24524344

Chiang, L., Chen, W., Dai, Y., & Ho, Y. (2012). The effectiveness of telehealth care on caregiver burden, mastery of stress, and family function among family caregivers of heart failure patients: A quasi-experimental study. *International Journal of Nursing Studies*, *49*(10), 1230–1242. doi:10.1016/j.ijnurstu.2012.04.013 PMID:22633448

Chiauzzi, E., Rodarte, C., & DasMahapatra, P. (2015). Patient-centered activity monitoring in the self-management of chronic health conditions. *BMC Medicine*, *13*(1), 77. doi:10.118612916-015-0319-2 PMID:25889598

Chien, E., Geffen, M., & Gordon, D. (2011). *Telehealth Benefits and Adoption: Connecting People and Providers Across Canada.* A Study Commissioned by Canada Health Infoway. Retrieved August 18, 2018, from https://blogs.dal.ca/distmeded/files/2012/08/telehealth_report_summary_2011_en.pdf

Chien, E., Geffen, M., & Gordon, D. (2011, May). *Telehealth Benefits and Adoption-Connecting People and Providers Across Canada.* A Study Commissioned by Canada Health Infoway.

Chininthorn, P., Glaser, M., Tucker, W. D., & Diehl, J. C. (2016). Exploration of deaf people's health information sources and techniques for information delivery in Cape Town: A qualitative study for the design and development of a mobile health app. *JMIR Human Factors*, *3*(2), e28. doi:10.2196/humanfactors.6653 PMID:27836819

Cima, R., Joore, M., Maes, I., Scheyen, D., Refaie, A. E., Baguley, D. M., Vlaeyen, J.W., & Anteunis, L. (2009). Cost-effectiveness of multidisciplinary management of tinnitus at a specialized tinnitus centre. *BMC Health Services Research*, *9*, 29-6963-9-29.

Cima, R. F., Vlaeyen, J. W., Maes, I. H., Joore, M. A., & Anteunis, L. J. (2011). Tinnitus interferes with daily life activities: A psychometric examination of the tinnitus disability index. *Ear and Hearing*, *32*(5), 623–633. doi:10.1097/AUD.0b013e31820dd411 PMID:21336139

Cochrane, A. (1972). *Effectiveness and efficiency: Random reflections on health services*. London: Academic Press.

Cockburn, A. (2012). *When half a million Americans died and nobody noticed.* Retrieved October 1, 2018, from http://www.theweek.co.uk/us/46535/when-half-million-americans-died-and-nobody-noticed

Coiera, E. (2015). *Guide to health informatics*. London, UK: Taylor Francis.

Connor, K., Brady, R. R. W., Beaux, A., & Tulloh, B. (2014). Contemporary hernia smartphone applications (apps). *Hernia, 18*, 557–561. PMID:23801277

Convery, E., Keidser, G., Dillon, H., & Hartley, L. (2011). A self-fitting hearing aid: Need and concept. *Trends in Amplification, 15*(4), 157–166. doi:10.1177/1084713811427707 PMID:22143873

Corry, M., Sanders, M., & Searchfield, G. D. (2017). The accuracy and reliability of an app-based audiometer using consumer headphones: Pure tone audiometry in a normal hearing group. *International Journal of Audiology, 56*(9), 706–710. doi: 10.1080/14992027.2017.1321791 PMID:28485673

Cox, R. M. (2003). *Assessment of subjective outcome of hearing aid fitting: getting the client's point of view. International Journal of Audiology*.

Cox, R. M., & Alexander, G. C. (2000). Expectations about hearing aids and their relationship to fitting outcome. *Journal of the American Academy of Audiology, 11*(7). PMID:10976498

Craig, P., Dieppe, P., Macintyre, S., Michie, S., Nazareth, I., Petticrew, M., & Medical Research Council Guidance. (2008). Developing and evaluating complex interventions: The new medical research council guidance. BMJ (Clinical Research Ed.), 337.

Cruikshank, J. (2010*). HealthCare without Walls: A Framework for delivering telehealth at scale.* Retrieved August 18, 2018, from http://www.2020health.org/2020health/Publications/Publications-2010/telehealth.html

Cuijpers, P., van Straten, A., & Andersson, G. (2008). Internet-administered cognitive behavior therapy for health problems: A systematic review. *Journal of Behavioral Medicine, 31*(2), 169–177. doi:10.100710865-007-9144-1 PMID:18165893

Davis, A., & Rafaie, E. A. (2000). Epidemiology of tinnitus. *Tinnitus Handbook,*, 1-23.

Davis, T. L., DiClemente, R., & Prietula, M. (2016). Taking mHealth Forward: Examining the Core Characteristics. *JMIR mHealth and uHealth*, *4*(3), e97. doi:10.2196/mhealth.5659 PMID:27511612

Day, S. X., & Schneider, P. L. (2002). Psychotherapy using distance technology: A comparison of face-to-face, video, and audio treatment. *Journal of Counseling Psychology*, *49*(4), 499–503. doi:10.1037/0022-0167.49.4.499

De Bronkart, D. (2013). *Let Patients Help*. CreateSpace Independent Publishing Platform. Retrieved April 10, 2018, from https://www.createspace.com/

de Graaff, F. I., Huysmans, E., Merkus, P., Goverts, S. T., & Smits, C. (2018). Assessment of speech recognition abilities in quiet and in noise: A comparison between self-administered home testing and testing in the clinic for adult cochlear implant users. *International Journal of Audiology*, 1–9. doi:10.1080/14992027.2018.1506168 PMID:30261772

de Graaff, F. I., Huysmans, E., Qazi, O. U., Vanpoucke, F. J., Merkus, P., Goverts, S. T., & Smits, C. (2016). The Development of Remote Speech Recognition Tests for Adult Cochlear Implant Users: The Effect of Presentation Mode of the Noise and a Reliable Method to Deliver Sound in Home Environments. *Audiology & Neuro-Otology*, *21*(1Suppl.), 48–54. doi:10.1159/000448355 PMID:27806354

De Raeve, L. (2016). Cochlear implants in Belgium: Prevalence in paediatric and adult cochlear implantation. *European Annals of Otorhinolaryngology, Head and Neck Diseases*, *133*(Suppl 1), S57–S60. doi:10.1016/j.anorl.2016.04.018 PMID:27246742

Deloitte Access Economics for the Hearing Care Industry Association. (2017). *The Social and Economic Cost of Hearing Loss in Australia*. Retrieved August 22, 2018, from http://www.hcia.com.au/hcia-wp/wp-content/uploads/2015/05/Social-and-Economic-Cost-of-Hearing-Health-in-Australia_June-2017.pdf

Deloitte Access Economics for the Hearing Care Industry Association. (2017). *The Social and Economic Cost of Hearing Loss in Australia.* Retrieved June 4, 2018 from http://www.hcia.com.au/hcia-wp/wp-content/uploads/2015/05/Social-and-Economic-Cost-of-Hearing-Health-in-Australia_June-2017.pdf

Deloitte Access Economics. (2017). *The social and economic cost of hearing loss in Australia*. Author.

Demidowich, A. P., Lu, K., Tamler, R., & Bloomgarden, Z. (2012). An evaluation of diabetes self-management applications for Android smartphones. *Journal of Telemedicine and Telecare*, *18*(4), 235–238. doi:10.1258/jtt.2012.111002 PMID:22604278

Department of Human Services. (2017). *Prioritising Mental Health — improving telehealth for psychological services in regional, rural and remote Australia*. Retrieved October 1, 2018, from. https://www.humanservices.gov.au/organisations/about-us/budget/budget-2017-18/health/prioritising-mental-health-improving-telehealth-psychological-services-regional-rural-and-remote

Department of Human Services. (n.d.). *MBS and telehealth*. Retrieved October 1, 2018, from https://www.humanservices.gov.au/organisations/health-professionals/services/medicare/mbs-and-telehealth

Derin, S., Cam, O. H., Beydilli, H., Acar, E., Elicora, S. S., & Sahan, M. (2016). Initial assessment of hearing loss using a mobile application for audiological evaluation. *The Journal of Laryngology and Otology*, *130*(3), 248–251. doi:10.1017/S0022215116000062 PMID:26781699

Desmet, P. (2002). *Designing Emotions*. Delft University of Technology.

Dillon, H. (2008). *Hearing aids*. London, UK: Hodder Arnold. doi:10.1201/b15118-293

Donahue, A., Dubno, J. R., & Beck, L. (2010). Accessible and affordable hearing health care for adults with mild to moderate hearing loss. *Ear and Hearing*, *31*(1), 2–6. doi:10.1097/AUD.0b013e3181cbc783 PMID:20040828

Donkin, L., & Glozier, N. (2012). Motivators and motivations to persist with online psychological interventions: A qualitative study of treatment completers. *Journal of Medical Internet Research*, *14*(3), e91. doi:10.2196/jmir.2100 PMID:22743581

Ear Foundation. (2014). *The real cost of adult hearing loss*. Retrieved October 1, 2018, from http://www.earfoundation.org.uk/research/current-research/the-real-cost-of-adult-hearing-loss

Economics, A. (2005). *Listen Hear!* The Economic Impact and Cost of Hearing Loss in Australia.

Eikelboom, R. H., & Swanepoel, D. W. (2016). International survey of audiologists' attitudes toward telehealth. *American Journal of Audiology*, *25*(3S), 295–298. doi:10.1044/2016_AJA-16-0004 PMID:27768191

Eldridge, S. M., Lancaster, G. A., Campbell, M. J., Thabane, L., Hopewell, S., Coleman, C. L., & Bond, C. M. (2016). Defining feasibility and pilot studies in preparation for randomised controlled trials: Development of a conceptual framework. *PLoS One*, *11*(3), e0150205. doi:10.1371/journal.pone.0150205 PMID:26978655

Elgoyhen, A. B., Langguth, B., De Ridder, D., & Vanneste, S. (2015). Tinnitus: Perspectives from human neuroimaging. *Nature Reviews. Neuroscience*.

European Patient Forum. (n.d.). Retrieved from http://www.eu-patient.eu/campaign/PatientsprescribE/

Eysenbach, G. (2008). Medicine 2.0: Social networking, collaboration, participation, apomediation, and openness. *Journal of Medical Internet Research*, *10*(3), e22. doi:10.2196/jmir.1030 PMID:18725354

Fabry, D., & Groth, J. (2017). Teleaudiology: Friend or Foe in the Consumerism of Hearing Healthcare? *The Hearing Review*. Retrieved September 30, 2018 from http://www.hearingreview.com/2017/04/teleaudiology-friend-foe-consumerism-hearing-healthcare/

Federal Communications Commission (FCC). (2012). *mHealth Task Force findings and recommendations*. Retrieved June 12, 2018, from http://www2.itif.org/2012-mhealth-taskforce-recommendations.pdf

Ferguson, M. A., Kitterick, P. T., Chong, L. Y., Edmondson-Jones, M., Barker, F., & Hoare, D. J. (2017). *Hearing aids for mild to moderate hearing loss in adults*. Retrieved 5 June, 2018 from https://www.cochrane.org/CD012023/ENT_hearing-aids-mild-moderate-hearing-loss-adults

Ferguson, M., & Henshaw, H. (2015). Computer and internet interventions to optimize listening and learning for people with hearing loss: Accessibility, use, and adherence. [PubMed]. *American Journal of Audiology*, *24*(3), 338–343. doi:10.1044/2015_AJA-14-0090

Fletcher, H. (1929). *Speech and Hearing*. New York: Van Nostrand.

Fokkinga, S., & Desmet, P. (2001). Ten Ways to Design for Disgust, Sadness, and Other Enjoyments: A Design Approach to Enrich Product Experiences with Negative Emotions. *International Journal of Design*, *7*(1).

Galster, J. A. (2012). Apps for audiology. *Audiology Practices*, *4*, 16–19.

Gander, P. E., Hoare, D. J., Collins, L., Smith, S., & Hall, D. A. (2011). Tinnitus referral pathways within the national health service in England: A survey of their perceived effectiveness among audiology staff. *BMC Health Services Research*, *11*(1), 1. doi:10.1186/1472-6963-11-162 PMID:21733188

Gartner. (2017). *Gartner Says 8.4 Billion Connected "Things" Will Be in Use in 2017, Up 31 Percent From 2016*. Retrieved June 1, 2017 from http://www.gartner.com/newsroom/id/3598917

Gill, M. A. (2011). *A National Telehealth Strategy For Australia - For Discussion*. Commissioned by Australian National Consultative Committee on Electronic Health (ANCCeH). Retrieved August 18, 2018, from http://www.who.int/goe/policies/countries/aus__support_tele.pdf

Glasberg, B. R., & Moore, B. C. (1988). Psychoacoustic abilities of subjects with unilateral and bilateral cochlear hearing impairments and their relationship to the ability to understand speech. *Scandinavian Audiology*, *1989*(32), 1–25. PMID:2711118

Glasgow, R. E., Lichtenstein, E., & Marcus, A. C. (2003). Why don't we see more translation of health promotion research to practice? rethinking the efficacy-to-effectiveness transition. *American Journal of Public Health*, *93*(8), 1261–1267. doi:10.2105/AJPH.93.8.1261 PMID:12893608

Glasgow, R. E., Vogt, T. M., & Boles, S. M. (1999). Evaluating the public health impact of health promotion interventions: The RE-AIM framework. *American Journal of Public Health*, *89*(9), 1322–1327. doi:10.2105/AJPH.89.9.1322 PMID:10474547

Goldstein, D. P., & Stephens, S. D. (1981). Audiological rehabilitation: Management model I. *Audiology*, *20*(5), 432–452. doi:10.3109/00206098109072713 PMID:7271594

Gosnell, J., Costello, J., & Shane, H. (2011). Using a clinical approach to answer "What communication apps should we use?" *ASHA SIG 12. Perspectives on Augmentative and Alternative Communication*, *20*(3), 87–96. doi:10.1044/aac20.3.87

Govaerts, P. J. (2016). Expert opinion: Time to ban formal CI selection criteria? *Cochlear Implants Intl.*, *17*(S1), 74-77.

Govaerts, P. J., Daemers, K., Yperman, M., De Beukelaer, C., De Saegher, G., & De Ceulaer, G. (2006). Auditory speech sounds evaluation (ASSE): A new test to assess detection, discrimination and identification in hearing impairment. *Cochlear Implants International*, *7*(2), 92–106. doi:10.1179/146701006807508106 PMID:18792377

Grantcharov, C. (2016). *Security of Internet-Connected Hearing Aids*. Retrieved June 1, 2017 from https://www.hearingtracker.com/blog/security-of-internet-connected-hearing-aids/

Grebel, K., Dang, D., Ma, L., Payne, D., & Cooper, B. (2015). iSound: A smartphone based intelligent sound fusion system for the hearing impaired. *Lecture Notes in Computer Science*, *9204*, 155–164. doi:10.1007/978-3-319-21837-3_16

Greenwell, K., Featherstone, D., & Hoare, D. J. (2015). The application of intervention coding methodology to describe the tinnitus e-programme, an internet-delivered self-help intervention for tinnitus. *American Journal of Audiology*, *24*(3), 311–315. PMID:26649537

Grenness, C., Hickson, L., Laplante-Lévesque, A., & Davidson, B. (2014). Patient-centred audiological rehabilitation: Perspectives of older adults who own hearing aids. *International Journal of Audiology, 53*(sup1), S68-S75.

Grewal, R., Spielmann, P., Jones, S., & Hussain, S. (2014). Clinical efficacy of tinnitus retraining therapy and cognitive behavioural therapy in the treatment of subjective tinnitus: A systematic review. *The Journal of Laryngology and Otology*, *128*(12), 1028–1033. doi:10.1017/S0022215114002849 PMID:25417546

Griffiths, F., Lindenmeyer, A., Powell, J., Lowe, P., & Thorogood, M. (2006). Why are health care interventions delivered over the internet? A systematic review of the published literature. *Journal of Medical Internet Research*, *8*(2), e10. doi:10.2196/jmir.8.2.e10 PMID:16867965

Griffiths, K. M., & Christensen, H. (2007). Internet-based mental health programs: A powerful tool in the rural medical kit. *The Australian Journal of Rural Health*, *15*(2), 81–87. doi:10.1111/j.1440-1584.2007.00859.x PMID:17441815

Grimshaw, J. M., Eccles, M. P., Lavis, J. N., Hill, S. J., & Squires, J. E. (2012). Knowledge translation of research findings. *Implementation Science; IS*, *7*(1), 1. doi:10.1186/1748-5908-7-50 PMID:22651257

Grol, R. (2001). Successes and failures in the implementation of evidence-based guidelines for clinical practice. *Medical Care*, *39*(8), II-46–II-54. PMID:11583121

Groshek, M. R., Oldenburg, J., Sarasohn-Kahn, J., & Sitler, B. (2015). *mHealth app essentials: patient engagement, considerations, and implementation*. Healthcare Information and Management Systems Society (HIMSS) News. Retrieved June 12, 2018 from http://www.himss.org/ResourceLibrary/genResourceFAQ.aspx?ItemNumber=39175

Hack and Hear. (2016). *Bits around hearing and acoustics*. Retrieved June 1, 2017 from http://www.hackandhear.com/

Hadjistavropoulos, H. D., Thompson, M. J., Klein, B., & Austin, D. W. (2012). Dissemination of therapist-assisted internet cognitive behaviour therapy: Development and open pilot study of a workshop. *Cognitive Behaviour Therapy*, *41*(3), 230–240. doi:10.1080/16506073.2011.645550 PMID:22428582

Hallam, R., Rachman, S., & Hinchcliffe, R. (1984). Psychological aspects of tinnitus. *Contributions to Medical Psychology*, *3*, 31–53.

Hall, D. A., Fackrell, K., Li, A. B., Thavayogan, R., Smith, S., Kennedy, V., ... Haider, H. F. (2018). A narrative synthesis of research evidence for tinnitus-related complaints as reported by patients and their significant others. *Health and Quality of Life Outcomes*, *16*(1), 61. doi:10.118612955-018-0888-9 PMID:29642913

Hall, D. A., Láinez, M. J., Newman, C. W., Sanchez, T. G., Egler, M., Tennigkeit, F., ... Langguth, B. (2011). Treatment options for subjective tinnitus: Self reports from a sample of general practitioners and ENT physicians within Europe and the USA. *BMC Health Services Research*, *11*(1), 302. doi:10.1186/1472-6963-11-302 PMID:22053947

Halperin, D., Heydt-Benjamin, T. S., Ransford, B., Clark, S. S., Defend, B., Morgan, W., . . . Maisel, W. H. (2008). Pacemakers and Implantable Cardiac Defibrillators: Software Radio Attacks and Zero-Power Defenses. In *Proceedings of the 2008 IEEE Symposium on Security and Privacy* (pp. 129-142). Washington, DC: IEEE Computer Society.

Harvey, G., & Kitson, A. (2015). Translating evidence into healthcare policy and practice: Single versus multi-faceted implementation strategies–is there a simple answer to a complex question? *International Journal of Health Policy and Management*, *4*(3), 123–126. doi:10.15171/ijhpm.2015.54 PMID:25774368

Hayes, S. C., Wilson, K. G., Gifford, E. V., Follette, V. M., & Strosahl, K. (1996). Experiential avoidance and behavioural disorders: A functional dimensional approach to diagnosis and treatment. *Journal of Consulting and Clinical Psychology*, *64*(6), 1152–1168. doi:10.1037/0022-006X.64.6.1152 PMID:8991302

Hedman, E., El Alaoui, S., Lindefors, N., Andersson, E., Rück, C., Ghaderi, A., ... Ljótsson, B. (2014). Clinical effectiveness and cost-effectiveness of internet-vs. group-based cognitive behavior therapy for social anxiety disorder: 4-year follow-up of a randomized trial. *Behaviour Research and Therapy*, *59*, 20–29. doi:10.1016/j.brat.2014.05.010 PMID:24949908

Heinrich, S., Rozental, A., Carlbring, P., Andersson, G., Cotter, K., & Weise, C. (2016). Treating tinnitus distress via the internet: A mixed methods approach of what makes patients seek help and stay motivated during internet-based cognitive behavior therapy. *Internet Interventions*, *4*, 120–130. doi:10.1016/j.invent.2016.04.001 PMID:30135798

Heiss, L. (2018). *Designing Emotional Technologies - Collaborating across design, health and engineering to humanise wearable health technologies* (Ph.D. thesis). RMIT University.

Helf, C., & Hlavacs, H. (2016). Apps for life change: Critical review and solution directions. *Entertainment Computing*, *14*, 17–22. doi:10.1016/j.entcom.2015.07.001

Henry, B. A., McDermott, H. J., McKay, C. M., James, C. J., & Clark, G. M. (1998). A frequency importance function for a new monosyllabic word test. Australian Journal of Audiology, November, 20(2), 79-86.

Henry, J. L., & Wilson, P. H. (2001). *The psychological management of chronic tinnitus: A cognitive-behavioral approach*. Allyn & Bacon.

Henshaw, H., & Ferguson, M. A. (2013). Efficacy of Individual Computer-Based Auditory Training for People with Hearing Loss: A Systematic Review of the Evidence. *PLoS One*, 10. PMID:23675431

Hesser, H., Weise, C., Westin, V. Z., & Andersson, G. (2011). A systematic review and meta-analysis of randomized controlled trials of cognitive–behavioral therapy for tinnitus distress. *Clinical Psychology Review*, *31*(4), 545–553. doi:10.1016/j.cpr.2010.12.006 PMID:21237544

Hill, J. W., & Powell, P. (2009). The national healthcare crisis: Is eHealth a key solution? *Business Horizons*, *52*(3), 265–277. doi:10.1016/j.bushor.2009.01.006

HIMSS Media. (2017). *Healthcare IT News*. Retrieved June 1, 2017 from http://www.healthcareitnews.com/

Hoare, D. J., Kowalkowski, V. L., Kang, S., & Hall, D. A. (2011). Systematic review and meta-analyses of randomized controlled trials examining tinnitus management. *The Laryngoscope*, *121*(7), 1555–1564. doi:10.1002/lary.21825 PMID:21671234

Huckvale, K., Adomaviciute, S., Prieto, J. T., Leow, M. K., & Car, J. (2015). Smartphone apps for calculating insulin dose: A systematic assessment. *BMC Medicine*, *13*(1), 106. doi:10.118612916-015-0314-7 PMID:25943590

Hussain, M., Al-Haiqi, A., Zaidan, A. A., Zaidan, B. B., Kiah, M. L., Anuar, N. B., & Abdulnabi, M. (2015). The landscape of research on smartphone medical apps: Coherent taxonomy, motivations, open challenges and recommendations. *Computer Methods and Programs in Biomedicine*, *122*(3), 393–408. doi:10.1016/j.cmpb.2015.08.015 PMID:26412009

IMS Institute for Healthcare Informatics. (2013). *Patient Apps for Improved Healthcare: From Novelty to Mainstream*. Retrieved June 12, 2018 from http://moodle.univ-lille2.fr/pluginfile.php/128248/mod_resource/content/0/patients%20apps%20for%20improved%20healthcare%20IMS.pdf

International Organization for Standardization. (2004). *ISO/TR 16056-1:2004*. Retrieved October 1, 2018, from https://www.iso.org/standard/37351.html

Jacobs, P. G., Saunders, G. H., Jacobs, P. G., & Saunders, G. H. (2014). New opportunities and challenges for teleaudiology within Department of Veterans Affairs. *Journal of Rehabilitation Research and Development*, *51*(5), vii–xii. doi:10.1682/JRRD.2014.04.0093 PMID:25334005

James, J. A. (2013). *Patient engagement: People actively involved in their health and health care tend to have better outcomes--and, some evidence suggests, lower costs*. Project HOPE.

Jasper, K., Weise, C., Conrad, I., Andersson, G., Hiller, W., & Kleinstaeuber, M. (2014). Internet- based guided self-help versus group cognitive behavioral therapy for chronic tinnitus: A randomized controlled trial. *Psychotherapy and Psychosomatics*, *83*(4), 234–246. doi:10.1159/000360705 PMID:24970708

Jastreboff, M. M. (2007). Sound therapies for tinnitus management. *Progress in Brain Research, 166*, 435–440. doi:10.1016/S0079-6123(07)66042-7 PMID:17956808

Jelonek, S. (1994). NOAH/HI-PRO system offers industrywide standard for fitting programmables. *The Hearing Journal, 47*, 21–21.

Jenstad, L., & Moon, J. (2011). Systematic review of barriers and facilitators to hearing aid uptake in older adults. *Audiology Research, 1*(1), 91–95. PMID:26557310

Jerram, J. C., & Purdy, S. C. (2001). Technology, expectations, and adjustment to hearing loss: Predictors of hearing aid outcome. *Journal of the American Academy of Audiology, 12*(2), 64–79. PMID:11261460

Johansson, R., & Andersson, G. (2012). Internet-based psychological treatments for depression. *Expert Review of Neurotherapeutics, 12*(7), 861–870. doi:10.1586/ern.12.63 PMID:22853793

Kaandorp, M. W., Smits, C., Merkus, P., Goverts, S. T., & Festen, J. M. (2015). Assessing speech recognition abilities with digits in noise in cochlear implant and hearing aid users. *International Journal of Audiology, 54*(1), 48–57. doi:10.3109/14992027.2014.945623 PMID:25156097

Kaldo-Sandström, V., Larsen, H. C., & Andersson, G. (2004). Internet- based cognitive-behavioral self-help treatment of tinnitus: Clinical effectiveness and predictors of outcome. *American Journal of Audiology, 13*(2), 185–192. doi:10.1044/1059-0889(2004/023) PMID:15903144

Kaldo, V., Cars, S., Rahnert, M., Larsen, H. C., & Andersson, G. (2007). Use of a self-help book with weekly therapist contact to reduce tinnitus distress: A randomized controlled trial. *Journal of Psychosomatic Research, 63*(2), 195–202. doi:10.1016/j.jpsychores.2007.04.007 PMID:17662757

Kaldo, V., Haak, T., Buhrman, M., Alfonsson, S., Larsen, H., & Andersson, G. (2013). Internet-based cognitive behaviour therapy for tinnitus patients delivered in a regular clinical setting: Outcome and analysis of treatment dropout. *Cognitive Behaviour Therapy, 42*(2), 146–158. doi:10.1080/16506073.2013.769622 PMID:23432207

Kaldo, V., Levin, S., Widarsson, J., Buhrman, M., Larsen, H. C., & Andersson, G. (2008). Internet versus group cognitive-behavioral treatment of distress associated with tinnitus: A randomized controlled trial. *Behavior Therapy, 39*(4), 348–359. doi:10.1016/j.beth.2007.10.003 PMID:19027431

Kaltenthaler, E., Sutcliffe, P., Parry, G., Beverley, C., Rees, A., & Ferriter, M. (2008). The acceptability to patients of computerized cognitive behaviour therapy for depression: A systematic review. *Psychological Medicine*, *38*(11), 1521–1530. doi:10.1017/S0033291707002607 PMID:18205964

Kaplan, K., Salzer, M. S., Solomon, P., Brusilovskiy, E., & Cousounis, P. (2011). Internet peer support for individuals with psychiatric disabilities: A randomized controlled trial. *Social Science & Medicine*, *72*(1), 54–62. doi:10.1016/j.socscimed.2010.09.037 PMID:21112682

Kaspersky. (2017). *Cyberthreat Real Time Map*. Retrieved June 1, 2017 from https://cybermap.kaspersky.com/

Kaufman, D. R., Pevzner, J., Hilliman, C., Weinstock, R. S., Teresi, J., Shea, S., & Starren, J. (2006). Redesigning a Telehealth Diabetes Management Program for a Digital Divide Seniors Population. *Home Health Care Management & Practice*, *18*(3), 223–234. doi:10.1177/1084822305281949

Keach, E. E. (2013). *Investigation of hearing aid provision via the first-fit efficacy of three adaptive dynamic range optimisation (ADRO) fitting methods* (Master thesis). University of Auckland.

Keidser, G., & Convery, E. (2016). Self-Fitting Hearing Aids: Status Quo and Future Predictions. *Trends in Hearing*, *2016*, 20. PMID:27072929

Keidser, G., Dillon, H. R., Flax, M., Ching, T., & Brewer, S. (2011). The NAL-NL2 prescription procedure. *Audiology Research*, *1*(1), 24. PMID:26557309

Kelly, J., & Matthews, B. (2014). Displacing use: Exploring alternative relationships in a human-centred design process. *Design Studies*, *35*(4), 353–373.

Kenner, A. (2016). Asthma on the move: How mobile apps remediate risk for disease management. *Health Risk & Society*, *17*(7-8), 510–529. doi:10.1080/13698575.2015.1136408

Khedr, E. M., Ahmed, M. A., Shawky, O. A., Mohamed, E. S., El Attar, G. S., & Mohammad, K. A. (2010). Epidemiological study of chronic tinnitus in Assiut, Egypt. *Neuroepidemiology*, *35*(1), 45–52. doi:10.1159/000306630 PMID:20389124

Khoza-Shangase, K., & Kassner, L. (2013). Automated screening audiometry in the digital age: Exploring uHear™ and its use in a resource-stricken developing country. *International Journal of Technology Assessment in Health Care*, *29*(1), 42–47. doi:10.1017/S0266462312000761 PMID:23298579

Killion, M. (1985). The noise problem: There's hope. *Hearing Instruments*, *36*(11), 26–32.

Killion, M. C., Niquette, P. A., Gudmundsen, G. I., Revit, L. J., & Banerjee, S. (2004). Development of a quick speech-in-noise test for measuring signal-to-noise ratio loss in normal-hearing and hearing-impaired listeners. *The Journal of the Acoustical Society of America*, *116*(4), 2395–2405. doi:10.1121/1.1784440 PMID:15532670

Kim, B. Y., & Lee, J. (2017). Smart Devices for Older Adults Managing Chronic Disease: A Scoping Review. *JMIR mHealth and uHealth*, *5*(5), e69. doi:10.2196/mhealth.7141 PMID:28536089

Kimball, S. H. (2008). Inquiry into online hearing test raises doubts about its validity. *The Hearing Journal*, *61*(3), 38–46. doi:10.1097/01.HJ.0000314717.42321.4a

Kim, J., & Moon, J. Y. (1998). Designing towards emotional usability in customer interfaces—trustworthiness of cyber-banking system interfaces. *Interacting with Computers*, *10*(1), 1–29. doi:10.1016/S0953-5438(97)00037-4

Knudsen, V., Öberg, M., Nielsen, C., Naylor, G., & Kramer, S. E. (2010). Factors Influencing Help Seeking, Hearing Aid Uptake, Hearing Aid Use and Satisfaction With Hearing Aids: A Review of the Literature. *Trends in Amplification*, *14*(3), 127–154. doi:10.1177/1084713810385712 PMID:21109549

Kochkin, S. (2000). MarkeTrak V: "Why my hearing aids are in the drawer" The consumers' perspective. *The Hearing Journal*, *53*(2), 34–36. doi:10.1097/00025572-200002000-00004

Kochkin, S. (2007). MarkeTrak VII: Obstacles to adult non-user adoption of hearing aids. *The Hearing Journal*, *60*(4), 24–51. doi:10.1097/01.HJ.0000285745.08599.7f

Kochkin, S., Beck, D. L., Christensen, L. A., Compton-Conley, C., Fligor, B. J., Kricos, P. B., & Turner, R. G. (2010). MarkeTrak VIII: The impact of the hearing healthcare professional on hearing aid user success. *Hearing Review*, *17*(4), 12–34.

Kreuter, M. W., Strecher, V. J., & Glassman, B. (1999). One size does not fit all: The case for tailoring print materials. *Annals of Behavioral Medicine*, *21*(4), 276–283. doi:10.1007/BF02895958 PMID:10721433

Krupinski, E.A. (2015). Innovations and possibilities in connected health. *Journal American Academy Audiology*, *26*, 761-767.

Krupinski, E. A. (2015). Innovations and possibilities in connected health. *Journal of the American Academy of Audiology*, *26*(9), 761–767. doi:10.3766/jaaa.14047 PMID:26415969

Kuzovkov, V., Yanov, Y., & Levin, S. (2014). Remote programming of MED-EL cochlear implants: users' and professionals' evaluation of the remote programming experience. *J. Acta Oto-Laryngologica*.

Kuzovkov, V., Yanov, Y., Levin, S., Bovo, R., Rosignoli, M., Eskilsson, G., & Willbas, S. (2014). Remote programming of MED-EL cochlear implants: Users' and professionals' evaluation of the remote programming experience. *Acta Oto-Laryngologica*, *134*(7), 709–716. doi:10.3109/00016489.2014.892212 PMID:24773208

LACE. (2018). Retrieved from https://www.neurotone.com/lace-interactive-listening-program

Landgrebe, M., Azevedo, A., Baguley, D., Bauer, C., Cacace, A., Coelho, C., ... Langguth, B. (2012). Methodological aspects of clinical trials in tinnitus: A proposal for an international standard. *Journal of Psychosomatic Research*, *73*(2), 112–121. doi:10.1016/j.jpsychores.2012.05.002 PMID:22789414

Landoll, D. (2011). *The Security Risk Assessment Handbook: A Complete Guide for Performing Security Risk Assessments* (2nd ed.). Boca Raton, FL: CRC Press. doi:10.1201/b10937

Langguth, B. (2011). A review of tinnitus symptoms beyond 'ringing in the ears': A call to action. *Current Medical Research and Opinion*, *27*(8), 1635–1643. doi:10.1185/03007995.2011.595781 PMID:21699365

Laplante-Lévesque, A., Brännström, K. J., Andersson, G., & Lunner, T. (2012). Quality and readability of English-language internet information for adults with hearing impairment and their significant others. *International Journal of Audiology*, *51*(8), 618–626. doi:10.3109/14992027.2012.684406 PMID:22731921

Larrosa, F., Rama-Lopez, J., Benitez, J., Morales, J. M., Martinez, A., Alañon, M. A., ... Rey-Martinez, J. (2015). Development and evaluation of an audiology app for iPhone/iPad mobile devices. *Acta Oto-Laryngologica*, *135*(11), 1119–1127. doi:10.3109/00016489.2015.1063786 PMID:26144548

Lazard, D. S., Vincent, C., Venail, F., Van de Heyning, P., Truy, E., Sterkers, O., ... Blamey, P. J. (2012). Pre-, per-and postoperative factors affecting performance of postlinguistically deaf adults using cochlear implants: A new conceptual model over time. *PLoS One*, *7*(11). doi:10.1371/journal.pone.0048739 PMID:23152797

Lekowski, R. (2016). *Bluetooth: Just How Secure Is It?* Retrieved June 1, 2017 from http://www.lawtechnologytoday.org/2016/05/bluetooth-how-secure-is-it/

Lewis, T. L. (2013). A systematic self-certification model for mobile medical apps. *Journal of Medical Internet Research*, *15*(4), e89. doi:10.2196/jmir.2446 PMID:23615332

Liao, G. Y., Chien, Y. T., Chen, Y. J., Hsiung, H. F., Chen, H. J., Hsieh, M. H., & Wu, W. J. (2017). What to Build for Middle-Agers to Come? Attractive and Necessary Functions of Exercise-Promotion Mobile Phone Apps: A Cross-Sectional Study. *JMIR mHealth and uHealth*, *5*(5), e65. doi:10.2196/mhealth.6233 PMID:28546140

Li, C., Raghunathan, A., & Jha, N. K. (2011). Hijacking an Insulin Pump: Security Attacks and Defenses for a Diabetes Therapy System. In *Proceedings of the 2011 IEEE 13th International Conference on e-Health Networking, Applications and Services* (pp. 150-156). Washington, DC: IEEE Computer Society.

Lin,, F.R., Yaffe,, K., & Xia,, J., Lie, X., Satterfield, S., Ayonayon, H.N., … Simonsick, E.M. (2013). Hearing Loss and Cognitive Decline in Older Adults. *American Medical Association Internal Medicine.*, *173*(4), 293–299.

Lin, F. R., Yaffe, K., Xia, J., Xue, Q., Harris, T. B., Purchase-Helzner, E., ... Simonsick, E. M. (2013). Hearing Loss and Cognitive Decline in Older Adults. *Journal American Medical Association Internal Medicine*, *173*(4), 293–299. PMID:23337978

Lin, Y., Lai, Y., Chang, H., Tsao, Y., Chang, Y., & Chang, R. Y. (2018). SmartHear: A smartphone-based remote microphone hearing assistive system using wireless technologies. *IEEE Systems Journal*, *12*(1), 20–29. doi:10.1109/JSYST.2015.2490104

Livshitz, L., Ghanayim, R., Kraus, C., Farah, R., Even-Tov, E., Avraham, Y., ... Gilbey, P. (2017). Application-based hearing screening in the elderly population. *The Annals of Otology, Rhinology, and Laryngology*, *126*(1), 36–41. doi:10.1177/0003489416672873 PMID:27913721

Lloyd, C., King, R., Bassett, H., Sandland, S., & Savige, G. (2001). Patient, Client or Consumer? A Survey of Preferred Terms. *Australasian Psychiatry*, *9*(4), 321–324. doi:10.1046/j.1440-1665.2001.00358.x

Lopez-Lorca, A. A., Miller, T., Pedell, S., Mendoza, A., Keirnan, A., & Sterling, L. (2014, November). One Size Doesn't Fit All: Diversifying "The User" using Personas and Emotional Scenarios. *6th International Workshop on Social Software Engineering*, pp. 25-32, Hong Kong, China.

Louw, C., Swanepoel, D. W., Eikelboom, R. H., & Myburgh, H. C. (2017). Smartphone-based hearing screening at primary health care clinics. *Ear and Hearing*, *38*(2), e93–e100. doi:10.1097/AUD.0000000000000378 PMID:27764002

Lustria, M. L. A., Noar, S. M., Cortese, J., Van Stee, S. K., Glueckauf, R. L., & Lee, J. (2013). A meta-analysis of web-delivered tailored health behavior change interventions. *Journal of Health Communication*, *18*(9), 1039–1069. doi:10.1080/10810730.2013.768727 PMID:23750972

Lutz, W. (2003). Efficacy, effectiveness, and expected treatment response in psychotherapy. *Journal of Clinical Psychology*, *59*(7), 745–750. doi:10.1002/jclp.10169 PMID:12808581

Lyall, F. C., Clamp, P. J., & Hajioff, D. (2016). Smartphone speech-to-text applications for communication with profoundly deaf patients. *The Journal of Laryngology and Otology*, *130*(1), 104–106. doi:10.1017/S0022215115003151 PMID:26611260

Mahomed-Asmail, F., Swanepoel, D. W., Eikelboom, R. H., Myburgh, H. C., & Hall, J. III. (2016). Clinical validity of hearScreen™ smartphone hearing screening for school children. *Ear and Hearing*, *37*(1), e11–e17. doi:10.1097/AUD.0000000000000223 PMID:26372265

Manchaiah, V., Danermark, B., Ronnberg, J., & Lunner, T. (2014). Importance of "process evaluation" in audiological rehabilitation: Examples from studies on hearing impairment. *International Journal of Otolaryngology*, *2014*, 168684. doi:10.1155/2014/168684 PMID:25276135

Mandavia, R., Lapa, T., Smith, M., & Bhutta, M. F. (2017). A cross-sectional evaluation of the validity of a smartphone otoscopy device in screening for ear disease in Nepal. *Clinical Otolaryngology*, *43*(1), 31–38. doi:10.1111/coa.12898 PMID:28485038

Mantovani, E., & Quinn, P. (2014), mHealth and data protection – the letter and the spirit of consent legal requirements. *International Review of Law, Computers and Technology, 20*(2), 222-236.

Martinez, C., Wallenhorst, C., McFerran, D., & Hall, D. A. (2015). Incidence rates of clinically significant tinnitus: 10-year trend from a cohort study in England. *Ear and Hearing, 36*(3), e69–e75. doi:10.1097/AUD.0000000000000121 PMID:25470370

Martínez-Pérez, B., de la Torre-Díez, I., Candelas-Plasencia, S., & López-Coronado, M. (2013). Development and evaluation of tools for measuring the quality of experience (QoE) in mHealth applications. *Journal of Medical Systems, 37*(5), 9976. doi:10.100710916-013-9976-x PMID:24014255

Martínez-Pérez, B., de la Torre-Díez, I., & López-Coronado, M. (2013). Mobile health applications for the most prevalent conditions by the World Health Organization: Review and analysis. *Journal of Medical Internet Research, 15*(6), e120. doi:10.2196/jmir.2600 PMID:23770578

Martínez-Pérez, B., de la Torre-Díez, I., López-Coronado, M., & Herreros-González, J. (2013). Mobile Apps in Cardiology [Review]. *JMIR mHealth and uHealth, 1*(2), e15. doi:10.2196/mhealth.2737 PMID:25098320

Masalski, M., Kipiński, L., Grysiński, T., & Kręcicki, T. (2016). Hearing tests on mobile devices: Evaluation of the reference sound level by means of biological calibration. *Journal of Medical Internet Research, 18*(5), e130. doi:10.2196/jmir.4987 PMID:27241793

Matthews, C. (2012, April 12). The Top Ten Fastest-Growing Industries in America. *Time Magazine*.

McCormack, A., & Fortnum, H. (2013). Why do people fitted with hearing aids not wear them? *International Journal of Audiology, 52*(5), 360–368. doi:10.3109/14992027.2013.769066 PMID:23473329

McFerran, D., Hoare, D. J., Carr, S., Ray, J., & Stockdale, D. (2018). Tinnitus services in the united kingdom: A survey of patient experiences. *BMC Health Services Research, 18*(1), 110. doi:10.118612913-018-2914-3 PMID:29433479

McKenna, L., Baguley, D., & McFerran, D. (2010). *Living with Tinnitus and Hyperacusis*. Sheldon Press.

Meder, A. M., & Wegner, J. R. (2015). iPads, mobile technologies, and communication applications: A survey of family wants, needs, and preferences. *Augmentative and Alternative Communication, 31*(1), 27–36. doi:10.3109/07434618.2014.995223 PMID:25685882

Medtronic plc. (2011). *Medtronic CareLink® Network Remote Monitoring Helps Improve Patient Care and Reduce Healthcare Costs*. Retrieved October 1, 2018 from http://newsroom.medtronic.com/phoenix.zhtml?c=251324&p=irol-newsArticle&ID=1771836

Meister, H., Walger, M., Brehmer, D., von Wedel, U. C., & von Wedel, H. (2008). The relationship between pre-fitting expectations and willingness to use hearing aids. *International Journal of Audiology, 47*(4), 153–159. doi:10.1080/14992020701843111 PMID:18389410

Mendoza, A., Miller, T., Pedell, S., & Sterling, L. (2013). The role of users' emotions and associated quality goals on appropriation of systems: two case studies. In *24th Australasian Conference on Information Systems (ACIS)*. RMIT University.

Meskó, B. (2018). *Health IT Or Digital Health? The Gary-Rule Helps!* Retrieved September 28, 2018 from https://www.linkedin.com/pulse/health-digital-gary-rule-helps-bertalan-mesk%C3%B3-md-phd/

Michie, S., van Stralen, M. M., & West, R. (2011). The behaviour change wheel: A new method for characterising and designing behaviour change interventions. *Implementation Science; IS, 6*, 42. doi:10.1186/1748-5908-6-42

Michikawa, T., Nishiwaki, Y., Kikuchi, Y., Saito, H., Mizutari, K., Okamoto, M., & Takebayashi, T. (2010). Prevalence and factors associated with tinnitus: A community-based study of japanese elders. *Journal of Epidemiology, 20*(4), 271–276. doi:10.2188/jea.JE20090121 PMID:20501961

Mielke, M., & Brueck, R. (2015). Design and evaluation of a smartphone application for non-speech sound awareness for people with hearing loss. In *Proceedings of the 2015 Annual International Conference of the IEEE Engineering in Medicine and Biology Society (IEEE EMBC 2015)*. IEEE Press.

Mielke, M., & Brueck, R. (2016). A home automation based environmental sound alert for people experiencing hearing loss. In *Proceedings of the 2016 Annual International Conference of the IEEE Engineering in Medicine and Biology Society (IEEE EMBC 2016)*. IEEE Press.

Mielke, M., Grunewald, A., & Brueck, R. (2013). An assistive technology for hearing-impaired persons: analysis, requirements and architecture. In *Proceedings of the 2013 Annual International Conference of the IEEE Engineering in Medicine and Biology Society (IEEE EMBC 2013)*. IEEE Press.

Miller, G. A., & Nicely, P. E. (1955). An analysis of perceptual confusions among some English consonants. *The Journal of the Acoustical Society of America*, *27*(2), 338–352. doi:10.1121/1.1907526

Miller, T., Pedell, S., Lopez-Lorca, A., Mendoza, A., Sterling, L., & Keirnan, A. (2015). Emotionally-driven models for people-oriented requirements engineering: The case study of emergency systems. *Journal of Systems and Software*, *105*, 54–71. doi:10.1016/j.jss.2015.03.044

Misra, S., Lewis, T. L., & Aungst, T. D. (2013). Medical application use and the need for further research and assessment for clinical practice: Creation and integration of standards for best practice to alleviate poor application design. *JAMA Dermatology*, *149*(6), 661–662. doi:10.1001/jamadermatol.2013.606 PMID:23783150

Molini-Avejonas, D. R., Rondon-Melo, S., de la Higuera Amato, C. A., & Samelli, A. G. (2015). A systematic review of the use of telehealth in speech, language and hearing sciences. *Journal of Telemedicine and Telecare*, *21*(7), 367–376. doi:10.1177/1357633X15583215 PMID:26026181

Moore, B.C. (2006). Speech mapping is a valuable tool for fitting and counseling patients. *Hearing Journal*, *59*(8), 26-8.

Moore, G., Audrey, S., Barker, M., Bond, L., Bonell, C., Hardeman, W., … & Baird, J. (2015). Process evaluation of complex interventions. *Complex Interventions in Health: An Overview of Research Methods,* 222 - 231.

Moore, B. C. (2006). Speech mapping is a valuable tool for fitting and counseling patients. *The Hearing Journal*, *59*(8), 26–28. doi:10.1097/01.HJ.0000286371.07550.5b

Morrison, L. G., Yardley, L., Powell, J., & Michie, S. (2012). What design features are used in effective e-health interventions? A review using techniques from critical interpretive synthesis. *Telemedicine Journal and e-Health*, *18*(2), 137–144. doi:10.1089/tmj.2011.0062 PMID:22381060

Mosa, A. S. M., Yoo, I., & Sheets, L. (2012). A systematic review of healthcare applications for smartphones. *BMC Medical Informatics and Decision Making*, *12*(1), 67. doi:10.1186/1472-6947-12-67 PMID:22781312

Muessig, K. E., Pike, E. C., LeGrand, S., & Hightow-Weidman, L. B. (2013). Mobile phone applications for the care and prevention of HIV and other sexually transmitted diseases: A review. *Journal of Medical Internet Research*, *15*(1), e1. doi:10.2196/jmir.2301 PMID:23291245

Muñoz, R. F. (2010). Using evidence-based internet interventions to reduce health disparities worldwide. *Journal of Medical Internet Research*, *12*(5), e60. doi:10.2196/jmir.1463 PMID:21169162

Murfin, M. (2013). Know your apps: An evidence-based approach to evaluation of mobile clinical applications. *The Journal of Physician Assistant Education: the Official Journal of the Physician Assistant Education Association*, *24*(3), 38–40. doi:10.1097/01367895-201324030-00008 PMID:24261171

Musiat, P., Goldstone, P., & Tarrier, N. (2014). Understanding the acceptability of e-mental health-attitudes and expectations towards computerised self-help treatments for mental health problems. *BMC Psychiatry*, *14*(1), 109. doi:10.1186/1471-244X-14-109 PMID:24725765

Na, N., & Suk, H.-J. (2014). The Emotional Characteristics of White for Applications of Product Color Design. *International Journal of Design*, *8*(2).

National Academies of Sciences, Engineering, and Medicine. (2016). *Hearing Health Care for Adults: priorities for improving access and affordability*. National Academies Press.

National Institute for Health and Care Excellent (NICE). (2009). *Cochlear implants for children and adults with severe to profound deafness*. Retrieved October 1, 2018, from https://www.nice.org.uk/guidance/ta166/chapter/4-evidence-and-interpretation

Na, Y., Joo, H. S., Yang, H., Kang, S., Hong, S. H., & Woo, J. (2014). Smartphone-based hearing screening in noisy environments. *Sensors (Basel)*, *14*(6), 10346–10360. doi:10.3390140610346 PMID:24926692

Newman, L. H. (2017). *Medical Devices Are the Next Security Nightmare*. Retrieved June 1, 2017, from https://www.wired.com/2017/03/medical-devices-next-security-nightmare/

Newswire, P. R. (2016). *Oticon Launches World's First Internet of Things Hearing Aid*. Retrieved from https://www.prnewswire.com/news-releases/oticon-launches-worlds-first-internet-of-things-hearing-aid-584077291.html

Noble, W. (2013). *Self-Assessment of Hearing* (2nd ed.). San Diego, CA: Plural Publishing.

Noor, A. K. (2015). Potential of cognitive computing and cognitive systems. *Ocean Engineering*, *5*(1), 75–88.

Norman, D. (2005). *Emotional Design: Why We Love (or Hate) Everyday Things*. Academic Press.

Nyenhuis, N., Golm, D., & Kröner-Herwig, B. (2013). A systematic review and meta-analysis on the efficacy of self-help interventions in tinnitus. *Cognitive Behaviour Therapy*, *42*(2), 159–169. doi:10.1080/16506073.2013.803496 PMID:23777192

Nyenhuis, N., Zastrutzki, S., Weise, C., Jäger, B., & Kröner-Herwig, B. (2013). The efficacy of minimal contact interventions for acute tinnitus: A randomised controlled study. *Cognitive Behaviour Therapy*, *42*(2), 127–138. doi:10.1080/16506073.2012.655305 PMID:22413736

O'Neill, S., & Brady, R. R. W. (2012). Colorectal smartphone apps: Opportunities and risks. *Colorectal Disease*, *14*(9), e530–e534. doi:10.1111/j.1463-1318.2012.03088.x PMID:22646729

Office of the Australian Information Commissioner (OAIC). (2017). *Business resource: Handling health information under the Privacy Act: A general overview for health service providers*. Retrieved June 1, 2017 from https://www.oaic.gov.au/engage-with-us/consultations/health-privacy-guidance/business-resource-handling-health-information-under-the-privacy-act-a-general-overview-for-health-service-providers

Olsen, W. O. (1998). Average speech levels and spectra in various speaking/listening conditions: A summary of the Pearson, Bennett, & Fidell (1977) report. *American Journal of Audiology*, *7*(2), 21–25. doi:10.1044/1059-0889(1998/012) PMID:26649514

Olson, A. D. (2015). Options for auditory training for adults with hearing loss. *Seminars in Hearing*, *36*(4), 284–295. doi:10.1055-0035-1564461 PMID:27587915

One Million Solutions in Health. (2018). Retrieved from http://www.onemillionsolutionsinhealth.org/

Organisation for Economic Co-operative Development (OECD). (2015). *Draft OECD Guide to Measuring ICTs in the Health Sector.* Retrieved August 18, 2018 from https://www.oecd.org/health/health-systems/Draft-oecd-guide-to-measuring-icts-in-the-health-sector.pdf

Ozdalga, E., Ozdalga, A., & Ahuja, N. (2012). The smartphone in medicine: A review of current and potential use among physicians and students. *Journal of Medical Internet Research, 14*(5), e128. doi:10.2196/jmir.1994 PMID:23017375

Paglialonga, A., Pinciroli, F., Barbieri, R., Caiani, E. G., Riboldi, M., & Tognola, G. (2017b). E-Health solutions for better care: Characterization of health apps to extract meaningful information and support users' choices. In *Proceedings of the 3rd IEEE International Forum on Research and Technologies for Society and Industry (IEEE RTSI 2017*). IEEE Press.

Paglialonga, A., Riboldi, M., Tognola, G., & Caiani, E. G. (2017d). Automated Identification of Health Apps' Medical Specialties and Promoters from the Store Webpages. In *Proceedings of the 6th IEEE International Conference on E-Health and Bioengineering* (*IEEE EHB 2017*). IEEE Press.

Paglialonga, A., Tognola, G., & Pinciroli, F. (2015a). Apps for hearing sciences and care. *American Journal of Audiology*, *24*, 293-298.

Paglialonga, A., Barbieri, R., Malgara, F., Rosati, R., Pinciroli, F., & Tognola, G. (2017c). Multidimensional characterization of mobile apps for hearing health care by using the ALFA4Hearing (At-a-glance Labelling for Features of Apps for Hearing health care) model combined with data visualization methods. In *Proceedings of the 2017 Medical Informatics Europe (EFMI MIE 2017).* IOS Press.

Paglialonga, A., Lugo, A., & Santoro, E. (2018). An overview on the emerging area of identification, characterization, and assessment of health apps. *Journal of Biomedical Informatics*, *83*, 97–102. doi:10.1016/j.jbi.2018.05.017 PMID:29852318

Paglialonga, A., Mastropietro, A., Scalco, E., & Rizzo, G. (in press). The mHealth. In G. Andreoni & G. Perego (Eds.), *Present, present continuous and future of mHealth: a reference grammar for next healthcare*. London: Springer.

Paglialonga, A., Pinciroli, F., & Tognola, G. (2017a). The *ALFA4Hearing* model (At-a-glance Labelling for Features of Apps for Hearing healthcare) to characterize mobile apps for hearing healthcare. *American Journal of Audiology*, *26*(3S), 408–425. doi:10.1044/2017_AJA-16-0132 PMID:29049624

Paglialonga, A., Schiavo, M., & Caiani, E. G. (in press). Automated Characterization of Mobile Health Apps' Features by Extracting Information from the Web: An Exploratory Study. *American Journal of Audiology*.

Paglialonga, A., Tognola, G., & Pinciroli, F. (2015b). Apps for hearing healthcare. *Studies in Health Technology and Informatics*, *210*, 666–668. PMID:25991233

Palmqvist, B., Carlbring, P., & Andersson, G. (2007). *Internet-delivered treatments with or without therapist input: Does the therapist factor have implications for efficacy and cost?* Academic Press.

Panahi, I., Kehtarnavaz, N., & Thibodeau, L. (2016). Smartphone-based noise adaptive speech enhancement for hearing aid applications. In *Proceedings of the 2016 Annual International Conference of the IEEE Engineering in Medicine and Biology Society (IEEE EMBC 2016)*. IEEE Press.

Pandey, A., Hasan, S., Dubey, D., & Sarangi, S. (2013). Smartphone apps as a source of cancer information: Changing trends in health information-seeking behavior. *Journal of Cancer Education*, *28*(1), 138–142. doi:10.100713187-012-0446-9 PMID:23275239

Păsărelu, C. R., Andersson, G., Bergman Nordgren, L., & Dobrean, A. (2017). Internet-delivered transdiagnostic and tailored cognitive behavioral therapy for anxiety and depression: A systematic review and meta-analysis of randomized controlled trials. [PubMed]. *Cognitive Behaviour Therapy*, *46*(1), 1–28.

Paxling, B., Lundgren, S., Norman, A., Almlöv, J., Carlbring, P., Cuijpers, P., & Andersson, G. (2013). Therapist behaviours in internet-delivered cognitive behaviour therapy: Analyses of e-mail correspondence in the treatment of generalized anxiety disorder. *Behavioural and Cognitive Psychotherapy*, *41*(03), 280–289. doi:10.1017/S1352465812000240 PMID:22717145

Peer, S., & Fagan, J. J. (2015). Hearing loss in the developing world: Evaluating the iPhone mobile device as a screening tool. *South African Medical Journal*, *105*(1), 35–39. doi:10.7196/SAMJ.8338 PMID:26046161

Perle, J. G., Langsam, L. C., Randel, A., Lutchman, S., Levine, A. B., Odland, A. P., ... Marker, C. D. (2013). Attitudes toward psychological telehealth: Current and future clinical psychologists' opinions of Internet-Based interventions. *Journal of Clinical Psychology*, *69*(1), 100–113. doi:10.1002/jclp.21912 PMID:22975897

Peterson, G. E., & Lehiste, I. (1962). Revised CNC lists for auditory tests. *The Journal of Speech and Hearing Disorders*, *27*(1), 62–70. doi:10.1044/jshd.2701.62 PMID:14485785

Pfleger, R. (2012). *Contract for a Healthy Future*. Presented at Innovation in Healthcare without borders, Brussels, Belgium. Retrieved October 1, 2018, from http://ec.europa.eu/research/health/pdf/event13/roland-pfleger_en.pdf

Pflug, J. (2011). Contextuality and computer-mediated communication: A cross cultural comparison. *Computers in Human Behavior*, *27*(1), 131–137. doi:10.1016/j.chb.2009.10.008

Philips, B., Smits, C., Govaerts, P. J., Doorn, I., & Vanpoucke, F. (in press). Empowering senior cochlear implant users at home via a tablet-computer application. *Journal of American Audiology.*

Piaggio, G., Elbourne, D. R., Pocock, S. J., Evans, S. J., Altman, D. G., & CONSORT Group. (2012). Reporting of noninferiority and equivalence randomized trials: Extension of the CONSORT 2010 statement. *Journal of the American Medical Association*, *308*(24), 2594–2604. doi:10.1001/jama.2012.87802 PMID:23268518

Pizer, S. D., & Prentice, J. C. (2011). What are the consequences of waiting for health care in the veteran population? *Journal of General Internal Medicine*, *26*(2), 676–682. doi:10.100711606-011-1819-1 PMID:21989621

Plomp, R. (1978). Auditory handicap of hearing impairment and the limited benefit of hearing aids. *The Journal of the Acoustical Society of America*, *63*(2), 533–549. doi:10.1121/1.381753 PMID:670550

Polisena, J., Coyle, D., Coyle, K., & McGill, S. (2009). Home telehealth for chronic disease management: A systematic review and an analysis of economic evaluations. *International Journal of Technology Assessment in Health Care*, *25*(3), 339–349. doi:10.1017/S0266462309990201 PMID:19619353

Prilleltensky, I. (2016). *The Laughing Guide to Well-Being: Using Humor and Science to Become Happier and Healthier*. Routledge and Miffllin.

Prime Minister's Science, Engineering and Innovation Council Working Group on Data in Science. (2006). *From Data to Wisdom: Pathways to Successful Data Management for Australian Science*. Retrieved October 1, 2018, from https://archive.industry.gov.au/science/PMSEIC/Documents/DataForScience.pdf

Privacy Rights Clearinghouse. (2016). *Mobile Health and Fitness Apps: What Are the Privacy Risks?* Retrieved June 12, 2018 from https://www.privacyrights.org/consumer-guides/mobile-health-and-fitness-apps-what-are-privacy-risks

Probst, T., Pryss, R., Langguth, B., & Schlee, W. (2016). Emotion dynamics and tinnitus: Daily life data from the "TrackYourTinnitus" application. *Scientific Reports*, *6*(1), 31166. doi:10.1038rep31166 PMID:27488227

Pross, S. E., Bourne, A. L., & Cheung, S. W. (2016). TeleAudiology in the Veterans Health Administration. *Otology & Neurotology*, *37*(7), 847–850. doi:10.1097/MAO.0000000000001058 PMID:27273404

Proynova, R., Paech, B., Koch, S. H., Wicht, A., & Wetter, T. (2011). Investigating the influence of personal values on requirements for health care information systems. In *Proceedings of the 3rd Workshop on Software Engineering in Health Care*. Honolulu, USA. ACM. 10.1145/1987993.1988004

Qiang, C. Z., Yamamichi, M., Hausman, V., Miller, R., & Altman, D. (2012). *Mobile applications for the health sector*. Washington, DC: World Bank. Retrieved June 12, 2018 from http://documents.worldbank.org/curated/en/2012/04/16742613/mobile-applications-health-sector

Ramos, I., & Berry, D. (2005). *Is emotion relevant to requirements engineering?* (Vol. 10). Requirements Engineering.

Reavley, N. J., & Jorm, A. F. (2011). The quality of mental disorder information websites: A review. *Patient Education and Counseling*, *85*(2), e16–e25. doi:10.1016/j.pec.2010.10.015 PMID:21087837

Rehman, H., Kamal, A. K., Morris, P. B., Sayani, S., Merchant, A. T., & Virani, S. S. (2017). Mobile Health (mHealth) Technology for the Management of Hypertension and Hyperlipidemia: Slow Start but Loads of Potential. *Current Atherosclerosis Reports*, *19*(3), 12. doi:10.100711883-017-0649-y PMID:28210974

Research2guidance. (2017). *mHealth app developer economics 2017 -The state of the art of mHealth app publishing*. Retrieved June 12, 2018 from https://research2guidance.com/product/mhealth-economics-2017-current-status-and-future-trends-in-mobile-health

Reynoldson, C., Stones, C., Allsop, M., Gardner, P., Bennett, M. I., Closs, S. J., ... Knapp, P. (2014). Assessing the quality and usability of smartphone apps for pain self-management. *Pain Medicine*, *15*(6), 898–909. doi:10.1111/pme.12327 PMID:24422990

Riach, E. (2003). The privacy and electronic communications directive. *The New Law Journal*, *1*(7071), 379–380.

Richards, J. R., Gaylor, K. A., & Pilgrim, A. J. (2015). Comparison of traditional otoscope to iPhone otoscope in the pediatric ED. *The American Journal of Emergency Medicine*, *33*(8), 1089–1092. doi:10.1016/j.ajem.2015.04.063 PMID:25979304

Rios, B., & Butts, J. (2017). *Security Evaluation of the Implantable Cardiac Device Ecosystem Architecture and Implementation Interdependencies*. Retrieved June 1, 2017 from https://drive.google.com/file/d/0B_GspGER4QQTYkJfaVlBeGVCSW8/view

Ritter, P., Lorig, K., Laurent, D., & Matthews, K. (2004). Internet versus mailed questionnaires: A randomized comparison. *Journal of Medical Internet Research*, *6*(3).

Roberts, K. (2005). *Love Marks: the future beyond brands*. Powerhouse Books.

Roland, J. T. Jr, Gantz, B. J., Waltzman, S. B., & Parkinson, A. J. (2016). United States multicenter clinical trial of the cochlear nucleus hybrid implant system. *The Laryngoscope*, *126*(1), 175–181. doi:10.1002/lary.25451 PMID:26152811

Ryan, R. M. (1982). Control and information in the intrapersonal sphere: An extension of cognitive evaluation theory. *Journal of Personality and Social Psychology*, *43*(3), 450–461. doi:10.1037/0022-3514.43.3.450

Ryan, R. M., & Deci, E. L. (2000). Self-Determination Theory and the Facilitation of Intrinsic Motivation, Social Development, and Well-Being. *The American Psychologist*, *55*(1), 68–78. doi:10.1037/0003-066X.55.1.68 PMID:11392867

Ryan, R. M., Patrick, H., Deci, E. L., & Williams, G. C. (2008). Facilitating health behavior change and its maintenance: Interventions based on Self- Determination Theory. *Eur. Health Psychology*, *10*, 2–5.

Sääksjärvi, M., & Hellen, K. (2013). How Designers and Marketers Can Work Together to Support Consumers' Happiness. *International Journal of Design*, *7*(3).

Sama, P. R., Eapen, Z. J., Weinfurt, K. P., Shah, B. R., & Schulman, K. A. (2014). An evaluation of mobile health application tools. *JMIR mHealth and uHealth*, *2*(2), e19. doi:10.2196/mhealth.3088 PMID:25099179

Sametinger, J., Rozenblit, J., Lysecky, R., & Ott, P. (2015). Security Challenges for Medical Devices. *Communications of the ACM*, *58*(4), 74–82. doi:10.1145/2667218

Sandström, J., Swanepoel, D. W., Carel Myburgh, H., & Laurent, C. (2016). Smartphone threshold audiometry in underserved primary health-care contexts. *International Journal of Audiology*, *55*(4), 232–238. doi:10.3109/14992027.2015.1124294 PMID:26795898

Saunders, G. (2014). *Teleaudiology: The future of audiology?* National Center for Rehabilitative Auditory Research. Retrieved August 22, 2018 from http://www.nationalacademies.org/hmd/~/media/Files/Activity%20Files/PublicHealth/HearingLossAging/1-13%20Saunders%20pdf.pdf

Saunders, R. P., Evans, M. H., & Joshi, P. (2005). Developing a process-evaluation plan for assessing health promotion program implementation: A how-to guide. *Health Promotion Practice, 6*(2), 134-147.

Saunders, E. (2015). *Sound of Silence*. New Holland Publishers.

Saunders, G. H., Lewis, M. S., & Forsline, A. (2009). Expectations, prefitting counseling, and hearing aid outcome. *Journal of the American Academy of Audiology*, *20*(5), 320–334. doi:10.3766/jaaa.20.5.6 PMID:19585963

Scherer, E. A., Ben-Zeev, D., Li, Z., & Kne, J. M. (2017). Analyzing mHealth Engagement: Joint Models for Intensively Collected User Engagement Data. *JMIR mHealth and uHealth*, *5*(1), e1. doi:10.2196/mhealth.6474 PMID:28082257

Schlee, W., Pryss, R. C., Probst, T., Schobel, J., Bachmeier, A., Reichert, M., & Langguth, B. (2016). Measuring the moment-to-moment variability of tinnitus: The TrackYourTinnitus smart phone app. *Frontiers in Aging Neuroscience*, *8*, 294. doi:10.3389/fnagi.2016.00294 PMID:28018210

Schneier, B. (2012). *The Big Idea: Bruce Schneier*. Retrieved June 1, 2017 from https://www.schneier.com/essays/archives/2012/02/the_big_idea_bruce_s.html

Schneier, B. (2004). *Secrets and Lies*. Indianapolis, IN: Wiley Publishing Inc.

Schroeder, S. A. (2007). Shattuck lecture. We can do better–improving the health of the American people. *The New England Journal of Medicine, 357*(12), 1221–1228. doi:10.1056/NEJMsa073350 PMID:17881753

Schulz, K. F., Altman, D. G., & Moher, D. (2010). CONSORT 2010 statement: Updated guidelines for reporting parallel group randomised trials. *BMC Medicine, 8*(1), 18. doi:10.1186/1741-7015-8-18 PMID:20334633

Scott, K. M., Lim, C., Al-Hamzawi, A., Alonso, J., Bruffaerts, R., Caldas-de-Almeida, J. M., ... Kessler, R. C. (2016). Association of mental disorders with subsequent chronic physical conditions: World mental health surveys from 17 countries. *JAMA Psychiatry, 73*(2), 150–158. doi:10.1001/jamapsychiatry.2015.2688 PMID:26719969

Shargorodsky, J., Curhan, G. C., & Farwell, W. R. (2010). Prevalence and characteristics of tinnitus among US adults. *The American Journal of Medicine, 123*(8), 711–718. doi:10.1016/j.amjmed.2010.02.015 PMID:20670725

Shore, J. H., Mishkind, M. C., Bernard, J., Doarn, C. R., Bell, I. Jr, Bhatla, R., ... Vo, A. (2014). A lexicon of assessment and outcome measures for telemental health. *Telemedicine Journal and e-Health, 20*(3), 282–292. doi:10.1089/tmj.2013.0357 PMID:24476192

Sindhusake, D., Mitchell, P., Smith, W., Golding, M., Newall, P., Hartley, D., & Rubin, G. (2001). Validation of self-reported hearing loss. The Blue Mountains Hearing Study. *International Journal of Epidemiology, 30*(6), 1371–1378. doi:10.1093/ije/30.6.1371 PMID:11821349

Singh, G., Pichora-Fuller, M. K., Malkowski, M., Boretzki, M., & Launer, S. (2014). Survey of the attitudes of practitioners toward teleaudiology. *International Journal of Audiology, 53*(12), 850–860. doi:10.3109/14992027.2014.921736 PMID:25017424

Sladen, D. P., Gifford, R. H., Haynes, D., Kelsall, D., Benson, A., Lewis, K., ... Westerberg, B. (2017). Evaluation of a revised indication for determining adult cochlear implant candidacy. *The Laryngoscope, 127*(10), 2368–2374. doi:10.1002/lary.26513 PMID:28233910

Smith, P., McKeon, A., Blunt, I., & Edwards, N. (2014). *NHS hospitals under pressure: Trends in acute activity up to 2022*. London, UK: Nuffield Trust.

Smits, C., Goverts, S. T., & Festen, J. M. (2013). The digits-in-noise test: Assessing auditory speech recognition abilities in noise. *The Journal of the Acoustical Society of America, 133*(3), 1693–1706. doi:10.1121/1.4789933 PMID:23464039

Smits, C., Kapteyn, T. S., & Houtgast, T. (2004). Development and validation of an automatic speech-in-noise screening test by telephone. *International Journal of Audiology*, *43*(1), 15–28. doi:10.1080/14992020400050004 PMID:14974624

Smits, C., Merkus, P., & Houtgast, T. (2006). How we do it: The Dutch functional hearing–screening tests by telephone and Internet. *Clinical Otolaryngology*, *31*(5), 436–440. doi:10.1111/j.1749-4486.2006.01195.x PMID:17014457

Stanley, F. (2010), Privacy or public good? Why not obtaining consent may be best practice. *Significance Magazine*, *7*(2).

Stay Smart Online Program. (2017). *Stay Smart Online*. Retrieved June 1, 2017 from https://www.staysmartonline.gov.au/

Stay Smart Online. (2017). *Small Business Guide*. Retrieved June 1, 2017 from https://www.staysmartonline.gov.au/get-involved/guides/smallbusinessguide

Steinhubl, S. R., Muse, E. D., & Topol, E. J. (2015). The emerging field of mobile health. *Science Translational Medicine*, *7*(283), 283rv3. doi:10.1126citranslmed.aaa3487 PMID:25877894

Stephens, D., & Kramer, S. E. (2009). Living with Hearing Difficulties: the process of enablement. Wiley-Blackwell.

Sterling, L., & Taveter, K. (2009). *Art of Agent-Oriented Modelling*. MIT Press.

Stinson, E. (2014). *This Guy's Hacked Hearing Aids Let Him Listen to Wi-Fi Networks*. Retrieved June 1, 2017 from https://www.wired.com/2014/12/guys-hacked-hearing-aids-let-listen-wi-fi-networks/

Stockdale, D., McFerran, D., Brazier, P., Pritchard, C., Kay, T., Dowrick, C., & Hoare, D. J. (2017). An economic evaluation of the healthcare cost of tinnitus management in the UK. *BMC Health Services Research*, *17*(1), 577. doi:10.118612913-017-2527-2 PMID:28830503

Stoyanov, S. R., Hides, L., Kavanagh, D. J., & Wilson, H. (2016). Development and validation of the user version of the Mobile Application Rating Scale (uMARS). *JMIR mHealth and uHealth*, *4*(2), e72. doi:10.2196/mhealth.5849 PMID:27287964

Stoyanov, S. R., Hides, L., Kavanagh, D. J., Zelenko, O., Tjondronegoro, D., & Mani, M. (2015). Mobile App Rating Scale: A new tool for assessing the quality of health mobile apps. *JMIR mHealth and uHealth*, *3*(1), e27. doi:10.2196/mhealth.3422 PMID:25760773

Swanepol, D. W., Koekemoer, D., & Clark, J. (2010). Intercontinental hearing assessment – a study in tele-audiology. *Journal of Telemedicine and Telecare*, *16*(5), 248–252. doi:10.1258/jtt.2010.090906 PMID:20457801

Teleaudiology, S. G. (n.d.). *Are patients and practitioners ready for it?* Retrieved from https://www.phonakpro.com/content/dam/phonakpro/gc_hq/en/events/2012/advances_in_audiology_lasvegas/Singh_G_Teleaudiology_Are_patients_and_practitioners_ready.pdf

Thabane, L., Ma, J., Chu, R., Cheng, J., Ismaila, A., Rios, L. P., ... Goldsmith, C. H. (2010a). A tutorial on pilot studies: The what, why and how. *BMC Medical Research Methodology*, *10*(1), 1. doi:10.1186/1471-2288-10-1 PMID:20053272

The Council for Public Health and Health Care. (2015). *Consumer e-Health*. Retrieved August 23, 2018 from https://www.raadrvs.nl/uploads/docs/Consumer_ehealth.pdf

Thomas, N., Farhall, J., Foley, F., Leitan, N. D., Villagonzalo, K. A., Ladd, E., ... Kyrios, M. (2016). Promoting Personal Recovery in People with Persisting Psychotic Disorders: Development and Pilot Study of a Novel Digital Intervention. *Frontiers in Psychiatry*, *7*, 196. doi:10.3389/fpsyt.2016.00196

Thompson, G. P., Sladen, D. P., Borst, B. J., & Still, O. L. (2015). Accuracy of a tablet audiometer for measuring behavioral hearing thresholds in a clinical population. *Otolaryngology - Head and Neck Surgery*, *153*(5), 838–842. doi:10.1177/0194599815593737 PMID:26183518

Thompson, P., Pryce, H., & Refaie, E. (2011). Group or individual tinnitus therapy: What matters to participants? *Audiological Medicine*, *9*(3), 110–116. doi:10.3109/1651386X.2011.604470

Thoren, E. S., Andersson, G., & Lunner, T. (2012). The use of research questionnaires with hearing impaired adults: Online vs. paper-and-pencil administration. *BMC Ear, Nose, and Throat Disorders, 12*.

Thorén, E. S., Öberg, M., Wänström, G., Andersson, G., & Lunner, T. (2014). A randomized controlled trial evaluating the effects of online rehabilitative intervention for adult hearing-aid users. *International Journal of Audiology*, *53*(7), 452–461. doi:10.3109/14992027.2014.892643 PMID:24749664

Titov, N., Andrews, G., Davies, M., McIntyre, K., Robinson, E., & Solley, K. (2010). Internet treatment for depression: A randomized controlled trial comparing clinician vs. technician assistance. *PLoS One*, *5*(6), e10939. doi:10.1371/journal.pone.0010939 PMID:20544030

Titov, N., Andrews, G., Schwencke, G., Solley, K., Johnston, L., & Robinson, E. (2009). An RCT comparing effect of two types of support on severity of symptoms for people completing internet-based cognitive behaviour therapy for social phobia. *The Australian and New Zealand Journal of Psychiatry*, *43*(10), 920–926. doi:10.1080/00048670903179228

Tognola, G., Paglialonga, A., Chiaramello, E., & Pinciroli, F. (2015). eHealth for Hearing – new views and apps practicalities. *European Journal of Biomedical Informatics*, *11*(3), en43–en49.

Tomlinson, M., Rotheram-Borus, M. J., Swartz, L., & Tsai, A. C. (2013). Scaling up mHealth: Where is the evidence? *PLoS Medicine*, *10*(2), e1001382. doi:10.1371/journal.pmed.1001382 PMID:23424286

Topol, E. (2015). *The Patient Will See You Now: The Future of Medicine Is in Your Hands*. New York: Basic Books.

Totten, A. M., Womack, D. M., Eden, K. B., McDonagh, M. S., Griffin, J. C., Grusing, S., & Hersh, W. R. (2016*). Telehealth: mapping the evidence for patient outcomes from systematic reviews*. Rockville, MD: Agency for Healthcare Research and Quality (US). Technical Briefs, No. 26. Available from: https://www.ncbi.nlm.nih.gov/books/NBK379320/

Tulbure, B. T. (2011). The efficacy of internet-supported intervention for social anxiety disorder: A brief meta-analytic review. *Procedia: Social and Behavioral Sciences*, *30*, 552–557. doi:10.1016/j.sbspro.2011.10.108

Tye-Murray, N. (2016). *A clEAR™ Solution to the Changing Climate of Hearing Healthcare*. Retrieved September 18, 2018 from https://www.clearworks4ears.com/static/media_relations/Audiology%20practices%20proofs.pdf

U.S. Department of Health & Human Services. (2003). *Research*. Retrieved October 1, 2018, from https://www.hhs.gov/sites/default/files/ocr/privacy/hipaa/understanding/special/research/research.pdf

U.S. Department of Health & Human Services. (n.d.). *Summary of the HIPAA Privacy Rule*. Retrieved October 1, 2018, from https://www.hhs.gov/hipaa/for-professionals/privacy/laws-regulations/index.html?language=en

U.S. Food and Drug Administration. (2016, December 7). *FDA takes steps to improve hearing aid accessibility*. Author.

UK Parliament. (1998). *Data Protection*. Retrieved 15 February 2016, from: http://www.legislation.gov.uk/ukpga/1998/29/contents

United States Department of Labor, Bureau of Labor Statistics. (2017). *Occupational Outlook Handbook*. Retrieved October 1, 2018, from http://www.bls.gov/ooh/healthcare/audiologists.htm

Vaerenberg, B., Smits, C., De Ceulaer, G., Zir, E., Harman, S., & Jaspers, N. (2014, February 4). …Cochlear implant programming: A global survey on the state of the art. *The Scientific World Journal*. PMID:24688394

Valente, M., Bentler, R., Seewald, R., Trine, T., & Van Vliet, D. (1998). Guidelines for hearing aid fitting for adults. *American Journal of Audiology*, *7*(1), 5–13. doi:10.1044/1059-0889.0701.05 PMID:26649513

van Beugen, S., Ferwerda, M., Hoeve, D., Rovers, M. M., Spillekom-van Koulil, S., van Middendorp, H., & Evers, A. W. (2014). Internet-based cognitive behavioral therapy for patients with chronic somatic conditions: A meta-analytic review. *Journal of Medical Internet Research*, *16*(3), e88. doi:10.2196/jmir.2777 PMID:24675372

van Kerkhof, L. W. M., van der Laar, C. W. E., de Jong, C., Weda, M., & Hegger, I. (2016). Characterization of apps and other e-tools for medication use: Insights into possible benefits and risks. *JMIR mHealth and uHealth*, *4*(2), e34. doi:10.2196/mhealth.4149 PMID:27052946

Vermeire, E., Hearnshaw, H., van Royen, P., & Denekens, J. (2001). Patient adherence to treatment: Three decades of research. A comprehensive review. *Journal of Clinical Pharmacy and Therapeutics*, *26*(5), 331–342. doi:10.1046/j.1365-2710.2001.00363.x PMID:11679023

Vieira Esteves, T., & Pacheco de Oliveira, S. (2015). Telehealth in Brazil: Contemporary Tool for Access to Health. *Studies in Health Technology and Informatics*, *216*, 995. PMID:26262297

Vize, W. (2017, September 8). The NHS must embrace digital services or risk being left behind. *The Guardian.* Retrieved August 22, 2018, from https://www.theguardian.com/healthcare-network/2017/sep/08/nhs-embrace-digital-services-risk-left-behind

VizeR. (2017). Retrieved from https://www.theguardian.com/healthcare-network/2017/sep/08/nhs-embrace-digital-services-risk-left-behin

Vlaescu, G., Alasjö, A., Miloff, A., Carlbring, P., & Andersson, G. (2016). Features and functionality of the iterapi platform for internet-based psychological treatment. *Internet Interventions*, *6*, 107–114. doi:10.1016/j.invent.2016.09.006 PMID:30135819

Vlaescu, G., Carlbring, P., Lunner, T., & Andersson, G. (2015). An e-platform for rehabilitation of persons with hearing problems. *American Journal of Audiology*, *24*(3), 271–275. doi:10.1044/2015_AJA-14-0083 PMID:26649528

Vogenberg, F. R., Barash, C. I., & Pursel, M. (2010). Personalized medicine: part 1: evolution and development into theranostics. *P&T*, *35*(10), 560.

Wachtler, C., Coe, A., Davidson, S., Fletcher, S., Mendoza, A., Sterling, L., & Gunn, J. (2018). Development of a Mobile Clinical Prediction Tool to Estimate Future Depression Severity and Guide Treatment in Primary Care: A User Centered Design. *JMIR mHealth and uHealth*, *6*(4), e95. doi:10.2196/mhealth.9502 PMID:29685864

Walker, E., & Nowacki, A. (2011). Understanding Equivalence and Noninferiority Testing. *Journal of General Internal Medicine*, *26*(2), 192–196. doi:10.100711606-010-1513-8 PMID:20857339

Wallhagen, M. I. (2009). The stigma of hearing loss. *The Gerontologist*, *50*(1), 66–75. doi:10.1093/geront/gnp107 PMID:19592638

Wallis, L. A., Fleming, J., Hasselberg, M., Laflamme, L., & Lundin, J. (2016). A smartphone app and cloud-based consultation system for burn injury emergency care. *PLoS One*, *11*(2), e0147253. doi:10.1371/journal.pone.0147253 PMID:26918631

Wang, A., An, N., Lu, X., Chen, H., Li, C., & Levkoff, S. (2014). A classification scheme for analyzing mobile apps used to prevent and manage disease in late life. *JMIR mHealth and uHealth*, *2*(1), e6. doi:10.2196/mhealth.2877 PMID:25098687

Ward, M. (2012). *Hearing-aid hackers fine-tuning their own devices*. Retrieved June 1, 2017 from http://www.bbc.com/news/technology-18690973

Weise, C., Kleinstauber, M., & Andersson, G. (2016). Internet-delivered cognitive-behavior therapy for tinnitus: A randomized controlled trial. *Psychosomatic Medicine, 78*(4), 501–510. doi:10.1097/PSY.0000000000000310 PMID:26867083

Wesarg, T., Wasowski, A., & Skarzynski, H. (2010). Remote fitting in Nucleus cochlear implant recipients. [PubMed]. *J. Acta Oto-Laryngologica, 130*(12), 1379–1388.

Wesarg, T., Wasowski, A., Skarzynski, H., Ramos, A., Falcon Gonzalez, J. C., Kyriafinis, G., ... Laszig, R. (2010). Remote fitting in Nucleus cochlear implant recipients. *Acta Oto-Laryngologica, 130*(12), 1379–1388. doi:10.3109/00016489.2010.492480 PMID:20586675

West, D. (2012). How mobile devices are transforming healthcare. *Issues in Technology Innovation, 18*(1), 1–11.

West, J. H., Hall, P. C., Hanson, C. L., Barnes, M. D., Giraud-Carrier, C., & Barrett, J. (2012). There's an app for that: Content analysis of paid health and fitness apps. *Journal of Medical Internet Research, 14*(3), e72. doi:10.2196/jmir.1977 PMID:22584372

Wicks, P., & Chiauzzi, E. (2015). 'Trust but verify'--five approaches to ensure safe medical apps. *BMC Medicine, 13*(1), 205. doi:10.118612916-015-0451-z PMID:26404791

Williams, C., & Whitfield, G. (2001). Written and computer-based self-help treatments for depression. *British Medical Bulletin, 57*(1), 133–144. doi:10.1093/bmb/57.1.133 PMID:11719913

Wise, K., Rief, W., & Goebel, G. (1998). Meeting the expectations of chronic tinnitus patients: Comparison of a structured group therapy program for tinnitus management with a problem-solving group. *Journal of Psychosomatic Research, 44*(6), 681–685. doi:10.1016/S0022-3999(97)00310-3 PMID:9678749

Wong, M. C., & Fung, K. (2015). Mobile applications in otolaryngology-head and neck surgery. *Otolaryngology - Head and Neck Surgery, 152*(4), 638–643. doi:10.1177/0194599815568946 PMID:25628367

World Health Organization (WHO). (2004). *Global Burden of Disease Report.* Retrieved October 1, 2018, from http://www.who.int/healthinfo/global_burden_disease/GBD_report_2004update_part4.pdf

World Health Organization (WHO). (2013). *Millions of People in the World have Hearing Loss that can be Treated or Prevented.* Retrieved October 1, 2018, http://www.who.int/pbd/deafness

World Health Organization (WHO). (2016). *Executive Board 139th Session: Resolutions and Decisions Annex.* Retrieved October 1, 2018. From http://apps.who.int/gb/ebwha/pdf_files/EB139-REC1/B139_REC1-en.pdf

World Health Organization (WHO). (2018). *Deafness and Hearing Loss.* Retrieved October 1, 2018, from: http://www.who.int/mediacentre/factsheets/fs300/en/

World Health Organization. (2011). *mHealth: New horizons for health through mobile technologies.* Retrieved June 12, 2018 from www.who.int/goe/publications/ehealth_series_vol3/en/

World Health Organization. (2011). Telemedicine - Opportunities and developments in Member States. Retrieved October 1, 2018, from http://www.who.int/goe/publications/ehealth_series_vol2/en/

World Health Organization. (2018). *Deafness and hearing loss.* Retrieved August 22, 2018, from http://www.who.int/mediacentre/factsheets/fs300/en/

Yoon, J. K., Pohlmeyer, A., & Desmet, P. (2016). When 'Feeling Good' is not Good Enough: Seven Key Opportunities for Emotional Granularity in Product Development. *International Journal of Design, 10*(3).

Zhao, J., Freeman, B., & Li, M. (2016). Can Mobile Phone Apps Influence People's Health Behavior Change? An Evidence Review. *Journal of Medical Internet Research, 18*(11), e287. doi:10.2196/jmir.5692 PMID:27806926

Ziebland, S., & Wyke, S. (2012). Health and illness in a connected world: How might sharing experiences on the internet affect people's health? *The Milbank Quarterly, 90*(2), 219–249. doi:10.1111/j.1468-0009.2012.00662.x PMID:22709387

About the Contributors

Elaine Saunders is co-founder and Executive Chairman of Blamey & Saunders Hearing Pty Ltd a profit-for purpose telehealth company. In her 40 year career, Elaine has been an advocate for people with hearing loss and aimed to reduce the barriers to quality hearing care and hearing aids. Elaine has a Master in Clinical Audiology from the University of Manchester and a PhD from the University of Southampton. She is a former member of the cochlear research team of Professor Graeme Clark; an outcome of this research was her co-founding of spin-off company Dynamic Hearing Pty Ltd (now part of Cirrus Logic), of which Elaine was CEO for 8 years. Elaine's awards include the American Academy of Audiology's Samuel F. Lybarger Award for Achievements in Industry and the Australia Academy of Technology and Engineering's Clunies Ross Medal for Entrepreneur of the Year. Elaine is an Adjunct Professor at Swinburne University and Chair of its Innovation Precinct Advisory Board. She is also a Non-Executive Director of the Australian National Fabrication Facility (ANFF), the Australian Innovation Research Group (AIRG), and the National Foundation for Medical Research and Innovation (NFMRI).

* * *

Eldré Beukes is a Clinical Scientist in Audiology. She received her BSc in South Africa and her MSc in Audiology from the University of Manchester, UK. She obtained her PhD for an Internet-based intervention for tinnitus in 2018 from Anglia Ruskin University, Cambridge. UK. The prestigious Shapiro prize was awarded by the British Tinnitus Association for research related to improving treatments for those with tinnitus in both 2017 and 2018. The British Society of Audiology provided an applied research grant to assist with this research. As a post-doctoral researcher she has continuing research in the field of Internet-interventions and teaches students. Following her training as a clinical scientist in Audiology, she was awarded the Richard May prize in 2009 as the best trainee and has worked in various clinical settings.

Peter Blamey has a PhD in Physics. He was the inventor and leader of the Combionic Aid team that initially developed the ADRO® signal processing strategy for the CRC for Cochlear Implant and Hearing Aid Innovation (CRC HEAR). During his career as a Principal Research Fellow at the University of Melbourne's Department of Otolaryngology, Peter has worked on the Bionic Ear, hearing aids and other devices for people with impaired hearing and was on the Bionic Eye psychophysics team for Bionic Vision Australia. He has published over 200 papers in physics, psychophysics, speech processing, speech perception and language development in children with impaired hearing. Peter is an inventor on 27 international patents or patent applications, including ADRO®, which was developed for the bionic ear. Peter was awarded the American Academy of Audiology's prestigious International Award in 2007 and a Clunies Ross Science and Technology Medal by the Australian Academy of Technological Sciences and Engineering (ATSE) in 2012. Peter is the former Deputy Director (Commercialisation and IP) of the Bionics Institute. He was the co-founder of Dynamic Hearing and was an Executive Director and Chief Technology Officer for 6 years, until leaving to found Blamey & Saunders Hearing Pty Ltd (the Australia Hears Pty Ltd), where he is the Director of Technology. (then Australia Hears Pty Ltd).

Alison Hardacre was named one of the Top 50 Australian and New Zealand Women in Tech in 2016, and in 2015 received the Victorian Pearcey Entrepreneur Award. Alison Hardacre and Lachlan Wheeler are the Co-Founders and Co-CEOs of HealthKit, a global health platform for practitioners, patients and people everywhere used in over 50 countries around the world, that makes healthcare efficient, effective and accessible. Before HealthKit, Alison was an accomplished general manager in health and banking, and a director of numerous health organisations. She holds an MBA from Melbourne Business School, and Law and Arts degrees from Monash University.

Rick Harvey (FACS, FIEAust, CEO Layer Security) is a successful technologist, executive and entrepreneur in both start-ups and multi-nationals. Over his thirty-year career, he has run international R&D labs, co-founded several successful companies and developed many world-class software products in security, privacy and large-scale distributed systems. Rick has filed over 40 patents and is broadly involved in industry as a presenter, judge, panellist, mentor, advisor and Board member.

Alessia Paglialonga received M.Sc. and Ph.D. degrees in Biomedical Engineering from Politecnico di Milano in 2005 and 2009. She is Research Scientist at the National Research Council of Italy (CNR), Institute of Electronics, Computer and Telecommunication Engineering (IEIIT). Her current research interests are in the areas of: technological developments in audiology (for screening, assessment, and rehabilitation), biomedical signal processing and modeling (speech processing, otoacoustic emissions analysis, sensory systems modeling, neural processing and coding), and eHealth and mHealth (digital applications for health and wellbeing; clinical data processing and analysis, mobile apps characterization and evaluation). She has authored 35 articles in peer-reviewed Journals, seven book chapters, and more than 80 communications in International Conferences.

Leon Sterling has had a distinguished academic career. After completing a PhD at the Australian National University, he worked for 15 years at universities in the UK, Israel and the United States. He returned to Australia as Professor of Computer Science at the University of Melbourne in 1995. He served as Head of the Department of Computer Science and Engineering for 6 years. After stepping down as Head, he took up the industry-sponsored Adacel Chair of Software Innovation and Engineering. In 2010, he moved to Swinburne University of Technology where he served as Dean of the Faculty of Information and Communication Technologies for 4 years and Pro Vice-Chancellor (Digital Frontiers) for two years. His current research is in incorporating emotions in technology development, where motivational models are an essential element.

Lachlan Wheeler leads global technology and operations at HealthKit, following a career in banking. He holds first class honours degrees in Arts and Business from Monash University, and is an Asialink Leadership Scholar and a graduate of the UC Berkeley Haas School of Business Entrepreneurship Executive Program. Alison Hardacre and Lachlan Wheeler are the Co-Founders and Co-CEOs of HealthKit, a global health platform for practitioners, patients and people everywhere used in over 50 countries around the world, that makes healthcare efficient, effective and accessible.

Index

G

H

I

L

M

O

P

R

S

T

U

V

www.ingramcontent.com/pod-product-compliance
Lightning Source LLC
LaVergne TN
LVHW081331300926
849161LV00008B/1938